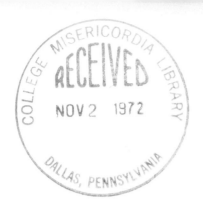

PERSONAL HEALTH IN ECOLOGIC PERSPECTIVE

Personal health in ecologic perspective

ROBERT H. KIRK, H.S.D.

Professor and Chairman, Health and Safety Department,
The University of Tennessee, Knoxville

CYRUS MAYSHARK, H.S.D., M.S.Hyg.

Associate Dean, College of Education, and Professor of Health Education,
The University of Tennessee, Knoxville

ROBERT PRESTON HORNSBY, M.D.

Internal Medicine, Allergy, and Clinical Immunology,
Knoxville, Tennessee

With 97 illustrations

The C. V. Mosby Company

SAINT LOUIS   1972

Preface

Maximum personal health has been a goal coveted by man for thousands of years. Because it must be earned, however, both individually and collectively, through advancing education and improving technology, the lip-service given to it has often been greater than the action expended to achieve it. Now the ecocatastrophe we have created causes the problems of personal health to pale against the more awesome possibility of human extinction. If we really are on the brink of total destruction, as so many claim, the here and now issue of health deserves little, if any, consideration.

But health as you and we would want it, in the ecologic perspective of today, is an undeniably necessary prerequisite to our existence. The following examples make clear this precursor relationship. To suffer from bronchitis now, as a consequence of uncontrolled air pollutants and do nothing to reduce them, may lead to our inability to breathe at all in the future. (The disasters in London, 1952, New York City, 1966, and others suggest greater eventual tragedy.) Lake Erie is "dead" now. Is this a preview of what will happen soon to Lake Michigan and eventually to the oceans? Is it possible that we could hard-surface (trade the chlorophyll molecule for a parking lot) ourselves out of oxygen? Many species suffer neurologic disintegration and death when their numbers increase exponentially. As the human population begins ascendency on its exponential curve, is the current epidemic spread of violence an early symptom of human disintegration?

Bronchitis, smog, impaired oxygen replenishment, a too-rapid increase in population, and violence all confront us today. Life on Earth will be in the balance tomorrow. To covet health but do nothing to achieve it is no longer possible. Our very lives and those of future generations demand that we seek it assiduously.

This text focuses on the individual in his environment. With matters of personal health and ecology it is no longer possible to consider either separately. If our message reaches you, we will have been only partially successful. What you do with this message, on behalf of yourself and others, will spell our ultimate success and, without question, contribute to the ultimate success—or failure—of mankind.

We are indebted to the following persons for significant contributions they made during the preparation of this text: Mary Rose Gram, Ph.D., Professor and Head, Department of Nutrition; David M. Lipscomb, Ph.D., Associate Professor of Audiology and Speech Pathology; Aaron J. Sharp, Ph.D., Professor of Botany; Mary Nelle Traylor, M.P.H., Assistant Professor of Nutrition; Hugh G. Welch, Ph.D., Assistant Professor of Physiology and Physical Education; all of The University of Tennessee, Knoxville. Also, we wish to thank Evalyn S. Gendel, M.D., Director, Division of Maternal and Child Health, State Department of Public Health, Topeka, Kansas; Mary Sharpe, Health Educator, Knox County Health Department, Knoxville, Tennessee; Richard E. Strain, M.D., Maryville, Tennessee.

Martin Webster, college student, skilled artist, and constructive critic, made many contributions. Several examples of his artistic interpretation are included in the pages that follow. His criticism of several chapters, while less evident, helped to mold the final product.

Our sincere appreciation is extended to Mrs. Gay Keenan, Mrs. Royce Hannah, and Mrs. Ruby Miller for their technical assistance in the preparation of the manuscript and in the many details of correspondence, and to Mrs. Mary Flanders, R.N., Mrs. Roenella Hornsby, B.S., R.N., and Margaret Lyon, all of Knoxville, Tennessee, for their technical advice and counsel.

Robert H. Kirk
Cyrus Mayshark
Robert Preston Hornsby

Contents

PART I

Introduction

The Simiadae then branched off into two great stems, the New World and Old World monkeys; and from the latter at a remote period, Man, the wonder of the Universe, proceeded.

CHARLES DARWIN

Thus man has evolved from primitive being to agrarian worker to industrial giant to technologic wizard.

Man's earliest antagonists were wild, ferocious animals that destroyed him in the fields, forests, and caves, but fortunately not to the point of extinction. In surviving, man learned to hunt, to kill, to plant, and to harvest. Gradually his numbers increased as he gained mastery over the larger organisms with whom he shared his environment. Less obvious foes, giving rise to disease in many forms, also challenged man's supremacy, often destroying or injuring him in tragic quantity. For centuries man's lot appeared hopeless, or at best a gamble over which he seemingly had little control. So it remained almost to modern times. But the scientific enlightenment brought with it relief from pestilence; in the past 300 years man has become master over most micro-organisms and other disease-producing entities, as he became master over macro-organisms in the dawn of his history. The eighteenth, nineteenth, and twentieth centuries have truly been the golden era of medicine, with man the grateful beneficiary.

Now a new plague girdles the earth. Our technology is at once miraculous and insidious, causing us to ask: "Is man but a planetary disease?" (Loren Eisley). Have we achieved a near millenium in individual health only to be mortally overwhelmed by the wastes of our brilliant achievements? Can it be that man's health, even his very life on this planet, will be sustained not because of, or in spite of, but only *without* the facts and truths of science that have brought him to this point? If life can continue only without these truths, survival is obviously impossible, and some people, therefore, are pessimistic of man's future on Earth. Optimism, however, tells us that whatever man can dream he can achieve. But to do so he must develop a perspective of himself in his world that he seemingly does not possess now.

Chapter 1 describes the ecologic perspective of personal health, which is the framework of this book.

Dealing in futures

"Our business is with life . . ." A short talk to a gathering of college students, faculty, and other interested persons, by George Wald, biologist and Nobel Laureate, on March 4, 1969, contained these words. They cut to the core of all human concern for life as we dream it should be on this planet Earth. No other words could state with greater clarity the focus and philosophy of the book you now hold in your hands. These words appear in the last paragraph of Wald's presentation.

> Our business is with life, not death. Our challenge is to give what account we can of what becomes of life in the solar system, this corner of the universe that is our home and, most of all, what becomes of men—all men of all nations, colors, and creeds. It has become one world, a world for all men. It is only such a world that can offer us life and the chance to go on.*

These words emphasize the importance of relationships, man to all other men, and man to his environment. They speak of the present and challenge us with the future. As the only men in the universe, we must rise to the challenge, or the bright promise of what we might have been will burn to nothingness.

PERSONAL HEALTH

This is a book about you and for you, a student of higher education in the last half of the twentieth century in the United States of America. These pages are concerned with events, discoveries, facts, behavior patterns, and individual and group decisions that affect health. On the personal level, they affect your health.

What do we mean by health? The World Health Organization defines health as the "state of complete physical, mental, and social well-being and not merely the absence of disease or infirmity." This seems to be a fairly adequate definition, but Christie and Newman* remind us that it is a linear definition that does not reveal the interrelationships of an ecologic application. Until the last 20 years or so we have been inclined to describe personal health with little or no reference to the interrelationships of the individual with other individuals or with his environment. We did so in part from ignorance of all the consequences of these interrelationships, but more because we didn't think, when our numbers were fewer and our alteration of the environment was minimal, that these interrelationships made much difference. Today we know better. Today we know that our health must be viewed in ecologic perspective if we—the human race—are to survive.

ECOLOGIC PERSPECTIVE

Ecology is that branch of biology concerned with the relations between organisms and their environment. The essence of our

---

*Wald, G.: A generation in search of a future, address at M.I.T., March 4, 1969; Boston Globe, March 8, 1969; New Yorker, March 22, 1969.

*Christie, T. G., and Newman, I. M.: A conceptual model for understanding the ecologic approach to health, The Health Education Journal **28:**2, May 1969.

ecologic perspective is the presentation and interpretation of physical, mental, and social transactions affecting health within and between people, and between people and their physical and biologic environment. (This is a paraphrase of the ideas presented by D. B. Shimkin; see p. 23.)

It is clear that interest in the environment is actually concern for human health and well-being. Advancing technology and increased industrialization have subjected the environment to a barrage of bacteriologic, chemical, physiologic, and psychologic insults. These impinge upon us so much that there no longer is any doubt that they threaten direct damage to everyone now living or who will be born in the future. Commoner made clear this relationship in a significant presentation.

For young people today have a very special relationship to the growing deterioration of the environment in which we all live. They are the first generation to carry strontium 90 in their bones, DDT in their fat, and asbestos in their lungs; their bodies will record the effects of these environmental insults on human health; they are the involuntary subjects of a huge world-wide experiment, which will, I believe, test the ability of human beings to survive on this planet.*

Toxic matter is being released into the air across the United States at a rate of more than 142 million tons a year. It comes from 90 million motor vehicles, from factories, power plants, municipal dumps, and backyard incinerators. The use of food additives has increased 50% in the past 10 years, and each of us now consumes about 3 pounds of these chemicals each year. Pesticides on food crops add to the chemical barrage. Over 2 million Americans are made ill each year by microbiologic contamination of food. We discard more than 3.5 billion tons of solid wastes every year that we haven't yet learned how to recycle. Automobile graveyards mar the landscape; foul-smelling dumps continue to prevail; and no-return bottles, cans, and other pack-

---

*Presented by Barry Commoner at the Annual Meeting of the American Public Health Association in Philadelphia, November 10, 1969.

aging line our highways and city streets. The garbage in urban areas, often irregularly removed, breeds rats and supports disease organisms. More than 500 new chemicals and related compounds are introduced into industry each year. Because industry, unions, and the government have failed to give adequate attention to these and other occupational hazards, thousands of persons suffer from cancer, lung disease, loss of hearing, dermatitis, and other preventable diseases. Chemical, viral, and bacteriologic wastes contaminate our rivers and lakes so that a water supply satisfactory for human consumption is increasingly difficult to find. Every year over 100,000 people die and over 12 million are injured in accidents in the home or on the highway. The accidental ingestion of poisons alone accounts for over 3,000 deaths each year. Add to all these the pressures and frustrations of urban and industrial life—the crowding and the noise, the monotony of repetitive, unchallenging work—and the complex impingement on our lives is awesome.

This then is our perspective. We have chosen to view personal health from an ecologic vantage point because it is obvious that to do otherwise would be unrealistic of today's situation. Man is not an island unto himself. He relates to others and to his environment in a continually reciprocal, dynamic way that influences all aspects of his being, including his health.

TRENDS IN AMERICAN HEALTH
General comparisons

The changing course of the health of Americans has been highlighted by many successes but also some failures. For example, we have developed a tremendous medical complex with the most sophisticated technologic advances known to man, but our delivery of health services is poor. Nearly 25 million Americans (approximately 13%), living in poverty pockets of the United States, receive minimal or no medical, dental, or psychiatric care. These wide geographic, economic, and secular disparities in health care give rise to the fact

Table 1-1. Changes in American life expectancies at birth, in years, by sex and race

Year	Total population			White population			Nonwhite population		
	Both sexes	Males	Females	Both sexes	Males	Females	Both sexes	Males	Females
1920	54.1	53.6	54.6	54.9	54.4	55.6	45.3	45.5	45.2
1930	59.7	58.1	61.6	61.4	59.7	63.5	48.1	47.3	49.2
1940	62.9	60.8	65.2	64.2	62.1	66.6	53.1	51.5	54.9
1950	68.2	65.6	71.1	69.1	66.5	72.2	60.8	59.1	62.9
1955	69.5	66.6	72.7	70.2	67.3	73.6	63.2	61.2	65.9
1960	69.7	66.6	73.1	70.6	67.4	74.1	63.6	61.1	66.3
1967	70.5	67.0	74.2	71.3	67.8	75.1	64.6	61.1	68.2

From U. S. Bureau of the Census: Statistical abstract of the United States: 1970, ed. 91, Washington, D. C., 1970, U. S. Government Printing Office.

Table 1-2. Expectation of life at birth in selected countries for year indicated, ordered by male rank

Country	Male	Female
Sweden (1967)	71.85	76.54
Norway (1961-65)	71.03	75.97
Netherlands (1967)	71.0	76.5
Iceland (1961-65)	70.8	76.2
Denmark (1965-66)	70.1	74.7
Israel (1968)	69.32	72.88
Ryukyu Islands (1965)	68.91	75.64
Japan (1967)	68.91	74.15
Bulgaria (1965-67)	68.81	72.65
Switzerland (1958-63)	68.72	74.13
East Germany (1965-66)	68.72	73.66
United Kingdom (1966-68)	68.48	74.65
New Zealand (1960-62)	68.44	73.75
Canada (1960-62)	68.35	74.17
France (1966)	68.2	75.4
Northern Ireland (1966-68)	68.19	73.45
Ireland (1960-62)	68.13	71.86
Australia (1960-62)	67.92	74.18
Belgium (1959-63)	67.73	73.51
Malta (1965-67)	67.53	71.64
Czechoslovakia (1966)	67.33	73.57
Spain (1960)	67.32	71.90
United States (1967)	67.0	73.8

Data from United Nations: Demographic yearbook, 1969, New York, 1970, Publishing Service.

that even though our average life expectancy is long (Table 1-1), at least 20 other countries have longer average life expectancies (Table 1-2).

An examination of the data in Table 1-1 makes real gains apparent if we look only at the extremes of the time continuums. Yet most of these gains were made in the first half of the twentieth century; in about the past 20 years our gains have been almost

miniscule. Environmental stresses and persistent deficiencies in the delivery and conduct of health services, especially to the nonwhite and poor segments of our population but to all segments to some degree, are the primary reasons for this halt in progress. Of additional influence are the facts that (1) we have reduced deaths from infectious diseases to the point, on an average, where further reduction, in relation to

Table 1-3. The ten leading causes of death per 100,000 in 1900 and 1969

	1900			1969	
Rank	**Cause**	**Rate**	**Rank**	**Cause**	**Rate**
1.	Influenza and pneumonia	202.2	1.	Heart diseases	364.1
2.	Tuberculosis	194.4	2.	Malignant neoplasms	160.1
3.	Gastroenteritis	142.7	3.	Cerebrovascular diseases	102.0
4.	Heart diseases	137.4	4.	All accidents	56.0
5.	Cerebral hemorrhage and other		5.	Influenza and pneumonia	34.7
	vascular lesions affecting CNS		6.	Certain diseases of early infancy*	20.9
	("stroke")	106.9	7.	Bronchitis, emphysema, and asthma	15.6
6.	Chronic nephritis	81.0	8.	Symptoms and ill-defined conditions	15.6
7.	All accidents	72.3	9.	Cirrhosis of liver	15.0
8.	Cancer and other malignant		10.	Congenital anomalies	8.7
	neoplasms	64.0			
9.	Certain diseases of early infancy*	62.6			
10.	Diphtheria	40.3			

Data from U. S. Public Health Service: Vital statistics report, annual summary for the United States, 1969, Rockville, Md., October 21, 1970, National Center for Health Statistics.
*Birth injuries, asphyxia, infections of the newborn, ill-defined infant diseases, and immaturity.

dollars spent, is virtually impossible; and (2) without the hoped-for breakthrough in heart disease and cancer research, these diseases take increasing numbers of lives each year.

In Table 1-3 the death rate statistics per 100,000 population are summarized. The serious problem that the infectious diseases presented in 1900 as compared with 1969 is made clear. In 1969 only one category in the first ten would be classified an infectious disease, and it ranked fifth with a death rate of 34.7, far below its rank and rate in 1900. In sharp contrast, in 1900 several infectious diseases were ranked in the first ten, including the first and second categories.

Death rate statistics by cause can be misleading if other considerations are not taken into account. For example, Table 1-3 indicates the number who died per 100,000 for designated reasons, but it does not reflect the total number of years lost to each cause of death based on remaining life expectancy at time of death. In relation to family welfare and gross national production this is an important statistic and would, if computed, cause a readjustment in the rankings. Likewise, three other variables are important: (1) number of days as inpatient, (2) num-

ber of days as an outpatient, and (3) days of restricted activity.

These variables and two constants have been included in the Health Problem Index developed by the staff of the Division of Indian Health of the Public Health Service. The index combines both mortality (deaths) and morbidity (illness) data in the same formula, which results in a Q value (a standardized score) that allows comparisons between health problems previously not possible. One Q value can be compared only with another Q value; the larger the Q value the more serious is that particular health problem. Table 1-4 indicates the top ten health problems based on Q value computations. Since the classification is based on the International Classification of Diseases, it is not possible to make direct comparisons with Table 1-3, but certain differences are clearly evident. For example, accidents advance from fourth position in Table 1-3 (mortality alone) to second position in Table 1-4 (mortality plus the other variables previously discussed).

The most important point to be derived from this brief presentation of the Health Problem Index is that there are many more variables in the assessment of health problems than deaths alone, and it is now pos-

Table 1-4. The health problem index of the United States for selected diseases, 1963-64

Major class of disease*	Q value
Diseases of the circulatory system	4,425
Accidents	2,781
Neoplasms	2,367
Diseases of the respiratory system	2,196
Diseases of the nervous system	1,344
Diseases of the digestive system	843
Infectious and parasitic diseases	575
Diseases of the genitourinary system	342
Complications of pregnancy	147
Diseases of bone and organs of movement	85

Adapted from Michael, J. M., Spatafore, G., and Williams, E. R.: A basic information system for health planning, Public Health Reports **83:**1, January 1968.
*From the International Classification of Diseases.

sible to use these other variables in making more accurate comparisons. Undoubtedly, health statisticians will do more of this in the future, and their findings will have an impact at the personal health level.

Specific comparisons

It is likely that the average health status of Americans during the past 20 years has remained static at best, but consideration of all factors reveals that it may have deteriorated to some degree. To illustrate this possible deterioration we look briefly at selected aspects of mental illness, homicide, suicide, accidents, and infant mortality. These represent only five of the many factors that could be similarly identified in such a discussion.

Mental illness. From many points of view, mental disease is the number one health problem in the United States. In 1970 an estimated 17 million people were suffering from some form of mental illness. Only a fraction of these were receiving treatment: approximately 2 million were given psychiatric care in hospitals or outpatient clinics. According to the National Institute of Mental Health, the annual cost of treating mental disease is almost 20 billion dollars.

Some dramatic changes have taken place, however, as Fig. 1-1 attests. The number of resident patients was increasing prior to 1956 at the rate of 10,000 to 12,000 a year. If this rate had continued, we would now need nearly 200,000 more hospital beds than we have. Prior to 1956 only a few drugs to treat mental illness were available: meprobamate (Miltown) to reduce anxiety; chlorpromazine (Thorazine) to treat psychoses; and iproniazid (Marsilid) to alleviate depression. Since that time, hundreds of new drugs have been developed and put into use despite the long time necessary for developing and testing each new drug. Still, the precise action of most of these drugs is not entirely clear. Today, 17 years after the introduction of chlorpromazine into therapeutic use, we still do not understand the mechanism by which this drug (and others like it) alleviates the psychotic state. Of greater concern, of course, is the fact that none of these drugs has an effect on the causation of mental illness. Little or no progress on this front has been made. Nonetheless, the use of these drugs has led to reducing the number of resident patients in mental hospitals. The steady decline in the number of these patients through 1967 is shown in Fig. 1-1. But mental illness, of the sort that does not require hospitalization but makes adequate coping with one's problems impossible, remains a continuing and increasing problem. A compounding problem is the fact that communities are not geared to handle the large numbers being released from psychiatric hospitals. Consequently, the readmission rate is tending to increase. Chapter 2 deals with this subject in detail.

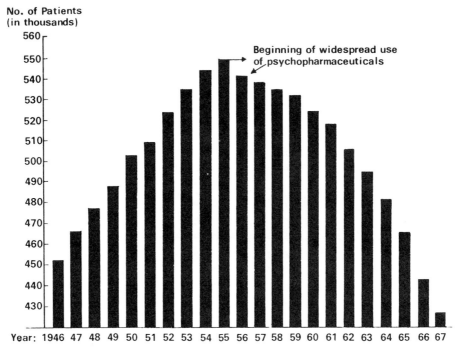

No. of Patients
(in thousands)

Beginning of widespread use
of psychopharmaceuticals

Year: 1946 47 48 49 50 51 52 53 54 55 56 57 58 59 60 61 62 63 64 65 66 67

Fig. 1-1. Number of resident patients in state and local mental hospitals in the United States. (From Maickel, R. P.: Psychopharmacology: new hope for treatment of mentally ill, Your University, 1969-1970, **1**:2, 1969, Indiana University, Bloomington; as modified from Psychopharmacology—a review of progress 1957-1967, National Institute of Mental Health, Public Health Service Publication #1836.)

Homicide. Homicides and suicides, although relatively minor contributors to total mortality, are significant indicators of social and mental health. While overall mortality declined, death rates by homicide rose from 1900 to 1933 to a high of 9.8 deaths per 100,000 population. They then declined to 4.8 per 100,000 in 1955 but again swung steadily up to 6.0 per 100,000 in 1964-65. In 1966 the homicide rate in cities was 6.3 per 100,000. In 1965 the highest rates in individual cities included St. Louis, 18.7; New Orleans, 16.7; Washington, D. C., 15.2; Houston, 12.8; Detroit, 11.7; and Philadelphia, 10.6. Deaths by homicide of nonwhite males were most responsible for these increases; these rates for nonwhites of all ages combined increased from 42.6 per 100,000 in 1955-56 to 47.1 in 1964-65. Table 1-5 summarizes homicide statistics by color and age for the 1955-56 and 1964-65 time periods.

There is a difference in the definitions of homicide in criminal and mortality statistics. Criminal homicides include only willful killings without due process of law and are recorded as such; in mortality statistics homicides also include homicides committed in self-defense, homicides by police officers in the performance of their duties, and legal executions. Of the 11,606 homicides in 1966, all but 300 were considered criminal homicides.

Suicides. American suicide rates have fluctuated widely since 1900, as is seen in Table 1-6. In 1966, 15,416 men and 5,865 women took their lives. These figures represent a 7% increase in the suicide rate among males and a 46% increase among females since 1930. Despite this increase for females, the general suicide rates today are little different from those of the 1920's, because of increased population.

Another change in the suicide statistics has taken place, this with regard to suicide rates for specific ages. From 1950 to 1964

Table 1-5. Trend in U. S. mortality from homicide per 100,000 population, 1955-56 to 1964-65, by color and age*

Age group	1964-65			1955-56			Percent increase		
	Total persons	White	Nonwhite	Total persons	White	Nonwhite	Total persons	White	Nonwhite
All ages†	6.0	3.1	29.0	4.9	2.4	26.1	22	29	11
Under 1	5.5	4.4	11.0	3.4	2.8	7.0	62	57	57
1-4	1.2	1.0	2.3	0.6	0.5	1.2	100	100	92
5-14	0.6	0.5	1.5	0.4	0.4	1.1	50	25	36
15-24	6.6	3.2	30.7	5.8	2.6	29.0	14	23	6
25-34	11.2	5.0	57.0	8.9	3.6	53.1	26	39	7
35-44	9.6	4.5	51.2	7.7	3.6	43.5	25	25	18
45-54	6.8	3.9	33.8	5.8	3.1	30.5	17	26	11
55-64	4.8	3.2	20.9	4.1	2.7	19.8	17	19	6
65-74	3.2	2.2	14.1	2.6	1.9	10.2	23	16	38
75-84	2.6	2.2	8.4	2.4	2.1	6.2	8	5	35
85 and over	2.8	2.4	6.6	2.7	1.8	12.7	4	33	‡

From Metropolitan Life Insurance Co.: Statistical Bulletin **49**:2, February 1968.

*The data in Tables 1-5 and 1-7, in Fig. 1-2, and in the accompanying discussion indicate the levels of health of whites and nonwhites in the United States today. As is most clear to those who study the American social scene, the nonwhite segment receives inadequate health care and so suffers comparatively in most health categories. If health care were equal for all segments of our population, there would be no significant differences in morbidity or mortality between these segments. Because differences do exist, however, it is important to recognize them so that sincere efforts to reduce these differences may continue.

†Adjusted on basis of the age distribution of the total U. S. population, 1940.

‡Less than 20 deaths in either period.

Table 1-6. American suicide rates per 100,000 for selected time periods

Year	Rate
1900	10
1908	17
1920	11
1932	17.4
1944	9.9
1950	11.4
1955	10.2
1960	10.6
1967	10.8

Data from U. S. Bureau of the Census: Statistical abstract of the United States: 1970, ed. 91, Washington, D. C., 1970, U. S. Government Printing Office.

the suicide rate of males at ages 55 to 74 declined over 20%. Among nonwhite males, ages 15 to 24, the rate rose by more than 80%; and the increase in suicide rate among all females, ages 15 to 24, was even greater.

The actual number of suicides cannot be precisely determined. The accuracy of suicide statistics is influenced by religious, social, and psychologic factors that often mask the real cause of death as opposed to the one reported on the death certificate. Also, many deaths reported as accidents include circumstances that make suicide suspect.

The rising number of suicides has led to its recognition as a major medical and public health problem. Existing suicide prevention centers have been successful in saving many lives in recent years. Many more can be saved if unusual depression or signs of mental illness are recognized and properly treated. The problem of suicides emphasizes the importance of viewing personal health in ecologic perspective.

Accidents. All accidents combined reflect the joint effects of personal errors and instabilities, and of environmental pressures such as speed, noise, inclement weather, darkness, and crowding. There is no question that these errors and pressures will increase in the years ahead, as will the numbers of moving vehicles of all types; and we must learn to cope more effectively with these problems if the accident rate is to be held steady.

Since 1950 the accident death rate per 100,000 population has dropped and then risen again: 1950, 60.6; 1955, 56.9; 1960, 52.3; 1966, 58.0. The increase since 1960 has been caused by a marked increase in automobile fatalities; of the 113,563 total fatalities in 1966, 53,041 occurred on the nation's highways.

Increasing trends in all fatal accidents since 1930 are more directly related to the automobile and the increased mechanization and productivity of our country. We have tried to counteract this increasing number of accidents, but with decreasing effectiveness, by better engineering, more stringent enforcement, and safety education.

Many people believe that the stress levels of our social behavior, such as traffic congestion, commutation distances, vehicular speeds, and work strains, have reached the point where engineering, enforcement, and education are no longer significant in their reducing effect on the accident rate. For example, between 1935 and 1955 the decline in automobile fatalities per 100 million vehicle miles was 40%. (Fatalities per 100 million vehicle miles provides a more precise measure than the rate per 100,000 population because it considers the population at risk, that is, those actually in cars on the nation's highways.) This reduction slowed, however, and in 1967 the motor vehicle fatality rate, 5.5 per 100 million vehicle miles, was only 10% less than the

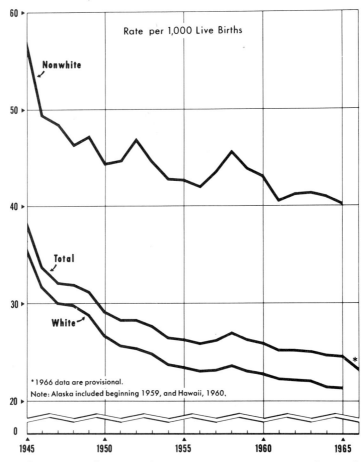

Fig. 1-2. Trend in U. S. infant mortality, 1945-1966. (From Metropolitan Life Insurance Co., Statistical Bulletin **48**:5, May 1967.)

rate of 1955. Are we adapting to the velocity of movement and work and to the rate of change in our society, or do these fatality figures portend a future disintegration of our ability to handle a stressful environment? We believe we can adapt; our outlook is positive and hopeful. Yours should be also. Chapter 5 deals with the problems of accidents in greater detail.

Infant mortality. In 1966 about 3,629,000 babies were born in the United States. Of this number 84,888 died in their first year of life. These deaths give a rate of 23.4 infant deaths per 1,000 live births, an all-time low for the nation to that date. However, the decreased rate of improvement in recent years, wide variations between segments of our population, and the better records of many other countries make it clear that we are not doing as well as we might.

It is apparent from Fig. 1-2 that the rate of improvement in infant mortality has decreased considerably since 1950. Four states, Rhode Island (+2), New Jersey (+1), Nevada (+1), and Mississippi (+6), and the District of Columbia (+14) had

increases in their total infant mortality during this period; and in four others, New York, Michigan, North Carolina, and Tennessee, the nonwhite segments of the population had increased infant death rates. Among the ten largest metropolitan areas, only Los Angeles and Houston had lower infant death rates in 1961 than in 1950; in six of these areas, the rates increased for both white and nonwhite infants, while in four, the increase was limited to nonwhite infants.

Our slow progress in reducing infant mortality in this country is magnified by the outstanding record of other countries. Half of the countries listed in Table 1-7 had higher rates than the United States in 1953-54; they all had lower rates by 1963-64. The trend since then has continued to our disadvantage.

Without question any death should be prevented if at all possible. For the baby who dies in his first year, the infant death rate is 100%. That so many should die in this country is tragic. At the very least we should be able to reduce infant death rates for all segments of our population to those of our more favored segments.

Table 1-7. Infant mortality in selected countries, 1963-64 and 1953-54

Country	Rates per 1,000 live births		Percent decline since 1953-54
	1963-64	1953-54	
United States	25.0	27.2	8
White	21.9	24.5	11
Nonwhite	41.3	43.4	5
Scotland	24.8	30.9	20
France	24.4	41.4	41
Israel	23.3	35.2	34
Japan	21.8	46.8	53
Czechoslovakia	21.7	41.3	47
England and Wales	20.5	26.2	22
Switzerland	19.8	28.5	31
Australia	19.3	22.9	16
Denmark	18.9	27.1	30
New Zealand	17.7	20.1	12
Finland	17.6	32.4	46
Norway	16.7	21.7	23
Netherlands	15.3	23.2	34
Sweden	14.8	18.7	21

From Metropolitan Life Insurance Co.: Statistical Bulletin, **48**:5, May 1967.

Table 1-8. Number of acute conditions per 100 persons, by age, sex, and condition group: United States, 1969

Condition group	All ages		Under 6		6-16		17-44		45 and over	
	M	F	M	F	M	F	M	F	M	F
Infective and para- sitic conditions	24.4	25.5	53.7	64.7	40.2	38.0	17.4	21.5	7.8	8.4
Respiratory condi- tions	104.1	115.8	189.9	187.0	140.4	163.8	83.8	110.6	63.2	64.8
Upper respiratory conditions	61.4	69.9	132.0	134.9	86.2	109.1	45.2	59.6	31.4	33.0
Influenza	37.3	41.5	41.1	42.2	48.1	50.7	35.4	46.9	29.2	28.6
Other	5.4	4.4	16.8	9.9	6.1	4.0	3.2	4.0	2.7	3.2
Digestive system conditions	10.1	10.3	10.0	14.8	16.2	14.0	8.8	9.9	6.9	6.6
Injuries	32.4	19.2	34.1	21.5	40.9	23.0	37.0	15.2	19.1	20.5
All other acute conditions	22.1	19.2	41.8	21.5	28.3	23.0	17.2	15.2	14.8	20.5
All acute condi- tions	193.1	208.0	329.4	341.7	266.1	271.2	164.2	204.0	111.8	124.0

Data from Vital and Health Statistics: Current estimates from the health interview survey, United States, 1969, PHS Publi- cation No. 1,000, Series 10, No. 63, Washington, D. C., June 1971, U. S. Government Printing Office.

Table 1-9. Days of restricted activity associated with acute conditions per 100 persons by age, sex, and condition group: United States, 1969

Condition group	All ages		Under 6		6-16		17-44		45 and over	
	M	F	M	F	M	F	M	F	M	F
Infective and para- sitic conditions	99.8	102.4	240.1	251.4	170.4	166.6	57.3	66.0	35.7	50.6
Respiratory condi- tions	362.6	449.0	619.1	595.8	419.2	516.4	253.0	380.7	344.1	433.4
Upper respiratory conditions	164.9	206.8	377.6	372.9	218.1	301.5	109.3	168.9	101.3	129.9
Influenza	158.0	202.2	142.0	166.0	164.9	181.7	118.1	181.3	207.8	253.0
Other	39.7	40.1	99.6	56.9	36.2	33.2	25.6	30.6	35.1	50.4
Digestive system conditions	38.6	39.2	21.8	38.5	35.8	28.7	36.9	39.2	50.1	46.6
Injuries	192.0	143.9	46.6	36.7	143.6	84.8	236.9	123.2	237.2	245.1
All other acute conditions	86.9	186.8	103.1	111.2	67.7	99.0	76.7	267.9	108.5	177.6
All acute condi- tions	853.3	921.3	1032.1	1033.5	865.7	895.5	775.0	877.1	871.3	953.3

Data from Vital and Health Statistics: Current estimates from the health interview survey, United States, 1969, PHS Publi- cation No. 1,000, Series 10, No. 63, Washington, D. C., June 1971, U. S. Government Printing Office.

THE NATIONAL HEALTH INTERVIEW SURVEY

In 1957 the National Center for Health Statistics was authorized by Congress to begin conducting a weekly survey of the health status of Americans. This is known as the National Health Interview Survey, and its findings have proved vitally important in analyzing up-to-date trends and needs in health matters.

We are reminded at this point of the World Health Organization's definition of health. Since most of the data reported from the National *Health* Interview Survey are reflections of deviations from health as it is defined, a more appropriate designation might be the National *Illness* Interview Survey. Although we recognize this discrepancy with our positive approach to health in this text, the data from the survey are most valuable: obviously those who are not ill by survey standards are well, and the best national estimate of this can only be gained from the National Health Interview Survey.

Each week since July 1957, a probability sample of households has been interviewed by trained personnel of the U. S. Bureau of the Census to obtain information about the health and other characteristics of each member of the household in the civilian, noninstitutional population of the United States. During the 52 weeks in 1969, the latest year for which complete data from this survey are available, the sample was composed of approximately 42,000 households containing about 134,000 persons living at the time of the interview. Since the survey follows a multistage probability design, it is possible to make estimates of the health of the total U. S. population with a high degree of statistical accuracy.

Acute conditions

During 1969 an estimated 396.5 million acute illnesses and injuries occurred that required either medical attention or reduced daily activity. The annual incidence rate per 100 persons was 200.8: Table 1-8 shows that the annual incidence for males was 193.1 per 100 males, whereas for females it was 208.0. Closer examination, however, reveals that there is generally little difference between the sexes at all ages with the exception of accidents, which tend to disfavor males. This difference is accounted for by the generally more hazardous work conditions that confront males and their tendency to take greater risks than females take. Most other acute conditions tend to disfavor females slightly, especially in the middle years. Since fewer women work, they may report reduced activity more readily than men who are inclined to continue work until an acute condition becomes relatively more severe. Table 1-9 relates acute conditions to days of restricted activity, and the data support the contrasts between injuries and other acute conditions in males and females.

Chronic conditions

Chronic conditions are all deviations from health that are not acute conditions as defined by the National Health Interview Survey. That is, a chronic condition is one that lasts more than three months and involves either medical attention or restricted activity. Conditions always classified as chronic, even though some symptoms of these might first appear within three months prior to the week of the interview, include the following.

Allergies
Arthritis or rheumatism
Asthma
Back or spine trouble (repeated)
Bronchitis (chronic)
Cleft palate
Club foot
Congenital conditions
Deafness or impaired hearing
Diabetes
Epilepsy
Gall bladder or liver trouble (chronic)
Hardening of the arteries
Heart trouble
Hemorrhoids or piles
Hernia or rupture
High blood pressure
Kidney stones or chronic kidney trouble
Mental illness
Missing fingers, hand or arm, toes, foot, or leg

Nervous trouble (chronic)
Palsy
Paralysis of any kind
Prostate trouble
Rheumatic fever
Sight impairment even when wearing glasses
Sinus trouble (repeated attacks)
Speech defects
Stiffness or deformity of the foot, leg, fingers, arm, or back (permanent)
Stomach ulcer and all other chronic stomach trouble
Stroke
Thyroid trouble or goiter
Tuberculosis
Tumor, cyst, or growth
Varicose veins

The data in Table 1-10 show that: (1) chronic conditions are rare prior to 17 years of age; (2) more men than women at all ages suffer from chronic conditions; and (3) chronic conditions increase

markedly with age and affect nearly 43% of the population over 65 years of age. Table 1-10 does not reveal the number of persons affected by one or more chronic conditions (estimated to be 53.9% in the 17 to 44 age group and 70.6% in the 45 to 64 age group), but only the percent of persons with limitations from such conditions.

Hospitalization

Some people do not consider themselves really ill unless they are admitted to a hospital. Although this appraisal is erroneous, the degree of hospitalization is, nonetheless, a valuable statistic in evaluating the health of the general population. Table 1-11 shows the number of discharges from short-term hospitals per 100 persons and the average stay in the hospital for each episode. Fe-

Table 1-10. Percent of persons with limitation of activity because of chronic condition, by degree of limitation, according to age, and sex: United States, 1969

Age group	Both sexes		Male		Female	
	With activity limitation	With major activity* limitation	With activity limitation	With major activity limitation	With activity limitation	With major activity limitation
All ages	11.6	9.1	12.2	9.6	11.0	8.7
Under 17 years	2.6	1.2	3.1	1.4	2.2	1.0
17-44	7.5	5.2	8.5	5.7	6.6	4.8
45-64	19.2	15.9	20.7	17.6	17.8	14.5
65+ years	42.4	37.5	45.8	41.8	39.9	34.3

Data from Vital and Health Statistics: Current estimates from the health interview survey, United States, 1969, PHS Publication No. 1,000, Series 10, No. 63, Washington, D. C., June 1971, U. S. Government Printing Office.
*Major activity refers to ability to work, keep house, or engage in school or preschool activities.

Table 1-11. Number of discharges from short-term hospitals and average length of stay by sex and age: United States, 1969

Age group	Number of discharges per 100 persons			Average length of stay		
	Both	Male	Female	Both	Male	Female
All ages	12.9	10.6	15.1	9.0	10.5	8.1
Under 17 years	6.5	6.9	6.0	5.6	5.4	5.8
17-24	15.5	8.2	21.8	6.1	9.9	4.9
25-34	16.4	7.6	24.4	6.2	9.3	5.4
35-44	12.9	10.7	15.0	8.9	10.8	7.7
45-64	14.8	14.2	15.4	10.8	11.8	10.0
65+	24.1	25.1	23.3	14.9	15.1	14.6

Data from Vital and Health Statistics: Current estimates from the health interview survey, United States, 1969, PHS Publication No. 1,000, Series 10, No. 63, Washington, D. C., June 1971, U. S. Government Printing Office.

males in the childbearing years have more hospital discharges than males in the same age categories. The average stay is less for females at all ages, but especially in the 17 to 24 age category. Table 1-12 provides additional data by number of episodes per person.

Caution is suggested in analyzing these data. Both Tables 1-11 and 1-12 refer only to short-term hospitals. Excluded are all hospitals for the chronically ill, convalescent, and mentally ill, and other facilities, such as nursing homes, that provide care for the disabled and sick.

Physician visits

The National Health Interview Survey defines a physician visit as any consultation with a doctor of medicine or an osteopath,

either in person or by telephone, for examination, treatment, or advice. The service may be rendered by the physician himself, or by a nurse or another person acting under the supervision of the physician.

During 1969 there were an estimated 839.6 million physician visits, excluding visits to hospital inpatients. Table 1-13 shows that 69.4% of the population saw or talked with a physician sometime in the previous year, 23.6% in the previous 1 to 4 years, 43% had not seen a physician in the past 5 years, and 2% either never had or did not know if they ever had seen a physician. There is little significant variation by age group.

Finally, Table 1-14 indicates the average number of physician visits each person makes a year.

Table 1-12. Percent distribution of persons with short-term hospital episodes, by number of episodes, age, and sex: United States, 1969

Age	Number of episodes							
	None		One		Two		Three and over	
	Male	Female	Male	Female	Male	Female	Male	Female
All ages	91.7	87.9	7.1	110.3	1.0	1.4	0.3	0.4
Under 17 years	94.0	95.1	5.4	4.3	0.5	0.5	*	*
17-24	93.1	81.2	6.2	16.9	0.6	1.7	*	*
25-34	93.3	79.3	6.0	17.8	0.6	2.3	*	0.5
35-44	92.1	87.2	6.7	11.2	1.0	1.3	*	*
45-64	89.1	88.4	8.9	9.6	1.6	1.5	0.4	0.5
65+	83.1	83.7	13.1	12.4	2.6	2.9	1.2	0.9

Data from Vital and Health Statistics: Current estimates from the health interview survey, United States, 1969, PHS Publication No. 1,000, Series 10, No. 63, Washington, D. C., June 1971, U. S. Government Printing Office.
*Not significant.

Table 1-13. Percent distribution since last physician visit, according to age: United States, 1969

Time since last physician visit	All ages	Under 17 years	17-24	25-44	45-64	65 and over
Less than 6 months	54.4	51.9	57.6	53.6	54.2	61.5
6-11 months	15.0	16.6	16.1	15.8	13.2	9.7
1 year	12.2	14.5	11.6	12.5	10.6	7.5
2-4 years	11.4	10.9	9.7	12.2	12.9	10.6
5 years and over	4.3	2.7	2.2	3.7	6.9	8.1
Never	0.7	1.4	0.7	0.2	0.2	0.3
Unknown	2.0	2.0	2.1	2.0	2.0	2.2

Data from Vital and Health Statistics: Current estimates from the health interview survey, United States, 1969, PHS Publication No. 1,000, Series 10, No. 63, Washington, D. C., June 1971, U. S. Government Printing Office.

Table 1-14. Number of physician visits per person per year, by age and sex: United States, 1969

Age group	Both sexes	Male	Female
All ages	4.3	3.7	4.7
Under 17 years	3.6	3.7	3.4
17-24	4.0	3.0	4.8
25-44	4.3	3.2	5.3
45-64	4.7	4.1	5.2
65-74	6.1	5.5	6.6
75 and over	6.2	5.5	6.7

Data from Vital and Health Statistics: Current estimates from the health interview survey, United States, 1969, PHS Publication No. 1,000, Series 10, No. 63, Washington, D. C., June 1971, U. S. Government Printing Office.

Implications for the young adult

But what meaning do these statistics from the National Health Interview Survey have for you? To answer this question we'll focus on the age categories that include you in Tables 1-8 through 1-14; these will be the 17 to 44, 17 to 34, 17 to 24 categories, depending on the tables being studied. First, if you are a man, you suffer from 1.64 acute conditions a year (Table 1-8) that cause an average of 7.75 days of restricted activity each (Table 1-9). If you are a woman, you suffer from 2.04 acute conditions a year that restrict your activity for nearly 8.8 days each. Injuries and upper respiratory conditions account for most of these difficulties in men; upper respiratory, influenza, and to a lesser degree injuries are the major sources of difficulty in women. At your age you probably are on the low side of the statistics that contribute to these averages. If so, enjoy your good fortune, because without positive action on your part, time will work against you, and you will tend toward the upper limits of these statistics. Note also that although the average acute conditions are fewer for the 45 and over age group, the days of restricted activity are greater.

Although acute conditions diminish after 45 years of age, chronic conditions increase markedly beyond the period in life you now enjoy. A little more than 7% in your age group suffer activity limitation because of a chronic condition (Table 1-10), men somewhat more than women. These statistics increase throughout life, tending always to disfavor males. Whatever you learn now about all chronic conditions in general may hold you in good stead in later years. Since we know how to cure few of these, knowledge that might help you to cope with them later in life, should you develop a chronic disease, will be immensely valuable.

More than 8% of males, ages 17 to 24, spend time in the hospital each year and average 9.9 days per visit (Table 1-11). The statistics for women, 21.8% discharged and 4.9 average days per visit, clearly indicate more discharges with shorter stays than those of men. Childbearing is undoubtedly the major reason for this difference, although there may be others: the incidence of acute conditions is more frequent in females than in males, and these conditions may lead to increased hospitalization; but also females are more apt to be at home for interviews and are more inclined to go to the doctor. The number of males going into the hospital only one time each year is steady up to 45 years of age and then increases gradually (Table 1-12). For women, the number of visits to a hospital increases during the childbearing years and then decreases after these years. The difference with increasing age is in the average length of stay in the hospital per episode (Table 1-11).

There is better than one chance in two that you have seen a physician in the last six months (Table 1-13), better than one chance in ten that you last saw one as long ago as two to four years, and one chance in twenty that your record is even poorer than that. Again, you probably tend toward the favorable end of the continuum. If dental information were available, however, we guess that the statistics for your age group would not be as good as those seen in Table 1-13. Table 1-14 indicates that if you have seen a physician in the last year, the chances are good that you have had several visits: if you are a male, you have averaged three visits; if a female, you have averaged nearly five.

Acute conditions, limitation of activity, hospitalization, and physician visits, singularly or combined, may not be of serious consequence for you personally, if in fact you belong in one or all of these categories. If you do, is the problem of a temporary nature? If it is, is there residual concern that might return? Does any part of your present behavior tend to extend or aggravate an existing subhealthy condition? Even if you do not see yourself in any of these statistics, and the chances are good that you do not, the fact that health is increasingly more difficult to maintain with age should encourage you to exercise every intelligent precaution in behalf of your health both now and in the future.

Up to this point we have talked about health mostly in the negative sense, that is in terms of mortality and morbidity statistics. These have been stage setters. They tell us that many people experience subnormal health, often temporary, sometimes permanent. But our primary subject is good health—yours, up to the limits of your potential—and how it might be maintained.

A FORMULA FOR HEALTH— THE ELEMENTS

A young girl visiting friends was asked if she wanted to prepare a dinner. She answered yes and decided upon macaroni and cheese. When she asked for a cookbook, her hostess exclaimed, "What! You need a cookbook to fix macaroni and cheese?" "Of course," the girl replied, "I don't want to make a mistake."

We choose to view health at this point as the girl did her macaroni and cheese. It would be easy for us to asume you know what health is, but we would rather not. There are many elements to health, and we need to discuss them all lest we overlook one that is important.

Heredity

A wag has said, "If you want a long life, choose long-lived grandparents." Obviously, choice is impossible, but the saying emphasizes the incontrovertible importance of heredity in our lives. Our heritage determines to a great degree our vision, dentition, height, body build, color of hair, and whether we keep our hair or not, intelligence or lack of it, and many other general characteristics. It also directly determines the presence or absence of many diseases or disorders including phenylketonuria (PKU), strabismus, Huntington's chorea, epilepsy, hemophilia, diabetes mellitus, migraine headaches, and to an unknown but influencing extent both cardiovascular disorders and cancer. Human beings have an estimated 10,000 pairs of genes, and each of the many characteristics we possess is controlled by a variety of genes that function not independently of each other but under the influence of other genes in a complex cellular environment.

Although you were not consulted when the male and female chromosomes were joined together to create you, you do have a most important decision to make about how the chromosomes of your germ cells are to be recombined. The decision you make in the choice of a marriage partner is personal health in ecologic perspective if you include eugenic principles in this decision. Part of Chapter 9 is devoted to this subject.

Early environment

Which is more influential on development, heredity or environment? We can't really say, but it is clear that each has considerable influence; and many experts believe environment to be as important as heredity. For example, babies born prematurely have a higher mortality than full-term babies. Similarly, babies born to Bantu mothers in

South Africa have a higher mortality than babies born to black mothers in the United States. These examples illustrate the influence of the environment rather than heredity, and the babies have very little more influence over the former than over the latter.

Once we are beyond infancy (statistically, the first year of life), we begin to shape our environment with increasing effect even as it continues to influence our development. For example, the more a child is read to in his early childhood years, the easier he is able to handle the entire process of language development. Children raised in families where one parent smokes have a 40% chance of developing the smoking habit; those raised in families where both parents smoke have an 80% chance. Most young people do not use drugs except perhaps during a brief period of experimentation, but some succumb to the "attraction" in the face of environmental pressures that they find overwhelming.

Although the correlation certainly is not perfect, the more satisfactory a person's early environment the more satisfactory will be his health. The effect of early environment on health is discussed in Chapter 9.

Understanding of physical self

An important element for health is an intelligent understanding of our physical self, our body with all its assets and limitations. As we strive to improve aspects of our physical self, our total health status tends also to be improved.

Accurate perception of status. Health status is enhanced when it is accurately perceived by its owner. Certainly, we would like to be free from all disease and disability, but few of us are. We know an Adonis who is a psychologic weakling because of a minor speech defect; we also know a 28-year-old political scientist (Ph.D.) at a leading state university, who is blind. These are both examples that are obvious to others as well as to the handicapped. Many other circumstances are more subtle. For example, glaucoma develops in the third and fourth decade

of life and is a prime cause of blindness. Yet its progressive nature need never terminate in blindness if early symptoms are recognized and the appropriate preventive action (see p. 67) is taken. This can only be done, of course, when we obtain current, accurate information about our status. Regular medical examinations (at least once every two years to age 30 and yearly thereafter, and specific examinations if necessary) must become routine.

Hypochondria. Routine examination by a qualified general practitioner or specialist does not always indicate an overconcern for our health status. Unfortunately, too many Americans have developed a hypochondriasis that is completely unrealistic with their true physical state, yet as they perpetuate a morbid concern for their physical being they very often do become ill. Such an illness is termed psychosomatic because of its emotional or psychogenic origin. Nutrition quacks (Chapter 4), cancer charlatans (Chapter 11), and many others feed like parasites on those who are mentally insecure about their health. Health can become a fetish; don't let it.

Ability to relax. It is important to learn to take time out at regular intervals each day and simply "let go." This can be done effectively in a quick break that lasts only a few minutes or in 10 to 20 minutes of sleep at mid-day. Another approach is to change activities; as one task begins to wear and prove difficult, set it aside and move to something else. When you recreate, forget your work and study problems. It is surprising how much easier a task becomes when you return to it after a period of relaxation or change.

The ability to relax extends to the sleeping period as well. Adequate sleep that normally follows a prebedtime routine is most conducive to desired accomplishment during the waking hours. Irregularity in your sleep patterns can only lead to reduced accomplishment and eventually poorer health.

Sufficient energy and proper nutrition. Any activity requires sufficient energy. If you have ever said, "I just don't feel like it; I don't have the energy," you may be reflecting normal fatigue; but if you use this excuse too often, there may be something physically wrong, and you should consult a physician. If your energy level is consistently low, and there is no underlying medical reason, you most likely have neglected a basic physical need. The direct cause is inadequate nutrition. Perhaps no aspect of health is so thoroughly and scientifically understood and yet so universally abused as that of nutrition. Despite the claims of faddists and quacks, there is no substitute for a balanced and adequate diet if good health is to be maintained. To believe and practice otherwise can only be deleterious to health. Chapter 4 covers this topic extensively.

There is a tendency for many American youth to develop an energy-less syndrome. This is caused by poor nutrition compounded by lack of activity and inadequate rest. This leads to depression and anxiety, which leads to continued poor nutrition, which leads to less activity, which leads to deeper depression, and so the cycle continues. The direct consequence is continually poor health in general, but the more tragic consequence is incomplete accomplishment of important life objectives.

Wise use of leisure time. It is predicted that by the year 2000 three persons in every ten will be able to provide all the goods and services needed by our society. How to use leisure time wisely may be a major challenge of the future and is fast becoming a challenge today. We are not succeeding in meeting this challenge, when the average life expectancy of males after retirement is approximately two years. We must learn to find purpose and meaning in other things besides work. This is a particular need for men. Those who do this more successfully early in life appear to enjoy longer, healthier lives.

Constant weight. Our weight at age 25 should be the weight we hold throughout the remainder of life. Too often, the young adult rides a roller coaster of pounds off,

pounds on, and then as a maturing adult, gradually adds insidious poundage with each passing decade. Both these practices are harmful to all body systems and result in premature death. Ideally, weight should gradually increase to its appropriate maximum for the height, sex, and structural development of the individual and should remain at this level thereafter. In the middle and late years predictable and uncontrollable change will be a slight loss in weight coincidental with the aging process. As part of aging, cells lose their ability to retain water, and weight loss is the observed consequence.

Appropriate behavior patterns

Homo sapiens is a complex species that is little more than primitively understood even by our most astute scientists. On the physical-chemical-medical level, the brain is still a mystery even though we can explain in a limited way how it functions biochemically. Difficult transplants (cornea, kidney, heart, lungs) have been attempted with varying success, but the problems of tissue compatability between human beings still remain.

On the social-behavioral level the interrelations of one person with another are perplexing and are becoming increasingly traumatic. The institution of marriage and family has had many variations everywhere over time, and we are still far from certain which variation is the most viable, or if in fact there is only one. Our social and political institutions—schools, hospitals, city councils, state legislatures, universities, neighborhood civic groups, churches—the formal and informal organizations we have developed to order our lives according to what we believe is meaningful and important, are subject to serious criticism from all quarters. There is general agreement that new organizational patterns are needed, but whether we are capable and flexible enough to develop them is not yet clear.

To each of us, our person seems to be in the center of all this activity, and in a sense it is. From one perspective, each person is the complex, beautiful consequence of billions of cells working together with some degree of efficiency and effectiveness. From another perspective, each person is as one cell in the complex, combined activity of all living organisms on this planet. Each of us copes with the myriad of interactions taking place at both these levels with a behavior pattern, which is, in fact, our personality.

Our ability to cope is shown in all matters that directly and indirectly affect health. Those of a direct nature are the most obvious and most traditional: cross only with the green light; hold suspect a painless lump in the breast; the drug habit is tough to kick, and drugs should be avoided. Those of an indirect nature are less obvious, but nonetheless relevant to individual health: a vote for fluoridation, a letter to a Congressman protesting endless atmospheric wastes from a nearby industrial plant, preventive maintenance of our automobile's exhaust system, responsible concern for the genetic possibilities as a consequence of the choice of marriage partner. The health behavior patterns that you reflect now and might develop in the future are important ingredients in your formula for health.

Relevancy—the being and belonging of life

Whatever our physical gifts and deficiencies, our ability to cope with and enjoy life is based on our attitudes. Our mental outlook, our ability to find purpose in our lives and to relate to other human beings and to our environment, is a final element for health. Like the perfect balance of several tasty spices, the following qualities, in satisfactory balance, are necessary to good health.

Acceptance and appreciation of self. We have talked of the need for understanding our physical self. But much more besides understanding is needed if we are to achieve and maintain health. We must accept and appreciate our physical self. For many people this is not always easy, and poor mental health is often caused by dissatisfaction or serious unhappiness with the self-image, par-ticularly its physical component. You are unique. There is no one else exactly like you alive today, nor will there ever be. You should accept, appreciate, and be proud of this fact.

Confidence tempered by insight. An acceptance and appreciation of self should be followed by confidence that we can perform well within our limitations. Obviously, a deaf person cannot aspire to become a skilled musician, nor can a person with only one arm become a surgeon. But the deaf, the amputees, all handicapped, and equally so, all human beings, need to develop confidence through achievement.

One approach is to identify a task or skill at which you are especially good and work to become even better at it. Whenever you feel frustrated by new challenges, return to this activity for a brief respite. Don't use it as a crutch that you never leave, but carry the confidence you build there to new tasks.

All people doubt themselves to some degree when they step out to meet a new challenge. The more confidence they carry with them from previous successful experiences, the more apt are they to be successful in the new experience.

Discipline. Dreams are easy to conjure. We see ourselves as successful businessmen, dancers performing before large audiences, or noted scientists perhaps winning a Nobel prize. But none of these desirable goals is achieved by dreams alone. Successful goal achievement is hard work that requires much self-discipline to do the small daily tasks well with confidence that the larger goals will eventually come about. As Thomas Carlyle said, "Our duty is not to see what lies dimly in the distance, but to do what lies clearly at hand."

Order. What is your life plan? By now you should be developing one even if it is not yet completely clear. Do your daily activities contribute to your life plan? They should. The fact that you desire an education beyond high school is a clear indication that you are developing a life plan, however vague it still may be. Your daily experiences—classes, study, small group meetings, drama, local politics, community action groups—should fit this life plan, and you should be committed to them. Have you studied the important social issues of our time, and have you committed yourself to one or more of them with personal involvement? What is the depth of your concern (Fig. 1-3)? What and who you become is being determined to no small measure right

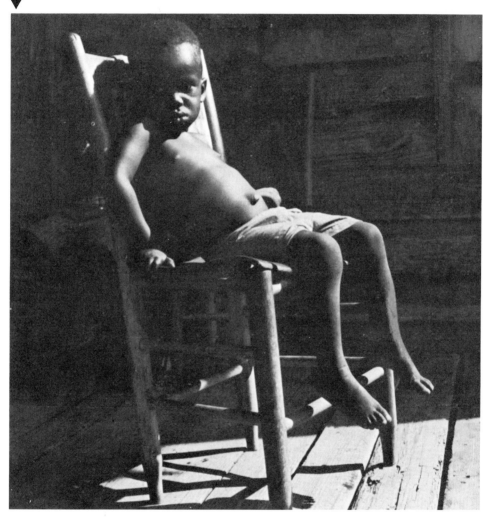

Published by
THE GREATER KANSAS CITY
CONFERENCE OF STUDENT
PROFESSIONAL ORGANIZATIONS

Fig. 1-3. The front cover from an early issue of **Concern,** a magazine reporting on the activities of one group of socially motivated students.

now by how you use your time. It should be ordered and purposeful, with time for fun and relaxation but not in disproportion to your other important activities.

Responsibility. The need to face responsibilities is obvious, but to do so is not always easy. Some responsibilities are thrust upon us by society. As a family member we have certain responsibilities to our parents, siblings, grandparents, and others. As a member of a campus community we have certain responsibilities to roommates, fellow resident hall members, instructors, and others. As a producer of goods or services in a community we have certain responsibilities to help maintain law and order, to improve unsafe conditions, to be concerned about local government, and to vote. Other responsibilities we assume voluntarily. In accepting a job, marrying, and conceiving a new life, we take on new responsibilities that we must not turn from lest we lose the respect of others as well as of ourselves. The degree to which we accept these responsibilities will reveal, in part, the quality of health we possess.

Courage. Adversity is a part of life. Some people are fortunate to be challenged by relatively little; others have the misfortune to be challenged by a great deal. Some are defeated by a single tragic event; others overcome recurrent tragedies and lead meaningful lives despite them—or maybe because of them. How will you react to a major traumatic event in your life, one that demands courage to face new events despite the loss or defeat? We are never certain until the challenge faces us. We hope our health, particularly our mental health, and our philosophy and prior experience are sufficient for us to handle the situation successfully.

Interest in others. Basically, we are ego-centered individuals, and we demonstrate this characteristic in varying degrees and forms of selfishness. Within normal and controlled limits, selfishness has certain values, but too many people manifest this characteristic to a detrimental excess. When they do, their circle of friends is usually small and tends to be composed of similar types of persons. Sincere interest in other people is an important aspect of the healthy personality. As you are able to develop a concern for others, you will improve the quality of your interpersonal relationships. Your circle of friends, exciting, different kinds of people, will increase markedly.

Sense of humor. How seriously do you take yourself? Do you get angry when others catch you in a verbal slip or a behavior mannerism that proves embarrassing? You should be able to laugh at these situations. Enjoy the good fun at your expense, and then forget it. If you do, every one else will also. If you don't, you may be unhappy. Enjoy the temporary humor of others in similar situations, but then let the incident die. Continual recall lacks humor and rapidly becomes morbid.

A sense of humor permits you to overcome otherwise difficult circumstances. The English theme that comes back to you for a third and fourth time doesn't seem so bad if you can laugh and then try once more to improve it. The short story you believe is wonderful needs a laugh when it is returned for the fifth time from a potential publisher with the standard reject slip. Laughter, at ourselves, with others, and in the face of difficulty, is the balm that oils the track to eventual success.

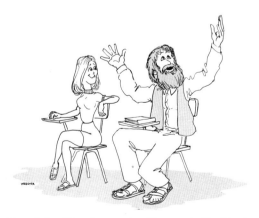

Fig. 1-4. "As I see it, 'Personal Health in Ecologic Perspective' means you should be aware of the interconnectedness of all existence —and think about it while brushing your teeth." (Courtesy Martin Webster.)

The joy and beauty of life. All previous elements are useless unless you can say, "How wonderful it is to be alive. Life is so beautiful, so joyous, and there is so much to be done. Let me get on with it *now.*" If you can do this, you have the final vital element for health.

A FORMULA FOR HEALTH—THE WORKING INSTRUCTIONS

Webster's Third New International Dictionary defines ecology as:

1: a branch of science concerned with the interrelationship of organisms and their environment esp. as manifested by natural cycles and rhythms, community development and structure, interaction between different kinds of organisms, geographic distributions, and population alterations . . . 2: the totality or pattern of relations between organisms and their environment . . .

Human ecology would be similarly described if we let the adjective simply restrict the field of discourse to man.

Earlier (p. 4) we paraphrased a definition of human ecology by Shimkin that is somewhat more specific than Webster's definition. In complete context, Shimkin's concept of human ecology is as follows.

Human ecology seeks to identify common elements, organizational systems, and processes in the vast array of human behavior. . . . The focus of human ecology, like that of ecology generally, is the interacting population in a specific framework of time, space, and habitat. The essence of ecological analysis is the measurement and interpretation of physical transactions within the population, and between the population and its physical and biological environment.*

To some degree these two definitions are divergent. Webster's general definition, restricted to man, signifies the totality or pattern of relation between men and their environment. Shimkin, expanding on his definition from *Introduction to Human Ecology,* tends to look at the parts first, suggesting we limit ourselves to identified elements and interrelationships, the use of

precise mathematical models, and the development of statistical procedures. Both these definitions are necessary to describe our ecologic perspective. We view the personal health of all men in the holistic manner that Webster describes, but we shall also show how the precision of Shimkin's approach is applicable to problems of cancer, viral diseases, behavioral disorders, traffic hazards, air and water pollution, as well as others. The principles of epidemiology, the most developed area of applied ecology, will be included, according to Shimkin's approach, when appropriate.

The crisis of crises

Are you inclined to believe the barrage of fearful predictions about the destruction of our vital ecologic balances? It might be easy to discount these warnings, especially when the predictions are more emotional than factual. After all, the world has existed for a long time, perhaps five billion years or more, and any talk about extinction in five, fifty, or even five hundred years is ridiculous. But is it? We may very well be at the point in time where it is our choice to turn down the road to the millenium or down the road to obliteration. A noted scientist, J. R. Platt, has indicated why this might be so. Writing in *Science,* Platt said:

There is only one crisis in the world. It is the crisis of transformation. The trouble is that it is now coming upon us in a storm of crisis problems from every direction. But if we look quantitatively at the course of our changes in this century, we can see immediately why the problems are building up so rapidly at this time, and we will see that it now becomes urgent for us to mobilize all our intelligence to solve these problems if we are to keep from killing ourselves in the next few years.*

Platt indicates that the human race is on the rising "S-curve" of change. We see new levels of technologic power being developed but do not appreciate how rapid

*From Shimkin, D. B.: Introduction to human ecology, ed. 2, Champaign, Ill., 1969, Center of Human Ecology and University of Illinois, p. 1.

*From Platt, J. R.: What we must do, Science **166**(3909):1115, November 28, 1969. Copyright 1969 by the American Association for the Advancement of Science.

Table 1-15. Classification of problems and crises by estimated time and intensity: United States

Grade	Estimated crisis intensity (number affected × degree of effect)		Estimated time to crisis*		
			1 to 5 years	5 to 20 years	20 to 50 years
1.		Total annihilation	Nuclear or RCBW escalation	Nuclear or RCBW escalation	*(Solved or dead)
2.	10^8	Great destruction or change (physical, biological, or political)	(Too soon)	Participatory democracy / Ecological balance	Political theory and economic structure / Population planning / Patterns of living / Education / Communications / Integrative philosophy
3.	10^7	Widespread almost unbearable tension	Administrative management / Slums / Participatory democracy / Racial conflict	Pollution / Poverty / Law and justice	?
4.	10^6	Large-scale distress	Transportation / Neighborhood ugliness / Crime	Communications gap	?
5.	10^5	Tension producing responsive change	Cancer and heart / Smoking and drugs / Artificial organs / Accidents / Sonic boom / Water supply / Marine resources / Privacy on computers	Educational inadequacy	?
6.		Other problems— important, but adequately researched	Military R & D / New educational methods / Mental illness / Fusion power	Military R & D	
7.		Exaggerated dangers and hopes	Mind control / Heart transplants / Definition of death	Sperm banks / Freezing bodies / Unemployment from automation	Eugenics
8.		Noncrisis problems being "over-studied"	Man in space / Most basic science		

From Platt, J. R.: What we must do, Science **166**(3909):1118, November 28, 1969. Copyright 1969 by the American Association for the Advancement of Science.

*If no major effort is made at anticipatory solution.

Table 1-16. Classification of problems and crises by estimated time and intensity: world

Grade	Estimated crisis intensity (number affected × degree of effect)		Estimated time to crisis*		
			1 to 5 years	5 to 20 years	20 to 50 years
1.	10^{10}	Total annihilation	Nuclear or RCBW escalation	Nuclear or RCBW escalation	*(Solved or dead)
2.	10^9	Great destruction or change (physical, biological, or political)	(Too soon)	Famines Ecological balance Development failures Local wars Rich-poor gap	Economic structure and political theory Population and ecological balance Patterns of living Universal education Communications-integration Management of world Integrative philosophy
3.	10^8	Widespread almost unbearable tension	Administrative management Need for participation Group and racial conflict Poverty-rising expectations Environmental degradation	Poverty Pollution Racial wars Political rigidity Strong dictatorships	?
4.	10^7	Large-scale distress	Transportation Diseases Loss of old cultures	Housing Education Independence of big powers Communications gap	?
5.	10^6	Tension producing responsive change	Regional organization Water supplies	?	?
6.		Other problems—important, but adequately researched	Technical development design Intelligent monetary design		
7.		Exaggerated dangers and hopes			Eugenics Melting of ice caps
8.		Noncrisis problems being "overstudied"	Man in space Most basic science		

From Platt, J. R.: What we must do, Science **166**(3909):1119, November 28, 1969. Copyright 1969 by the American Association for the Advancement of Science.
*If no major effort is made at anticipatory solution.

and large these changes are compared with all previous changes in history. For example, in the past 100 years, we have increased our speed of communication by a factor of 10^7, our speed of travel by 10^2, our speed of data handling by 10^6, our ability to control diseases by 10^2, and our rate of population growth by 10^3 from what they were a few thousand years ago.

But these technologic changes are now approaching certain natural limits. The "S-curve" is leveling off. It is likely that we shall never have faster communication, more powerful weapons, or more danger than we have now. If this prediction is true and if we could learn to live with ourselves in the next few years without causing near or complete destruction, we might develop new, adequate social and political structures that we could live with for many generations into the future.

The trouble, Platt cautions, is that we may not survive these next few years.

The human race today is like a rocket on a launching pad. We have been building up to this moment of takeoff for a long time, and if we can get safely through the takeoff period, we may fly on a new and exciting course for a long time to come. But at this moment, as the powerful new engines are fired, their thrust and roar shakes and stresses every part of the ship and may cause the whole thing to blow up before we can steer it on its way. Our problem today is to harness and direct these tremendous new forces through this dangerous transition period to the new world instead of to destruction. But unless we can do this, the rapidly increasing strains and crises of the next decade may kill us all. They will make the last 20 years look like a peaceful interlude.*

To document his concerns Platt has classified all problems on a gradation from those that could be most destructive (that is, total annihilation) to those least destructive but nonetheless serious; and for each rank, he has defined an estimated time and type of crisis if no effort is made at anticipatory solution. Table 1-15 shows Platt's classifica-

*From Platt, J. R.: What we must do, Science **166**(3909):1115, November 28, 1969. Copyright 1969 by the American Association for the Advancement of Science.

tion of problems by estimated time and intensity for the United States; the classifications in Table 1-16 are for the world.

Of most concern, of course, is nuclear or radiologic-chemical-biologic warfare (RCBW) escalation that might result in total annihilation; health, in a civilized sense, would be without meaning. At all grade levels below this, however, the magnitude of health problems, among all the problems cited, is awesome. And the items included in the tables are not exhaustive.

Each of these crises is serious in itself. What makes them still more dangerous is their combination. We usually manage to deal effectively with one, two, or even three crises; but when several converge simultaneously, the additive effect may overwhelm our administrative and individual coping processes. Large cities could become silent canyons if crises of garbage, crime, transportation, electricity, fire, and disease were all to peak at once, as was the case in New York City in 1968. If this should happen on a widespread scale and last for a significant period of time, both individual health and the total ecologic system could literally disintegrate. Platt has appropriately described this very possible situation as our "crisis of crises."

Our uncertain perspective

Platt's perceptive and disturbing presentation of a most complex situation reminds us that we have moved so fast that we do not realize how dangerous many of our crises are. W. D. McElroy explains our problem as follows:

The most serious problems listed [in Platt's article] present a common feature; they will be settled principally by political decision, by economic choice, and by the education of people. If such solutions are to be truly effective, however, they must be buttressed by sound knowledge and understanding. It is precisely at this point that the problems that confront us today differ from those that led to the massive scientific efforts during and following World War II. Thirty years ago much of the basic science was available and was used to devise urgently needed technologies; today, much of the requisite knowledge simply does not exist. We know far too little about the interactions that occur within any ecological system. We do not really understand the dynamics of our environment or the effects of the technology upon it. We know little about the more subtle effects of pollution. We cannot predict with confidence the behavior of individuals nor that of social groups and institutions. We are not in a position to assess adequately the relative costs and benefits to society of any technology or any course of action.*

In the face of this uncertainty we must maintain our perspective. We must continue to support science but also be certain that science examines its own priorities. Grades 5 and below in Platt's tables occupy the largest numbers of scientists. Consider, for example, the dramatic news of heart transplants and the many scientists and technicians occupied by this one problem. This work, however, will never help more than a few thousand of the six billion people on the earth in the year 2000. In another area, tens of thousands of our best scientists are tied up in space research—glorious morale-building for the whole nation, yes, but grossly overstudied in relation to our real crises.

Our perspective today is uncertain and probably somewhat distorted. As individuals and as a nation we must strive to refocus it on the issues, the problems, the crises, that are most important.

Open-ended men in a closed-system world

Man may be viewed as an open-ended system, constantly interacting with his environment in order to maintain his life and his functions as a member of the species. In centuries past he has interacted indiscriminantly with other species and the total ecosystem, but he has not suffered the consequences immediately because the world was his oyster and space was unlimited. In reality, of course, space was not unlimited, but appeared to be while the continents were being discovered and human numbers were few.

But the world *is* a closed system, our cautious steps toward outer space notwithstanding; and Dubos reminds us that we must achieve equilibrium if we are to maintain life and health.

All ecological systems, whether man-made or natural, must in the long run achieve a state of equilibrium and be self-regenerating with regard to both energy and materials. The ecology of highly industrialized nations has been in a state of disequilibrium for several decades. Furthermore, ecological instability is increasing at such an accelerated rate that disasters are inevitable if the trend continues. We cannot afford to delay much longer the development of a nearly "closed" system in which materials will retain their value throughout the system, by being recycled instead of discarded.*

Interaction between man and his environment must take on new dimensions. Endless quantitative growth has been the American philosophy for 300 years. Now it is important that we achieve an equilibrium for society just as we strive for it as individuals. If we fail in this, the predictions of men like Platt, McElroy, and Dubos will surely come true.

Mix gently, sample often

Our formula for health needs its working instructions. We can only caution at this point to "mix gently and sample often."

Maximum health potential is found in such key words as moderation, regularity, diversity, and relaxation. Each of these terms conveys the idea of slow mixing rather than fast agitation. Severe and rapid deviation from the normal balance of individual life processes will usually prove harmful. In the long run it is much easier and more healthful to identify deviation when it is small and to make the appropriate, equally small, correction required.

In addition, conditions in the world, and particularly in the industrialized, more affluent portion of it, are such that we damn well better examine what we are doing to

*From McElroy, W. D.: A crisis of crises, Science 167(3914):9, January 2, 1970. Copyright 1970 by the American Association for the Advancement of Science.

*From Dubos, R.: A social design for science, Science 166(3907):823, November 14, 1969. Copyright 1969 by the American Association for the Advancement of Science.

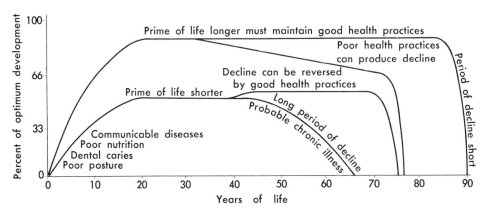

Fig. 1-5. Prime of life in relation to optimum development and longevity.

ourselves and discover fast what changes need to be made to maintain and ensure our continued viability. On the personal level this means medical and psychologic examinations as needed and conscientious follow-through on the advice received. On the community level this means concern, rationality, responsibility, involvement, and whatever else it takes to apply our intelligence to the improvement of our ecologic relationships. As "sample often" implies, these efforts, immediately personal but always couched in ecologic perspective, must be continuous.

DEALING IN FUTURES

In the commodity market the phrase "to deal in futures" means that someone expects the value of something, perhaps gold or silver, to increase in value in the future, and so he buys as much as he dares and can obtain. If the price does go up, he is able to sell at a profit; if the price goes down, he can sell only at a loss.

You are dealing in futures right now whether you want to or not. The commodity is yourself, and what you "buy" today, tomorrow, this year, and beyond will determine the long-run value of your investment. Fig. 1-5 depicts this concept clearly. Will your prime of life be close to your maximum health potential? How long will you maintain your prime of life? Answers to these questions are being recorded now with or without your conscious influence. We hope your current investment is both conscious and considerable; if not, perhaps it will be by the time you finish this book.

PART II
Personal health

But do your own work and I shall know you. Do your work and you shall reinforce yourself. A man must consider what a blind-man's-buff is this game of conformity.

RALPH WALDO EMERSON

Emerson's essay "Self-Reliance," written in 1841, speaks cogently to us today. In the language of the present he tells us to "do our own thing"; to assess our goals; to evaluate the distractions; and to make rational decisions in all matters of life, including those that directly affect our health and well-being. For example, Emerson would find the current drug craze, much of it perpetuated by follow-the-leader behavior, abhorrent. He would wonder what goals a drug addict could hold to play such "blindman's-buff," and thereby seriously jeopardize his life, not to mention his health.

A person's values determine his behavior; Emerson might have a struggle analyzing the values held by youth, were he living today. Our culture is complex whether we view the inner city or suburbia, and even rural living offers conflicts and problems not present a hundred years ago. But we dare not transfer the responsibility for personal value assessment to others; each person must define his own values and determine his behavior accordingly.

Part II is a potpourri of many subjects that constantly demand decisions by all of us. How do I view my world and respond to it (Chapter 2); what physical image do I want to project to others (Chapter 3); what is the most ideal balance of food and activity for me (Chapter 4); can I really be safe in an increasingly dynamic environment (Chapter 5); should I allow tobacco, alcohol, drugs, and related substances to directly influence my personality and my life (Chapter 6); are diseases, either acute or chronic, really a problem today (Chapter 7)? As you read Part II harken back to Emerson's admonition. It takes greater courage to be your own master than it does to conform.

CHAPTER 2

Healthy personality

Mental illness is America's worst social problem. One out of every twelve Americans needs treatment for mental illness; only a fraction of these are receiving it. More than one half of those who visit physicians with physical complaints are actually plagued by mental and emotional problems. One out of every twelve persons will be hospitalized for mental illness in his lifetime. About 480,000, or nearly a third, of all hospital beds in America are occupied by mentally ill patients. It is estimated that over 7 billion dollars are spent for treatment, care, and time lost because of the illness. These are just a few of the quantitative facts that are used to demonstrate the dimensions of the mental health problem. The source of the problem is the personality of people. Broadly interpreted, personality is the functioning of the whole person as a unique organization that distinguishes him from other people.

College students show great concern for the many factors that contribute to their mental health. A recent study by Kirk, designed to ascertain the health priorities in a course such as this, revealed that college students believe that mental health is the most important. The students were asked to indicate their priorities for twenty-one different areas. Only the first five are shown in Table 2-1.

GOOD MENTAL HEALTH

Many a college student has, in a moment of unfulfillment, asked himself, "How can I tell when I am emotionally disturbed?" Invariably, the student's real question is,

"What is good mental health?" The problem is that there are varying degrees of mental and emotional health. Actually, there are often very fine lines of difference between mental health and mental illness. But good mental health, although not fully understood, can be described as the complete state of mental well-being; it includes the ability to manage one's self and to cope with one's external environment in an effective and self-satisfying manner. One's feelings about himself are the basic parameters of mental health. Self-acceptance, insight, and self-esteem included makes the definition of mental health more explicit. When a practical perception of self is combined with a realistic perception of one's environment, the possibility of a satisfactory interaction is reasonably assured.

Relevance to total health

Your mental health relates specifically and directly to your total state of health. When you are physically ill, the chances are better than 50% that your illness was induced or influenced by your state of mental and emotional health. The two terms most generally used to describe these relationships are psychosomatic and somatopsychic. A psychosomatic state is one in which the physical health of the body is influenced by one's mental and emotional state. Psychosomatic medicine uses the principles and methods of psychology in the diagnosis and treatment of physical illness that is thought to be psychomatic in nature. Some conditions that are apt to have psychosomatic overtones are various

Table 2-1. Summary of health priorities of college students

Subject	Female rank	Male rank	Female and male rank
Mental health	1	1	1
Communicable diseases	2	3	2
Community health	3	5	4
Safety	4	2	3
Chronic and degenerative diseases	5	8	6

kinds of pains, weakness, cramps, asthma, high blood pressure, and peptic ulcers.

A somatopsychic condition is one in which one's state of mental health is influenced by one's physical state. Some conditions believed to be somatopsychic in nature are fear, anxiety, and hopelessness. The correlation between the body and mind is vitally important; they are indissolubly welded together in the study of physical and mental disease. But there is also much to be said about the effect of mental health upon social well-being. Social well-being must be accepted as an essential ingredient of total health to which the other two states contribute. You don't accomplish much while studying when you are extremely nervous, afraid, or depressed. College students rarely participate in social activities if they are excessively introverted. Life tends to have little meaning for one who does not value it totally.

Interpretations of normality and abnormality

Standards of mental health vary greatly from one society, culture, or ethnic group to another. Mental and emotional behavior that is acceptable in one culture may be significant enough to have one confined to a mental hospital in another. To say that one's mental state is normal or abnormal requires more than a simple explanation. The term normal is derived from the Latin root *norma,* which literally means a rule or pattern. Thus *normal* behavior is theoretically described in terms of norms that are assumed, adjudged, or categorically derived. If the behavior is abnormal, it is assumed to

be a deviation from behavior that adheres to some norm. Young adults are expected to prepare for a livelihood, to be interested in members of the opposite sex, not to marry one of another race, and to marry and live happily ever after. How is behavior that is contrary to the above expectations classified? What is abnormal about a fellow wearing his hair to the waist? What about the antibathers? Is draft dodging an abnormal behavior? The concept of what is normal varies not only with the setting but also within the same setting at different times. The concept of normality and abnormality is, in addition, decided by the approval or disapproval of certain standards of behavior within a particular group that imposes these attitudes upon its members.

Persons may indeed deviate from the average without being abnormal in the clinical sense. A man who has the opportunity of earning $100,000 a year on a particular job but turns it down in favor of another job with an annual salary of $30,000 may be mentally and emotionally abnormal, or he may simply be acting as a good husband and father by not allowing known excessive pressures of the higher paying job to overwhelm the mental and emotional stability of home and family life.

Many normal people settle for a great deal less than they want out of life. You know the history of this quite well. Life does not always present easy circumstances for all people. It is difficult to find persons whose lives are, or have been, without some crucial frustration or some profound grief. There are few ways out of frustration and grief except living through them and surviving in some manner that allows one to maintain a tolerable life. For example, to be average is to be angry with one's son several times during the week, yet make it up with a fishing trip on the weekend. It is to fail to study assignments that are made throughout the term but cram for a final examination. It is to drink enough with your peers until the drinking of alcoholic beverages becomes a habit, then "get a divine call," cease drinking, and start preaching. Most of these examples are of borderline behavior—normal or abnormal—which are ultimately categorized according to the concept of normality or abnormality to which one subscribes. There are two basic concepts: a concept based on statistical frequency (average), and a concept that relates to a standard (norm) of mental health.

Basic characteristics of a healthy personality

The mentally healthy personality is that which is exemplified in a person adhering to the description of mental health covered earlier in this chapter. It is the personality of one who demonstrates the ability to feel comfortable about himself, feel comfortable about other people and his environment, and meet reasonably well the usual and unusual circumstances of life.

In order to feel comfortable about oneself, one has to: understand and accept one's own handicaps and other shortcomings—physical, mental, and spiritual; endure the frustrations of life; live with oneself on workable terms; deal constructively with reality; and dictate positive change on one's own terms.

Consider a few simple questions. Are you a human being or a robot? Are you brilliant, borderline, or ignorant? Are you white, black, or some other color? Are you an active agent or a passive one? Are you an open system or a closed system? Why are you in this college? If you were to ask yourself "Who am I, and how do I feel about my mental and emotional state," you would probably answer male or female, son or daughter, father or mother, good student

or poor student, etc. But all of these descriptions would still be incomplete. Who are you, and how do you feel about your image of yourself? Herein lies the essence of how one approaches the true feeling within oneself about oneself. The mentally healthy person learns to construct the real image of himself, the one with which he comfortably lives. He learns to accept his shortcomings if he finds he cannot improve them, but he is also willing to extend his capabilities to the maximum potential.

The mentally healthy person in his quest for stability feels comfortable about other people and the environment in which he lives. He has a meaningful sense of responsibility to his family, neighbors, and others. He is able to sublimate his ego so that he can feel and function as a part of society in general and assume social responsibility on occasions. He is not overly aggressive in his relationships with people, nor does he allow other people to be overly aggressive with him.

Your family and other persons and groups around you constitute those with whom you interact socially. They provide the major models for you to use in deciding how you feel in relation to other people. If you have chosen college, then one in your family may have gone to college, or someone you think is important wants you to be here. You may have decided to come of your own free will. Nonetheless, you probably hold in your mind an image or personal need that commits you to a long-term set of goals. The chances are that your image or feeling is hazy. The greatest task necessary to realize the healthy personality is to clearly define these feelings about what other people expect and what your environment demands. Until you know what your social and economic relations are and where you are ultimately going and for what purposes, you will be unable to differentiate yourself from your environment and other people. You will be lost in the crowd, and it won't be the crowd that suffers; it will be your healthy personality. If you are white, be white and proud; if you are black, be black and proud. If you want to belong to a fraternity or sorority but cannot, be proud to be independent. If you can maintain your image of yourself, be your own person as related to others, and still survive with a healthy personality, you will become capable to relating to others and feel comfortable about it.

The mentally healthy person is able to meet the normal and abnormal circumstances of life in general. He possesses no excessive fears about his ability to handle most problems. How do you adjust to the death of a close relative or friend? What happens to you if finances or grades prevent your continued attendance in college? Are you subject to being drafted? The mentally healthy person is able to make decisions about the critical problems of life after having taken into account the many ramifications involved. Formulating alternative interpretations of life situations can help you create choice conditions. In choosing alternatives, however, priorities must be established. The mentally healthy person confronts and solves his problems in terms of his priorities.

A healthy personality is found in one who has shed the cloak of childhood. A person's mentally healthy state does not stop developing. This implies that you have passed beyond the infantile stage of behavior, that you have not brought to your current stage of development remnants of childish behavior that have become impossible to change and that will remain a permanent burden to you, and that you can expect dynamic development throughout life.

Misconceptions of mentally healthy and unhealthy persons

Mental health is basically a matter of degree. As previously discussed, there is no absolute line between mental health and mental illness. For example, it is an absurd idea that a person is mentally ill if he appears odd or different under certain circumstances (for example, if he talks to himself). Nonetheless, people are often accused of being ill or healthy on the basis of this crude criterion. Several of the many misconceptions of the mentally healthy person are:

1. The mentally healthy person is completely free from tension and anxiety.
2. He conforms explicitly to the status quo.
3. He reduces his mental output to avoid overextending his mental processes.
4. He does not possess personal idiosyncrasies.
5. He is comfortably acclimated under all circumstances.
6. He is absolutely free from dissatisfaction.
7. He rebels against authority and older persons who naturally threaten his stability.
8. He never gets angry.
9. He opposes fundamental philosophical and religious values.
10. He possesses constant and complete happiness.

Some of the misconceptions of the mentally unhealthy person are:

1. The mentally unhealthy person can snap out of his problem by himself.
2. He always needs to be hospitalized.
3. When he enters the mental institution, he never leaves.
4. His condition is mostly inherited.
5. He is usually dangerous to other people.
6. His condition is a disgrace to society.
7. His mental illness will clear up if he can be "brought to his senses" or can get away from all outside pressures for a while.

The above misconceptions are quite simply stated. Within this simplicity, however, reside some of our major misunderstandings of good mental health.

EMOTIONAL HEALTH

There are many requisites for mental health in the form of interrelated emotional needs just as there are requisites for physical health in the form of exercise, rest, relaxation, and nutrition. Emotions are responses to stimuli. For example, remembering certain lyrics to an old song may call forth the same sensation of pleasure as when they were first heard. Tears and sobs are often part of the emotion of sorrow or grief. Excessive fear may be expressed by an increased heart rate. Even though most of our goals, ambitions, and drives are emotionally based, we frequently fail to recognize either our emotions or their stimuli. Emotionally healthy response patterns have much to do with success in dealing with emotional problems. It naturally follows that if a state of negative emotional response is allowed to continue for a long period of time, it may harm both mind and body.

Emotions

As defined above, an emotion is a mental state or process accompanied by bodily responses that occur in expectation or realization of unfulfillment or satisfaction of basic needs. In essence, it is an inner personal turbulence with some outward expression. It is also an aroused state of the body caused by the threat of danger, real or imagined; by some event resulting in strong and frequently poorly coordinated thought and action; or by an unfulfilled desire. Rarely, if ever, does man react in a completely rational manner to events and problems. How often are your decisions and actions at least partly determined by emotional states that are variously referred to as prejudices, feelings, and attitudes? There would be very little action in many endeavors without emotions to furnish the motivation.

Emotions come in many forms: passion, fear, rage, anxiety, love, hate, elation, depression, fascination, pleasure, sympathy, admiration, amusement, and a host of others. The normally healthy personality experiences these states in varying degrees and manifests reasonable and controlled responses to them as they occur in the varied situations of daily life. The person with abnormal emotions demonstrates behavior that is excessive, inadequate, or otherwise inappropriate to his personal life situation or problems. How many times have you heard

that a man isn't supposed to cry? Socially, this is generally accepted as an abnormal emotional act on the part of the male. Why isn't a man supposed to cry if crying will alleviate the problem or conflict facing him? Crying is often the natural emancipatory and satisfying response to alleviate the problem or the tension.

Emotional development

"Once an adult and twice a child." Man is born dependent upon his parents or guardians. Through various stages he assumes an independence and interdependence that exist throughout most of his life. If he lives the expected 70 years or longer, he ultimately reverts to some state of dependence. As an infant you were totally dependent upon others to satisfy your basic needs. During your preschools days you began to learn about your immediate environment and to explore the ways you related to it. As the sequence evolved you became familiar with the implications of socialization versus autonomous thoughts and deeds. At your present stage of emotional development you are faced with the need to accept responsibility for failure or success, establish realistic goals, and develop self-awareness as a young adult. As you cope successfully with these challenges you will prepare yourself to handle better the emotional states related to occupational tensions, marriage, middle age, retirement, and old age.

As you emotionally progress through subsequent stages, normal development in each stage greatly depends on what occurred in the preceding ones. The degree of the influence of previous experiences in the development of emotions is uncertain; but it is known that your potential for full emotional development depends upon the constitutional factors, heredity and environment.

Physiologic needs

Although physiologic needs are often overemphasized, they are nevertheless important. Some of the basic needs that must be satisfied are sleep, hunger, thirst, sex, and elimination of pain and fatigue. Anyone who cannot satisfy these needs probably desires to fulfill them much more strongly than any of the higher-level needs. Most of the physiologic needs of man are normally and automatically satisfied. That some of these needs may not have been met, may have been influenced by the individual's environment, his heredity, his social relationships, or his emotional health status. Of all the physiologic needs, hunger and sex are probably the two most significant for college men and women.

Although there are major differences in the two, hunger and appetite needs are considered as being somewhat similar in terms of emotional problems. The former is basically organic, whereas the latter is mostly psychic in origin. What drives one to eat too little, whereas another is driven to eat too much? The need to gain or lose weight may be one reason; another reason might be the emotional tension that activates or inhibits the practice. The pleasure of eating may be substituted for other pleasures that are desired but that are unavailable. One may overeat because he feels insecure. His uninterpreted reason for overeating will likely add another cause of emotional and physiologic trauma, that of excessive self-consciousness because of overweight. A more comprehensive discussion of the causes of this problem is covered in Chapter 4. Conversely, one who refuses to eat may be responding to the stigma of gaining weight, or he may have learned that by not eating he can coerce other individuals into granting certain demands. The prisoner who goes on a hunger strike probably understands that his jailers are sensitive to this physiologic need and do not wish that even the prisoner should die from lack of food.

It is well known that the sex drive is a significant force in one's overall emotional well-being. The innumerable taboos and social restrictions added to this primary physiologic need may cause a major emotional health problem. Millions of college students still live in continual emotional conflict over the problem of homosexual and heterosexual activities. The satisfaction of sex needs, which occurs in evolutionary states from birth throughout life, is essential to the development of a healthy personality. Several of the means of satisfying this need and its related problems are more comprehensively discussed in Chapter 9.

Psychosocial needs

You came into this world as an individual. You acquired a status or position in society, and at the same time you became a unique person. Ultimately, you are an individual within a group and within your environment. Your social needs are determined to a great degree by the rules set for personal guidance in the sphere of morality, law, social relationships, business, education, religion, or recreation.

Each individual has a role to play, and he learns early in life that it is necessary to play it in a manner that will be acceptable to the social groups of which he is a part. The ever increasing participation of college men and women in the antiwar movements, the civil rights movements, free speech movements, and other movements of social protest is an indication of the variability of group involvement that youth face today. Identification with a protest movement is one way some people use to identify with a cause and to belong to a group.

Status implies acceptance and recognition of a member by the other group members. Just belonging, on the other hand, simply identifies you with the group. To have status means that you describe others in the social system as extensions of yourself, that you would adopt the "us" concept rather than "they." As a member of such a group, as long as you feel you belong, you want to remain a part of it. If you are a member of a minority group, you may have serious problems conceptualizing your status within segments of the majority group.

What is it that makes you feel that you have status whether in a school, corporation, race, family, movement, or a church? Conversely, what makes you feel you do not have status? The answers are not simple in many instances, but the best are those that allow you satisfactorily to meet your personal needs.

The magnitude to which your need for emotional security is gratified or thwarted is influential in determining your mentally healthy personality. From early childhood to old age you need a feeling of emotional security. But this need must be held in check. Emotional security is a relative matter, and you should not allow this desire to dominate your plans to the point of crowding out the promise of other achievements. No person can tolerate endlessly the strain placed upon him by the prolonged depletion of energy resources used to combat a perceived threat to his emotional security.

You study hard, hopefully, to achieve high grades in all of your courses, including this one. Why? There are many reasons, but the most important is the need to satisfy your drive for achievement. The same elementary drive might be applied to athletics, band, debating team, student government, and any number of endeavors. In your quest for achievement, you will at times be successful, and at other times unsuccessful. The need to achieve is real, but because of marked differences in individuals some may encounter limitations of ability. College students should understand their assets and limitations and set their goals accordingly. All too often students attempt to do things that are far above their level of attainment. In other instances the reverse is true. We are cheered by worthwhile achievement whenever our sense of personal worth is strengthened by our knowledge that we have done well or when our success is recognized by others. A sincere compliment to a student about his academic, athletic, or other achievement tends to boost his morale. The desire for achievement is a significant force in promoting human progress. But if it becomes too strong, it may lead to undesirable or unethical behavior.

COMMON MENTAL AND EMOTIONAL PROBLEMS OF OUR TIME

Entering college certainly produces changes in your mode of living. Many new

pressures arise. Your independence increases whether you live on campus or commute from home. One of the major hazards confronting you is your ability to handle the degree of independence you have. The problems you face are those that are a part of the late twentieth century college environment. As a modern college student you must project yourself into a new setting among peers of differing abilities, ages, ethnic backgrounds, and beliefs. You are under a different type of authority and are confronted with new guidelines of behavior. You must plan an academic or technical program that is directed toward your main objectives but that allows time to do many other things.

Self-concept

Whitman wrote in his poem "Song of Myself":

I have said that the soul is not more than the body,
And I have said that the body is not more than the soul,
And nothing, not God, is greater to one than one's self is.

Even though the self is dynamic as it changes in response to environmental pressures, it is at the same time striving toward equilibrium. Whatever your self-concept, it is learned. It is learned from yourself, family, friends, and others of your world. In spite of all the influences, there is much consistency in your behavior based on your self-concept. The "who am I?" discussion earlier in this chapter relates to identifying this self-concept. In a fairly nonthreatening environment, you may display one of two possible responses: you may reach out for new and meaningful experiences, or you may develop an excessive sense of superiority. Conversely, resistance to change with accompanying rigidity in behavior is increased when the individual believes that his self-concept is threatened. The self-concept is subject to change when certain conditions or circumstances warrant change. But some people refuse to adjust, and they employ defense mechanisms allegedly to protect or support their self-concept. The search for the self-concept and the defense of the self-concept is an ongoing process. The following are some of the mechanisms frequently used, inadvertently and sometimes fallaciously, in reacting to threats.

Denial is the refusal to acknowledge the existence of a threat to one's self-concept, as when you put out of your mind an impending examination or simply assume that the examination will not be difficult.

Displacement is the transfer of antagonistic emotions to a person other than the one who caused the antagonism, as when you develop hostility toward one of your college instructors but take it out on your younger brother.

Identification is the process by which one gains some relief from the threat to his self-concept by ascribing to himself the characteristics of some other person, as when you assume yourself to be the professor of your class.

Projection is an act in which one ascribes his own feelings to others, as when you explain your hostility to a classmate simply by feeling that your classmate harbors ill will toward you.

Provocation is a process of defense in which one deliberately stimulates aggressive action in order that one's own aggressive action may appear merely as a reaction, as when you provoke a classmate until he takes the first action in degenerating the interpersonal relations between you and himself.

Rationalization occurs when one assumes false reasons for his behavior or actions. You may conclude that your professor has taken advantage of you because he gave you an extremely time-consuming home assignment rather than realizing that you did not care to exert as much effort as was required by the assignment.

Regression is the process of returning to a form of behavior that was acceptable in an earlier situation involving a threat to your self-concept, as when you have completely recovered from a malady but because of academic pressures revert to a state of helplessness.

Sublimation is channeling the energy that might be used for one form of behavior into a more socially acceptable form of behavior, as when you channel your anger into social activity or your personal discontent into some creative activity.

Relationships to those of significantly different ages

This is not a period in which the aged are necessarily considered wise; yet it is a period in which the aged are ever with us, demanding to be heard. The so-called generation gap usually develops in the family first. At the turn of this century, at least one parent was likely to have died before the last child was married. Today, parents will probably live approximately fifteen years after their youngest child is married. Not only will they live longer, but they will also live healthier and more intelligent lives; and like everyone else, they are not zealous to give way to new eras or to keep their opinions to themselves.

Many young people feel that there are political, philosophic, and social differences that cause part of the problems between child and parent, young and middle-aged, and young and old. These young people feel that their generation is qualitatively different from all previous generations. Vast educational and social chasms often do separate the old from the young, but in some instances the blunt attack by a young person on an older person's values may be no more than an attempt to verify that the young person is a member in good standing of the "new" generation. They are apparently engaging older persons in combat that was unconditionally declared in childhood. The combat continues with neither side the victor. Ironically, the goal of the combat on both sides of the battle line is to compel the adversary, by any technique possible, to demonstrate concern, love, and compassion.

In every case, the old-young relationship goes through significantly different stages. In some enjoyable situations a relationship that had been pleasant in childhood and turbulent in adolescence can, and often does, become pleasant again at the end of the teen-age years. The original feelings or relationships never change completely but are modulated on both sides by mature sympathy and mutual respect. In relationships of this kind, young people give what they can because of love and respect and not because of shame or compunction. They take what they want to take without feeling pressured or controlled. There can be a healthy, wholesome, and mature relationship between the old and young; it takes two mature persons —one on each side of the age continuum— to make it thrive.

Social uneasiness

There are students who have too few dates, not enough friends, or who are involved in too few student activities. Some of these men and women would be welcomed into more social activities but often withdraw because they are extremely timid or feel a self-defeating sense of uneasiness. Some become so caught up in the maelstrom of social uneasiness and turmoil that they lose their perspective or interest in life itself. They tend to produce further uneasiness to the degree that their nonsocial conduct results in excessive deviation from the norm. In spite of all the additional information that might be shed on uneasiness, the genesis of this type of response is difficult to uncover.

In developing an approach to eliminating or reducing the uneasiness, one must look for the qualities of social adeptness. The people who experience the least social uneasiness are outgoing and friendly; they seek opportunities to make and nurture new friendships; they are objective with criticism; they are open-minded, not prejudiced. Most of all, they have a realistic sense of their own goals and personal worth and rarely misrepresent them.

Response to authority and systems

We are social beings who need the warmth and encouragement of our society. We cannot live without conflict and at the same time ignore rules of the society in which we desire to live and function. Rebellious as we may be during contemporary times, we cannot continue to live without some sanction of our conduct from our society. Authority or various kinds of checks and balances keep people together. These media may be intrinsically imposed. They may be legal or illegal. The authorities or systems may be personal, social, religious, governmental, military, or industrial in nature.

How do you respond to authority or certain systems? If you are committed to a complete reassessment and restructuring of these systems, your response has taken a decided form, actively or passively. If you rebel, you rebel against someone or something, and your actions may be well within the boundaries of normality. Such actions are a normal process of growth and development. The tiny infant learns to resist some things that are imposed upon him. He may refuse to take the bottle according to the time regimen that has been suggested by the physician and enforced by the mother. We all develop this sense of autonomy extremely early in life, even without a sophisticated background of knowledge and experience to conceptualize alternatives.

Independence of thought and action is taught to many children before they develop the needed maturity. All too often, however, the paradox between what adults do and what they consciously try to teach their children to do reinforces the rebellious attitude. Dad speeds beyond the posted speed limits, and his child observes this. Mother is not always authentic in her actions. Politicians may be imprudent in their dealings with certain segments of the public. Because of examples such as these, as children progress toward adulthood their respect for authority and systems may be deflated.

Your generation is accused of being a severe threat to authority and established systems: the forceful rebellion of a few is considered typical of all young people. Consider the example of an atypical student who went to extremes in rebelling. Nathaniel is an 18-year-old sophomore in a southern college. His home is in the Midwest, and he has not returned there since he left just prior to his freshman year. He led a protest movement against his college administration that was successful in forcing the president to resign and leave the state. Nathaniel is a good student and a popular athlete. Several conversations with him reveal that he possesses a strong resistive attitude toward most forms of authority. He feels that the administration of the former president blatantly imposed its authority on the students and faculty of the college. More significantly, however, he reflects upon his relations with his dad, which according to him have been quite negative since he was a senior in high school. Nathaniel's degree of rebellion is atypical of the masses of your generation.

There are thousands of college men and women who have similar types of grievances against authority but who respond covertly rather than overtly. For the most part, those with a healthy personality attempt to work within normal channels to present their grievances and to establish a dialogue with the authorities and managers of the systems. Obviously there is much about authority to irritate and disturb young people, but even though severe provocation and various forms of protest have increased, it must not be overlooked that many constructive things are being done to bridge the gap. Young people have become more involved in the solution of the problems of the establishment. Community action programs, VISTA, the Peace Corps, the Teacher Corps, College and University Board of Trustee membership, and other experiences are providing many avenues to serve effectively as agents of change. In the final analysis, we must recognize that respect for authority and established systems is essential even for our right to protest what we collectively abhor. War, civil injustices, autocratic college administrations, autocratic parents, and needless inflation are problems for some of you now and others of you in the future. What kind of parent will you be? Will you be a government official who will relate in the best way to the needs of your constituency? Equitable authority and good systems are essential to a mentally healthy society.

Racism, prejudice, and mental health

How do you feel about interracial marriage? Would you want your child, sister, or brother to marry one of another race? What is your reaction to WASP? Do you feel strongly enough about the objectives of the Black Panthers to join them? What about the Ku Klux Klan? What is your opinion of the status of American Indians? What does the Confederate Flag mean to you? What happens to you when you know that someone dislikes you or feels uncomfortable around you because you happen to be of another ethnic origin?

The Kerner Report of 1968 asserted that our nation is moving toward two societies, one black, one white—separate and unequal —and that such a polarization will possibly destroy America's basic democratic values. The report further stated that the basic problem was racism. Racism or prejudice is a composite of stereotypes and myths in which a collective label or symbol is used to define, characterize, and classify a group or an individual considered as a whole. A white is referred to as a "honky," a black as a "nigger," an Italian as a "dago," a Polish man as a "Polack," a Japanese as a "Jap," a Korean as a "Gook." Rarely does the racist consider the individual as a human being in his own right with assets, shortcomings, or all of the other attributes that would be tolerated among those of his own race or ethnic origin.

The interpretation of the term prejudice is explicit in the word itself. It means to prejudge. It is basically a perversion of judgment by group-interest or self-interest. It is supported by vivid likes and dislikes of a particular "race." Racism and prejudice go hand in hand. The racist person is committed in his attachment to a particular creed, symbol, or group to the exclusion of all others. Ultimately prejudice is an explicit expression of conflict between the racist's group and the other group, primarily designed to keep the two separated. As has been brought to mind quite frequently in current times, racism is most dangerous when the status of the approving groups is in a state of flux.

We are not born racists or to be prejudiced. It is neither instinctive nor innate. It has to be taught, experienced, and learned. Nonetheless, the racist attitudes of many of us seem so natural that we tend to take them for granted and believe that we were born with a dislike for some people. But when parents and other adults refrain from interfering with the social relations of children of different races, it is often found that racial prejudices are at least postponed until negative conditioning occurs.

Deeply entrenched prejudice usually depicts an immature form of opposition and conscious or unconscious emotional insecurity and conflict that are projected upon the victims of the racist. Traditionally, it was also felt that the oppressed readily developed a fear of his oppressor, which inhibited his reactions and forced him into a state of retreat. Those with a healthy personality do not possess an excessive sense of oppression. When the threat is imminent, they either reduce it or eliminate it in a positive manner.

The Mexicans, Orientals, Jews, Christians, Catholics, whites, blacks, conservatives, liberals, and the whole range of a cosmopolitan American population must find some means of implementing the forward together theme. Not only does your healthy personality depend upon it but so does that of your college, community, state, and nation. Democracy is, mentally and emotionally, one of the most challenging patterns of psychosocial systems on earth, for it requires a sensibility, a live-and-let-live existence, that runs counter to racism and prejudice. The practice of democracy is an excellent measure of mental and emotional maturity.

Anxiety

Anxiety is primarily a negative reaction to a threat. It may also be thought of as an intrinsic pain that causes worry or tension and disrupts mental or emotional stability. It is often a factor that stimulates one to find ways of meeting an imminent threat successfully. All of us possess some anxiety. In many respects it is operational in stimulating growth and development in individuals. It is learned usually as the result of some childhood or earlier experiences but quite often as an end product of some later experiences, experiences similar to those you may have now. There are many sources of anxiety that may cause various degrees of severity. Some attention will be given to a more serious kind, known as anxiety neurosis, in a following section. The minor anxieties for most people probably take the form of fear or worry. They may arise, for example, because the student fails to have a functional time schedule. He does not have enough time for recreation, study, sleep, and work. He may ultimately feel that all is in vain and become extremely hurried and disjointed. He may become afraid and worried because he can't concentrate well or because he does not know how to study effectively. He may even assert that he doesn't have the compositional ability to do what has to be done. At times the anxious student may give way to states of the "blues" or severe introversion. The healthy personality is surely threatened when anxiousness centers around long-range choices of an occupation or profession and the assumed possibilities of failure.

Suicide

Suicide is a major mental health problem among college students and citizens of our country in general. It robs us of some of our most potentially productive members of society. In America in recent years about 3,000 deaths each year have been attributed to suicide among the 15- to 24-year-old age group. This includes college students. It is the fourth leading cause of death for this age group, following accidents, homicide, and cancer. Men commit suicide more often than do women. Approximately 4 out of every 100,000 young women who die do so by suicide, whereas 11 out of every 100,000 men take their own lives. The rate of men committing suicide is 2.5 to 3 times that of women.

The difference in this rate may be explained by several factors. It may be postulated that the man's inability to bear sustained pain, his incapacity to put up with the minor stresses of life, and other physiologic and psychosocial factors are possible reasons. The social attitudes imposed by the role that each sex plays in our culture have certainly had some effect in determining the difference in the suicide rate. Traditional formal and informal education of the two sexes has dictated the aggressiveness of the male and the passivity of the female. With the current developing equality of the status of women the traditional roles may change. It is important to remember that many more women attempt suicide, but many more men are successful in their pursuit of death. On the basis of past history the white male is the most likely candidate to commit suicide. He is followed, in order, by the white female, the nonwhite male, and the nonwhite female.

The contemplation of such an act could be the result of terror and anguish that cause one to prefer death to mental and emotional trauma. Very few kinds of emotional behavior have received as much attention as suicide, but the major focus of attention has to be to prevent the actions, rather than simply to explain the implications.

A Texas student shot himself because he was caught stealing. An Ohioan attempted to commit suicide because she had been left standing at the altar without a groom. In New York, a young man burned himself to death because of an alleged protest against the Vietnam conflict. Another young college woman in Kentucky for no known reason jumped to her death from the top of a tall dormitory. These incidents are representative of the approximately 3,000 that are reported each year. The direct or indirect cause in each of the above cases could be called absurd. But the announced motive may have been only the superficial one. The underlying cause that led to each in-

dividual's death had probably developed over a period of time.

Suicide attempts are caused by many factors. The basis of existence appears to be beyond the realm of life itself. One may possess a lack of self-control that relates to his frustrations and suffering. Some individuals may decide that there is no reason for living. Other individuals find that their world is disintegrating and that they do not have the strength to sustain themselves. Serious suicide attempts often take place in a condition of dire loneliness. Young people who are extreme introverts tend to be quite susceptible. The obsessive desire to join a loved one in death or the attempt to escape or forget the feeling of the unresolved loss may be a motive; or a permanent, overwhelming sense of failure may be another.

Most suicides stem from a sense of loneliness and from feelings of intolerable emotional trauma. In essence, suicide is an attempt to stop or prevent a personally intolerable existence. Each person defines intolerability according to his own terms. Stresses, disappointments, or other problems that might be easy for one person to handle might well be intolerable for someone else in his frame of mind. Any precipitating cause may be intolerable for a particular young man or woman and may lead to suicidal behavior. In order to anticipate and prevent this type of behavior one must understand what the breaking point means to another person.

The methods of suicide are unlimited; however, there are several conditions that may determine the method the man or woman will use. Availability and accessibility of agents is the paramount factor. A steeplejack would tend to jump from some high structure. A physician would tend to consume some lethal drug. The policeman would tend to shoot himself. In addition to the availability of agents, the stress state of the potential self-killer is important. Some use a means to dramatize a cause, such as the young man from New York who became a torch. Other persons prefer to end it all in seclusion, with or without a note of explanation. Women tend to use gas and poisons, whereas men tend to shoot themselves. Women tend to use less violent means that allow for follow-up activities by another party, such as time for rescue or resuscitation. The usual methods of suicide, in order of those most frequently used, are firearms and explosives, gases and poisons, hanging and strangulation, cutting or piercing devices, drowning, and jumping from high places.

Suicidal behavior has no conspicuous, overt warning signals, but there are several basic indications that are fairly constant in most known suicide cases. Contrary to popular belief, many persons who talk excessively about committing suicide actually do it. Suicide is not usually an impulsive act. It often culminates a long history of neurotic problems in which the person has given many clues of his intentions. Most of these individuals are not fully dedicated to killing themselves; rather, they are pleading for some reduction of the intolerable stress that has gone beyond the breaking point of their personality structure.

SPECIAL PSYCHONEUROTIC PROBLEMS

Psychoneurosis is a functional nervous disorder. In lay language, a psychoneurosis is the same as a neurosis. A person who has a psychoneurosis is called psychoneurotic or neurotic. Of all the major mental diseases, the etiology of psychoneuroses is the most obscure. They are generally recognized by the manner in which a person attempts to deal with a threat that is felt in his conscious personality but that germinates in the unconscious. The kinds of neuroses vary in severity. Though very rare, some may be so serious as to prevent one from carrying on with a normal life, ultimately requiring hospitalization. Others may be less serious, permitting one to carry on his work with reduced efficiency. Although the symptoms of psychoneurosis frequently appear first in the late teens or early twenties, the disease may have been cultivated in early infancy. Temper tantrums, sleepwalking, bed wetting, and nail biting are called

childhood neurotic traits. Most often they will be outgrown. But in some cases, although they may disappear, the underlying problems that caused them linger to become the forerunners of more problems later.

The largest group of mental illnesses are the psychoneuroses. Approximately 10% of all admissions to mental hospitals are diagnosed as neurosis. However, most persons with psychoneurotic problems are never admitted to mental hospitals or clinics. The neurotic person often exhibits a variety of symptoms, which are rarely severe enough to require hospitalization. He may feel that he is worthless, inadequate, inferior, and helpless. He may become angry too frequently and inappropriately and remain so for a long period of time. He must be reassured at incongruous times of another's love or affection. He may be so afraid of losing his independence that he shuns any kind of dependence. He allows his desire for security to cloud his pleasure of life.

Several types of psychoneurotic reactions are recognized. Some of the more common ones are reviewed in the following sections.

Conversion reaction

Conversion reaction is one of the more dramatic neurotic symptoms. It is a form of hysteria that is psychogenic in nature. It is generally produced by suggestion and might be removed by various degrees of persuasion. A person attempts to resolve a mental or emotional problem by literally adopting the symptoms of some organic disease. The major characteristic of conversion reaction is the faulty synthesis of personality. Some persons lose their sight, become deaf, lose their ability to walk, or sustain some other psychogenic disorder. Often the conditions are temporary and will disappear without any apparent explanation or with therapeutic persuasion.

Neurasthenia

Neurasthenia, or nervous exhaustion, is a functional nervous condition marked by extreme fatigue and a variety of subjective symptoms without evidence that an organic disease is present. As with conversion reaction, neurasthenia appears to be largely psychogenic in origin. The most prominent symptom is that of excessive fatigue on slight exertion. Mentally and emotionally, one is unable to concentrate, is restless, has a poor memory, and is irritable. The neurasthenic generally makes himself the center of all his thoughts and has extreme difficulty throwing off his frustrations. He has too little interest in people and life around him and too much interest in his own thoughts and actions.

Hypochondriasis

Hypochondriasis is a condition characterized by excessive worry about one's health even though there may be no reasonable cause for worry or anxiety. At times, fatigue or other minor variations in body activity or chemistry may provoke an attack of anxiety. This anxiety of ill health relates essentially to the functioning of the genital structures, the heart, or the intestinal canal. Some hypochondriacs display little faith in a physician but stock their medicine cabinets with everything in the drugstore. Some will continually sit in the physician's office looking for a cure for a disease or disorder that does not exist. Some become devoted physical and/or diet faddists. Meaningful treatment of these cases is often very difficult, for the hypochondriac usually does not cooperate fully.

Anxiety neurosis

Anxiety neurosis is a condition in which one experiences occasions of anxiety that may vary from a slight uncomfortableness to extreme panic. The occurrence is basically one of anticipation, as if something disastrous is about to occur, except that there is no visible proof of what the disastrous experience might be. The responses are frequently expressed in the form of agitation, insomnia, palpitations of the heart, or the fear of death. Excessive fatigue, occasional confusion, and chronic physical complaints may also appear as complica-

tions. It is, like other neuroses, an exaggeration of behavior that if less severe might be considered normal.

Phobias

Phobias are to some extent similar to anxiety neuroses in that the person's reaction is fear or even panic. A phobia is an unusual fear of someone or something for which there is no apparent sound reason or explanation. Fear has many interpretations. Some are hesitation, awe, consternation, or horror. In these days of increased crime rates and the accelerated pace of competition, no one escapes the experience of some fear. The late President Franklin D. Roosevelt in a national appeal to all Americans, speaking of the challenge of confrontation from other powers, asserted that the greatest thing we had to fear was fear itself. As related to phobias, that assertion holds great significance. What do you fear? How much do you fear what you fear? Fear is a normal phenomenon. We fear losing our jobs, losing a very ill parent by death, not doing well in college, not being able to meet financial obligations, or not making the right professional or occupational decision. But most of us are not obsessively shackled even by our major fears.

Persons with phobias are obsessed by irrational fears of people, things, and events. Their fear is generally derived from unconscious sources, such as desires of an aggressive and sexual nature and other allegedly forbidden impulses. The fear is transferred to an object that is symbolic of the fulfillment of the threatening desire. Some of the more common phobias are acrophobia (high places), agoraphobia (open space), aichmophobia (sharp objects), anthropophobia (people), astrophobia (storms), batophobia (falling objects), claustrophobia (close space), climacophobia (falling down stairs), dromophobia (crossing wide streets), hypnophobia (sleep), kleptophobia (stealing), monophobia (being alone), necrophobia (death), syphilophobia (syphilis), xylophobia (forest), and zoophobia (animals).

MAJOR PSYCHOTIC PROBLEMS

The psychotic individual loses contact with reality. The illness renders the person of unsound mind and judgment. As a result, when the severity of the psychosis is interpreted as insanity (the legal term) the court will give someone, usually a member of the family, the legal authority to make decisions for the psychotic.

Psychoses are customarily classified as (1) organic and (2) functional. Organic psychoses are mental illnesses resulting from organic lesions that include the type of disorders accompanying physical deterioration, trauma, or diseases that destroy brain tissue. In this type of psychosis, an organic condition of the body may be identified as a specific cause. Among the functional psychoses are mental and emotional abnormalities that are probably the result of unconsciously learned behavior patterns. The functional psychoses have no observable physical or organic basis; the etiology is not known. It is often assumed that functional psychoses are curable, whereas those of organic origin are not. Some types of functional psychoses recur and become progressively worse even after apparent successful treatment. Conversely, some organic abnormalities of the brain may occasionally be corrected, and the person improves.

The major psychotic problems are schizophrenia, manic-depressive psychosis, paranoia, and involutional psychosis.

Schizophrenia

Schizophrenia leads all of the psychoses, organic or functional, in frequency. It accounts for more than 50% of all the patients in mental hospitals today. It is also one of the most difficult functional psychoses to treat. Schizophrenia literally means splitting of the mind and is most generally interpreted as a "split personality." The term is somewhat misleading, however, because the "splitting" is actually a separation of self from society. The schizophrenic person has no interest in adjusting to reality; thus the schizoid or autistic state is characterized by extreme social withdrawal, emotional disturbances of a magnitude negatively affecting relationships with other people, and disturbances of thinking. There are several types of schizophrenic reactions: simple, hebephrenic, catatonic, paranoid, acute undifferentiated, schizoaffective, childhood, and residual. This illness is not inherited. There are many findings, however, that demonstrate that an individual may inherit a predisposition to it. Its development is influenced by many factors, most of which are incapable of specific description.

Manic-depressive psychosis

Manic-depressive psychosis is the most frequent of the psychotic affective reactions. These reactions are mainly characterized by an excessive disturbance of mood. The mood is marked by emotional oscillations of a recurrent type. Simply described, the manic-depression process is a transition from either a hyperexcited or elated state to an extreme state of depression or apathy. It may be either, or it may occur sequentially in the opposite direction. The manic state is associated with euphoria or elation. In the depressed state, the reactions are disorders of various thought processes characterized by retardation, accessory somatic dysfunction, feelings of melancholia, and usually some indication of psychomotor retardation. It tends to occur more commonly in males than in females. The average age of a person admitted to hospitals for treatment is thirty-three years.

All persons experience changes in mood. We have our "highs" and "lows." We may feel happy about what life offers us most of the time, but infrequently a sense of futility or discontent makes life appear dismal. We become moody, but this moodiness for the healthy personality does not persist in excessive degrees and is far from the state of psychosis described here.

Paranoia

Paranoia is characterized by systematized delusions of persecution or grandeur. This condition appears to be precipitated by other emotional disorders. Compared with schizophrenia and manic-depressive reactions, paranoid reactions are relatively rare. They develop slowly. One may experience them for a brief period of time and recover. On the other hand, they may become chronic and ultimately incurable. It is difficult to ascertain when a paranoid condition becomes serious enough for the person to be considered a threat to himself or society.

The paranoid's personality may actually be well integrated. His self-confidence may be so outstanding that it may appear abnormal. He knows who his adversaries are but does not really fear them. Basically, he feels that since he is persecuted, it is necessary to develop the defenses to thwart any threat to his well-being. He checks and double-checks people, things, and events.

Involutional psychosis

Involuntional psychosis generally does not occur at a young age. It usually occurs in women in their forties and in men in their fifties. It is covered here because the roots of this problem go back to childhood and young adulthood. It is characteristically an illness of biologic degeneration. The atrophy of the sex glands and degeneration of the sex function appear to be the major causes. Will you be excessively depressed when your biologic sex life comes to an end? This is admittedly an absurd question in terms of the objective answer that you might provide at this moment. Nonetheless, it remains an important question because individuals who do not understand the implications of the melancholia that can result may be potential candidates for suicide or paranoia.

SOME PSYCHOSOCIAL PROBLEMS

In this section attention is devoted to a dimension of personality breakdown that is difficult to define. This group of problems includes those in which the person, instead of utilizing symptoms expressed in mental, organic, or emotional terms in his efforts to effect proper adjustment, manifests socially deviant patterns of action or behavior.

These problems may be divided into three groups: (1) disturbance of personality pattern, (2) disturbance of personality traits, and (3) sociopathic personality disturbances. The majority of persons who sustain the type of personality disorders in question have been produced by our dynamic and sometimes unstable society. Much confusion and controversy surround personality disorders. Included in this group are those who rebel against authority (previously discussed), alcoholics (discussed in another section of this text), the criminal types, sex deviates, those who do not conform, and those who have extreme difficulty with self-control.

Criminality

The criminal is one who is guilty of a criminal offense. The nature of any crime is difficult to explain. Criminality is a condition in which the behavior of the person is subversive to society or is an act of moral and social turpitude. In an attempt to appraise criminal responsibility, courts of law divide criminals into two groups, sane and insane. Criminality, like other types of negative behavior, is one result of a learning process. Most often it is learned by the person from his antisocial environment. But the environment is not the only precipitator. The cause is the interaction of the environment with the personality or the impact of the person's environment upon his personality structure.

Interpretations of what actually constitutes a crime vary according to time and place. Ordinarily we think of murder, rape, theft, graft, or treason. These are in violation of public law. A variation of these, torts, is in violation of civil law. Practically all types of crime are punishable by prison sentences, fines, or loss of civil rights.

The acts of the healthy personality are devoid of strict criminal association. Nonetheless, when the dimensions of a comprehensive interpretation of crime are explored, it is found that few individuals are completely devoid of all criminal-like behavior. Probably few people have never stolen anything, not cheated in some endeavor, or in some fleeting emotional escapade not dreamed for the destruction of some other person; but most people are not classified as criminal types.

Generally the concept of the psychotic person as a potentially criminal type is not valid. For example, very few psychotics commit murder; those who do commit acts of violence usually commit suicide. The psychotic is usually so preoccupied and disorganized that his destructive actions are most often against himself.

Sexual problems

No phase of the personality is so fraught with the possibility of social condemnation, emotional disillusionment, and mental and physical illness as that of those who seek sexual satisfaction inside or outside society's accepted standards. Sex conflicts and frustrations often lead to serious personality disturbances. The sex needs are primarily psychogenic, and since they are very strong many people may experience sex practices that run counter to social standards. It may be expected that individuals will deviate in various ways—mentally, emotionally, socially, and biologically. The major problem for many young men and women is to develop acceptable self-control and to direct the sex drive in a manner that is conducive to a healthy personality and is so-

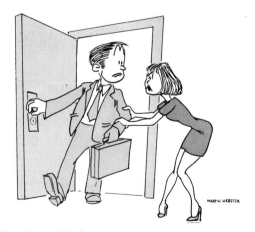

Fig. 2-1. "Work and status! Why couldn't you be addicted to something else?" (Courtesy Martin Webster.)

cially acceptable. The major aspects of sexuality are discussed in Chapter 9.

Status addiction

People who possess an insatiable desire for social position, professional or political recognition, or some other form of status are often addicted to the endeavor. A man may actually spend so much of his time improving his political status that other forms of wholesome interpersonal relations are slighted. Often this obsessive desire for status and the addictive process that accompanies it threaten the very fibers of a healthy personality. Status addiction is the type of personality disorientation that may be demonstrated, to a minor degree, in our everyday living habits.

The status addict has to be first or the best; he has to possess the biggest and best house in town; he has to send his children to the best schools; he has to be the highest ranking student of his class; his position has to be the top one in the corporation. The status addict is driven by a single purpose that is completely out of harmony with his general ability to accomplish the objective. Some economists reason that much of the rising rate of bankruptcy may be attributed to obsessive buying habits. Why does one obtain a $75,000 home mortgage when he can afford one of only $20,000? He probably needs the status of the house mortgage, along with all of the other status symbols that he assumes go with it.

Just as other forms of addiction may have disastrous emotional results, so may status addiction. The man who has financial commitments that divest him of his status symbols may be driven to serious negative emotional behavior or even to suicide. Many persons divorce their spouses simply because the spouse was never able to accomplish the degree of status desired. Most Americans, to be sure, will not become status addicts but nonetheless will experience many mental and emotional problems because of an excessive desire for some form of personal status. They may possess nothing more than a covetous desire for some advantage possessed by another. Accompanying the covetous desire may be the feeling of ill will toward the success or superiority of others. Envy is a natural phenomenon of human behavior, but it is a threat to the healthy personality when it becomes excessive and leads to status addiction.

Work addiction

Work addiction is a relatively new concept. A work addict is identified by an absolute commitment to his work. As some individuals live to eat, the work addict actually lives to work. As he continues to work, he develops an unusual appetite for more work. When he has to slow down or stop, his reactions are negative or he experiences withdrawal symptoms. He may use work as compensatory responses to emotional problems. Work may be simply described as activity. The housewife, because of poor relations with her husband, may have to be cooking, cleaning, transporting children, or doing anything else from rising until she is tired enough to sleep. Some of your college professors are so wound up in what they are doing for you and for their own self-improvement that they may have serious family problems. They may not have time for the other things necessary for a whole and meaningful life. Although it is rare that college students immediately become victims of this type of addiction, some young people become progressively addicted to studying in order to compensate for other personal inadequacies. This particular form of undertaking may or may not be related to status addiction.

GUIDELINES FOR MAINTAINING OR REGAINING A HEALTHY PERSONALITY

Our expanded concept of the healthy personality demands that we should not consider treatment of severe personality problems alone but should also consider preventing minor mental and emotional disturbances from developing into more serious ones. We should be constantly trying to understand ourselves and other people.

Sometimes we fail to take into account, as a part of the assessment, the stresses that are constantly at work in our environment. These stresses are ever present, sculpturing our thoughts, actions, responses, and general feelings. One of the most common stigmas in our society is that of being or having been mentally ill. But all too frequently some of us fail to take care of even the minor signs and symptoms of mental and emotional disturbances in ourselves. A healthy attitude toward mental illness is essential to maintaining a healthy personality.

General self-help guides

All of us develop negative feelings, fears, tensions, anxieties, and problems of other forms that must be reduced to a safe and sane level of adjustment. Many of the positive mechanisms for maintaining the healthy personality are capable of execution by ourselves. We can prevent some major problems from developing. This advice is simple and, most of all, well comprehended by the majority of us. There is, of course, no simple panacea for any particular problem. Even if it were available, the differences in the constitutional makeup of people would negate the solution to negligible significance. Nevertheless, there are some self-help guides that can be used to maintain a healthy personality.

Share your problems. No man should remain alone with his problems. Somewhere there is someone who will listen and interact. Often after a sincere conversation about your problems you may find that they are not so grave as you originally thought. Do you have serious financial or academic problems? Have you conversed with the person who may be in a position to help or are you a loner who automatically feels that only you can find the solution? It is often said of some of the seriously disadvantaged that they would rather remain in that state than to ask for assistance.

Face life realistically. Facing life realistically is one of the more difficult things for some individuals to do. The many conflicts and aspirations of life make reality difficult to adjust to. Earlier in this chapter, identification and status problems were discussed. You want to be uniquely identified with certain endeavors, and you also want to achieve a particular status. You must make decisions about conflicting values. You need to study on the one hand, but you also feel a great need to go to the dance. Normally, our desire to experience the more pleasant things of life is greater than our desire to experience the unpleasant. Going to the dance instead of studying, in itself, is not a negative action. As a single incident, the time could well be made up. But you should establish and keep as the focal point the values that are most important to you. Work to accomplish those you can; reevaluate those you assume can't be accomplished; and continue to work. Some of the values and objectives may be immediate; others may be remote. Nonetheless, they all should be reasonably capable of accomplishment— not too easy or too difficult.

Improve your relations with people. Many of the factors we have discussed about the healthy personality point up problems one has that relate to other people. Many of your attitudes have already been developed from your relations with other people. Most of these relations have been good; some have been poor. Do you have empathy for other people's problems? Can you project yourself into the role of persons who are mentally ill, poorer than you, crippled, blind, of a different religion or creed, of a different color or race than you, and those who you assume don't like you? Learn to put yourself in the place of other people and develop new friendships whether problems are involved or not. Don't let people expect too much from you; but don't expect too much of other people. Herein lies the basis for many poor interpersonal relations on college campuses. Your personal role should be a cooperating one that makes it easier for you to give other people an opportunity to do well, to criticize other people positively rather than negatively, and not to let anxieties and worries about your

relations cloud your contacts with other people.

Confront your problems squarely. Very few of our problems and responsibilities are so unique that others do not share the same kind. You are expected to have responsibilities and problems of various types and degrees. Procrastinating and worrying about responsibilities, without positive and timely action, can only lead to conflict. Why fight them? Ultimately, they will have to be faced. We have all had the experience of dreading a task or making a decision; but after having taken care of it promptly, we find our response quite satisfying. The more readily you confront problems, the more prepared you will be for the ones that will follow. If an academic assignment bothers you, complete it as directly and quickly as you can. Refusing to confront problems squarely can only lead to an accumulation of tensions. Through objectivity, you can become more capable in solving problems, in spite of how difficult it is to be objective about your own behavior.

Broaden your interests. If your interests, mentally, socially, and recreationally are too limited, you may ultimately be too restricted in terms of the positive response mechanisms available to you during moments of frustration. Even at this stage of your development you may be personally bankrupt in terms of the different things you can do. Broad interests add up to a more enriched life free of too many tensions. Some of the courses you take in college may seem boring, but by concentrating on them and working a little more diligently you may find them more interesting. Why don't you like sports, art, music, ballet, or certain types of food? The ability to relax from routine or to engage in recreational activities depends greatly on the different interests and abilities you have developed. In the search for constructive outlets to frustration or general tension, you will have at your disposal many positive avenues through varied interests.

The five self-help guides discussed above are only general approaches. There are many authoritative suggestions offered for the maintenance of the healthy personality, but space does not allow for others to be discussed. A few more specific guides are presented below. Some are more succinct statements of those previously presented, and others are simple variations and extensions. You may wish to discuss some of them with your instructor or a fellow student or friend.

Specific self-help guides

1. Excessive worry is unnecessary and nonfunctional in most cases, so reduce your worry and anxieties.
2. Strive to feel comfortable about yourself in spite of your alleged inadequacies.
3. Work toward feeling comfortable about other people.
4. Remember that negative criticism about other people often has a way of reverting to the criticizer.
5. Work to be a participant in life rather than a lonely spectator.
6. Don't cheat in your willingness to experience the discomforts as well as the pleasures of self-evaluation.
7. Strive to conform where conformity is absolutely necessary without developing a negative conscience about conforming. Alter values as changes dictate.
8. Recognize with true humility that you can't be best at every endeavor.
9. Smile and be gracious if things go well, but if things go poorly and you feel the urge to cry, cry. The traditional adage that a man isn't supposed to cry is hogwash.
10. Freely and genuinely grant to others their right to values and morals that are not identical to yours.
11. Don't let excessive forms of status-seeking overwhelm you.
12. Develop varied interests, and set aside time to pursue those you like best. A balanced life is necessary.
13. Give freely a helping hand to some-

one who needs it without expecting recompense.
14. Remember that your life will be long and will consist of many days. Try to live each day at a time while keeping sight of your long-range goals.
15. Accept the fact that you may not be able to understand all of your gravest problems. When the problem appears to be intolerable, seek professional assistance.

Guides for understanding others

There is much that we are capable of doing to understand people. The things you can do and should avoid doing are suggested below.

You can:

1. Let people know you are interested and care about their problems.
2. Be a good listener. Make yourself available when necessary.
3. Do more than simply be interested in the other person's problems. Try to help out with everyday, practical problems, for example, study problems, social problems, financial problems, and employment problems.
4. Become more informed by reading, in depth, to increase understanding.
5. Get help from a professional for the person if the disturbance indicates a serious problem. Persuasion may be necessary in order to motivate some people to receive treatment.
6. Be responsible for hospitalization of certain persons such as a spouse, child, or mother when necessary. You should make every effort to get other people to admit themselves voluntarily.

You should avoid:

1. Setting yourself up as a judge in the condemnation of a person.
2. Telling the troubled person to "snap out of it." The troubed person usually knows that he should, but his problem is so deep-seated that it requires more than a verbal demand.

3. Arguing with the troubled person.
4. Diagnosis and treatment. The layman does not have the professional education and experience that is necessary.

PROFESSIONAL ASSISTANCE FOR THOSE WITH MENTAL HEALTH PROBLEMS

On some occasions it may not be possible for you to work out or solve your problems. When this occurs, it is necessary for you to receive good professional assistance. Remember our discussion of the negative attitude of many people. Don't be diverted by any negative attitude you may have adopted. Don't wait until you are so troubled that much time and money will be needed to treat the problem.

There are many resources available to help those with mental and emotional problems. Your student health service, family physician, or counseling service may be in an excellent position to help. But such qualified personnel may not be immediately available. Frequently, when one waits too long, one has to take anyone available. Few college and family physicians have the expertise needed to treat mental and emotional problems themselves. They are, therefore, no better prepared to treat a problem of psychoneurosis or psychosis than any intelligent friend. But they do know who may help you, and they are available at least to make referrals.

The professionals

The clinical psychologist. The clinical psychologist is one who has earned a Ph.D. degree in clinical psychology. He has usually had extensive work in clinical psychology prior to the time he practices. He is an expert in psychologic techniques. He is thoroughly trained in the use of psychologic tests. He is also well prepared with knowledge of the learning process, which is essential to therapy of functional mental and emotional problems.

The psychiatrist. The psychiatrist is a medical doctor who has specialized in mental and emotional disorders. He is usually better prepared to treat people with mental disorders that have either an organic or psychosomatic origin rather than those with functional problems. He can also prescribe medication and use other medical techniques that are beyond the realm of a clinical psychologist. To some extent, these factors account for the general preference for a psychiatrist over the psychologist. But the psychiatrist is not necessarily a better practitioner than the psychologist in all cases. As previously mentioned, the well-qualified clinical psychologist specializes in caring for functional behavioral problems, which are most prevalent among college men and women. Also, the two different specialists often work together. Psychiatrists are not easily available: a recent survey of psychiatrists revealed that five states having one third of America's population have one half of the country's psychiatrists.

The psychoanalyst. A psychoanalyst specializes in psychoanalysis. Psychoanalysis is a technique that employs dream analysis, free association, catharsis, and transference. Most psychoanalysts are more comprehensive specialists than are psychiatrists. They are not necessarily of a higher professional status than psychiatrists.

The psychiatric social worker. The psychiatric social worker is a college graduate with graduate education in social work that stresses working with mental and emotional problems. He works with patients and their families and often does a follow-up after the patient is discharged to assist with readjustment.

Some treatments for major problems

No type of treatment for mental illnesses guarantees a successful outcome. As is true of many physical illnesses, treatment is specific to diagnosis. The limited discussion that follows reviews some of the major types of treatment used. The emphasis is devoted primarily to preventive measures and personal resources available to you. The following discussion points out, primarily for general information purposes, what is used to treat serious problems that are beyond the scope of the layman's expertise.

Psychotherapy. Psychotherapy is the most frequently used technique of treatment for mental illness. It is generally best suited for functional problems. It consists of many approaches. Some of them are individual psychotherapy, group psychotherapy, psychodrama, and psychoanalysis. Individual psychotherapy is a form that involves getting the patient to appraise his problems clearly instead of from a distorted point of view. The patient discusses and analyzes, on a one-to-one basis, his negative feelings and experiences that may be responsible for his problems. On the basis of the series of interactions, the psychotherapist attempts to assist him in finding solutions to the problems. Group psychotherapy includes several patients with a single psychotherapist. It is a supporting type of therapy from which different individuals, who may not have the same problems, generally benefit. Quite frequently group psychotherapy may be used in conjunction with individual therapy. Psychodrama is a special type of group psychotherapy in which the patients not only talk about their problems or feelings but also act their problems out through role playing or role taking. Although a patient usually acts out his own problems, others may take over his role. With the skilled psychotherapist as director, many personal problems are well interpreted even though the therapist, another clinical staff member, or another patient may have been the role-playing catalyst. Psychoanalysis is a more sophisticated form of individual psychotherapy. It is a long-term form of therapy in which the patient meets his psychoanalyst by appointment and talks about whatever comes to his mind. It seeks to uncover causes of mental and emotional illness by searching into the patient's early experiences. Successful treatment often takes a year or more.

Somatotherapy. The body is the focal point in this type of therapy. Somatotherapy means working with the nervous systems and the physiologic structure through means such as shock therapy, chemotherapy, and neurotherapy. Shock therapy is designed to bring about changes in the patient's nervous system that will bring him out of his state of excitement, depression, or withdrawal. Electroshock and insulin shock are the most common techniques employed. Insulin shock is caused by the injection of insulin, which produces a temporary coma. In electroshock, a light electric current is passed through the brain causing the patient to experience a short period of unconsciousness. Chemotherapy uses drugs to treat patients. Drug therapy has been found, in many instances, to control symptoms of mental and emotional illness so well that potential patients never have to be hospitalized. The time spent in hospitals has also been reduced in many cases. A number of different drugs are employed in chemotherapy. The most widely used are tranquilizers, such as reserpine (Chrystoserpine), chlorpromazine (Thorazine), and meprobamate (Miltown). Much attention has been given to the uses of these drugs. There is an indication that increasingly more Americans, who have no need for tranquilizers, are becoming more dependent upon the drugs for mental and emotional stability. Psychosurgery is no longer in vogue in the U. S.

Milieu therapy. Milieu therapy is an activity-oriented form of therapy that attempts to remove conditions that might aggravate negative behavioral problems. It includes occupational and recreational therapy. Another technique is to change the environment by providing the therapy in such places as special schools and rehabilitation centers.

SURVIVAL OF THE HEALTHY PERSONALITY

This chapter has only introduced you to a small part of the problem and has provided a few examples of what you and others can do. In your quest to become a health-educated person, the obligation to learn more is clear. The additional obligation is to use what you know to fight:

1. Ignorance. This is the worst enemy that threatens survival. Far too few people understand mental illness as a condition that can be treated.

2. Indifference. Mental illness can and

does develop in people. One in four people thinks that he has serious mental problems, but only one in seven seeks any professional assistance. You have an obligation to yourself and others to help improve the existing legislation. New and comprehensive programs are needed. Far too little is being done to reach the people who need help.

3. Poverty. The poverty-stricken or disadvantaged have more than their share of mental and emotional problems. They are also the most neglected segment of the American population with regard to good mental health programs. There are many reasons for the existence of this problem; two of the most outstanding are lack of edu-

cation and a poorly functioning economic system.

4. Inaction. Your contributions in talent, money, or time are direly needed. As a college student, some of your time might be well spent in working on a voluntary basis in a rehabilitation center or as a part-time employee in a mental institution. As a parent, you are obligated to care for children, if they have serious emotional problems. It is estimated that over 500,000 children under 18 years of age receive some treatment in a psychiatric facility each year. You may have been of this number. For those of you who are not yet parents, a dedication to the children you may have begins to develop early in your adult life—now!

CHAPTER 3

Healthy appearance

An anonymous traveller reacted in the following way to the experience of jet flight high above the earth's surface.

I gazed into the night as the huge jet hurtled me toward a distant point on the earth's surface far below. Clouds prevented any lights from rising to my eyes, and I knew a storm was lashing the countryside even as I flew smoothly on. Above, millions of jeweled stars looked down with an awesome unblinking beauty. I sensed that I was suspended between the real and the unreal—yet even in that moment of awareness I had to ask, "Which is which? When we land do I return to reality or do I return from it?"

Suddenly, I saw that I was not alone. Someone outside the window was gazing in directly at me. When I moved, so did he; when I frowned, so did he; when I smiled, so did he. And then it struck me—he was me—and he looked much better when he smiled.

My anxiety eased—but I still couldn't answer that question about reality.

On occasion we all ask the question, "Am I real?" How we respond to our environment with the aid of our senses and appearance will provide at least a partial answer, both for ourselves and for those with whom we come in contact.

THE SKIN AND ITS CARE

Everyone wishes to make a good appearance, and the skin is our body's most visible part. It is an important contributor to the development of an efficiently functioning body and is also the observable portion of our hidden emotional selves. The skin frequently mirrors our emotional selves by blushing or occasionally developing a rash.

Structure and function of the skin

The skin weighs an average of about eight pounds. It has more than 3,000 square inches of surface area. The skin is filled with thousands of nerve endings for pain, touch, heat, cold, and pressure. The skin is important in maintaining health and keeping us fit in several ways.

The skin has two major layers. The epidermis or outer portion is formed by layer after layer of stratified epithelial cells. Millions of these cells are sloughed off every day. This layer of stratified cells forms a barrier against invasion of infectious bacteria and protects underlying tissue from injury, heat, cold, and water loss. No blood vessels or other specialized structures exist in this portion of the skin, although hair and sweat gland ducts pass through this protective outer layer.

Besides the epidermis, the skin has a second major layer called the dermis. The dermis is a tough, fibrous, elastic living tissue that contains a germinal or growing area of epithelium. Beneath this germinal area are the capillaries, lymph vessels, nerve endings, sweat glands, sebaceous glands, and roots of hair.

Beneath the dermis is a layer of subcutaneous tissue, which serves as a connecting layer between the overlying skin and the deeper tissues of muscles and bones.

Together the skin and subcutaneous layer help the body maintain a constant temperature as the arteries of these layers dilate or constrict. Dilation leads to heat loss by radiation through increased blood flow and

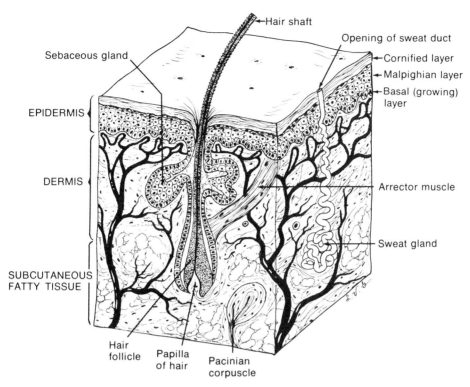

Fig. 3-1. Illustration of a section of human skin showing the several layers and many of the other structures appearing in skin. (From Tuttle, W. W., and Schottelius, B. A.: Textbook of physiology, ed. 16, St. Louis, 1969, The C. V. Mosby Co.)

evaporation of sweat. Sweat contains some salt (sodium chloride) and nitrogenous waste products of the body (urea). Sweat may have an odor depending on how much urea and other trace components are excreted, the extent of bacterial growth on the body's surface, and the state of emotions and health. Constriction of arteries of the skin leads to heat conservation with very little sweating and heat radiation, thus serving to maintain body warmth in cold weather.

Care of the skin

Instructions for the care of the skin are easily stated in four short sentences: Keep it clean. Keep it dry. Keep it free from injury. Protect its natural oils.

A daily bath or shower with a nonirritating soap will suffice to keep it clean. Soaps with hexachlorophene or other antiseptics reduce the bacterial count of the skin when used regularly. Presumably these antiseptic soaps help prevent skin infections. Occasionally a person may be allergic to a particular soap, which will irritate the skin. In such instances it may be difficult to find out what substance is causing the allergic irritation, since our skin daily contacts many different substances. A warm bath before bedtime is usually relaxing, whereas a brief warm shower followed by a cold one in the morning is stimulating and exhilarating.

Odors of the skin may be produced from the interaction of urea secreted by the sweat glands onto the skin with bacteria normally present on the skin. Sebum, which lubricates the skin, may also become rancid with age. Regular daily bathing will usually prevent such body odors. Skin under the arm pits and about the groin and rectum tends to be wet because of the constant secretion of sweat and opposing skin folds coming in contact with each other. These areas need careful, gentle cleansing daily with a mild soap. The liberal use of ordinary face (talcum) powder will help keep these areas dry. Excessive perspiration under the armpits can be prevented by deodorants, most of which contain aluminum chloride as the active chemical. Some people with heavy layers of fat rolled against themselves perspire excessively. In hot weather, as high as 8 or 9 quarts of sweat in 24 hours may be secreted. This fluid must be replaced by drinking water *during* the activity. This may be supplemented in some instances by salt pills or various drinks containing the necessary chemicals in a palatable balanced drink to meet the body's needs. Proper clothes, such as light-colored cotton or linens that are loosely woven, will aid in the heat of summer, whereas nylon, rayon, dacron, and other synthetic closely woven clothing are best avoided in summer and worn only in winter.

Sunbathing

Sunlight has visible light rays extending from 3,000 Angström units to 7,700 units. Sunlight has nonvisible rays also: ultraviolet rays of wavelengths from 136 to 4,000 Angström units. Some wavelengths tan the skin, whereas others burn it. In exposure to the sun one should remember that white reflects all wavelengths and black absorbs them.

Nearly everyone likes a fashionable tan. A sensible sunbathing procedure would be to start tanning with a 10 to 15 minute daily exposure before 10 A.M. or after 3 or 4 P.M. and gradually increase the time of the exposure. Sunburn is better prevented than treated. Water, white sand, and snow will, by reflection, frequently double the amount of exposure, so suitable measures should be taken for protection. Polaroid lenses, worn to protect the eyes, cut down on the glare of the sun and will prevent eye irritation. Excessive sun not only dries out and coarsens the skin, but is a factor, in later life, in the incidence of slow-growing skin cancers. "Tan in a bottle" is now supposed to produce a tan without exposure to sun. Most of these preparations contain dihydroxyacetone (DHA), a chemical that causes skin discoloration but no real tan. Real tanning occurs when there is more melanin in the skin. This is a protective reaction of the skin, which does not occur with "tan in a bottle."

Cold and freezing of the skin

Cold and freezing of the skin are common in winter climes. Again, prevention is better than treatment. Chilblains are mild reactions to cold, usually on exposed areas of the body. Frostbite is actually freezing of skin tissue. With both chilblains and frostbite gradual warming by warm water (100° F) is helpful. Rubbing the involved skin with snow or too rapid warming should be avoided.

Use of commercial preparations

Commercial preparations for the care of the skin, most in the form of cosmetics, are a major industry with over 1.5 billion dollars in sales annually. The word "cosmetics" comes from *kosmetikos* meaning "skill in decorating." Cosmetics have been used in all civilizations throughout recorded history.

Many creams, some with claimed "magical chemicals" or secret potions, are advertised to bring back youth and glamorize the user. In fact, cold cream, which contains lanolin for lubricating the skin, together with almond oil and beeswax in various forms, is really all that is needed or helpful in normal skin care. Vitamin and hormone creams for the most part are of no great value. If vitamins and hormones are needed, they are best prescribed by a physician. For those with certain kinds of allergic skin rashes, ointments containing corticosteroids for local application may be prescribed by a physician but *should be used only under prescription*. Finely ground talc with some perfume added has drying and deodorizing qualities that offset its mild irritant characteristics and make it almost a necessity for proper skin care. Lipstick and rouge add much color and are usually harmless. Some people who are allergic to various substances will find it necessary to use one of the hypoallergenic products that are readily available at very little extra cost.

The Food and Drug Administration is set up to protect the consumer. It has a never ending task to control extravagant, sometimes false claims made in the advertising of cosmetics. Unfortunately, the F.D.A. has a poor record for cosmetic control and has been virtually ineffective with control of those cosmetics not transported across state lines.

Common skin disorders

Acne, or pimples, is the common bane of young adults. Acne occurs more in people with oily skin. Keeping the skin clean and dry will do much to prevent acne. Occasionally elimination of chocolates, other sweets, nuts, or greasy foods from the diet may help. Acne usually starts when the pituitary gland, housed at the base of the brain, begins to produce a hormone at 12 to 15 years of age that stimulates production of estrogen from the ovaries of girls and androgens from the testes of boys. For some reason not clearly understood, this new hormonal stimulation at puberty causes an increase in the size and activity of the sebaceous glands of the skin, and may lead to a blackhead, the result of oxidized lipid from sebum. Infection, usually caused by staphylococcus bacteria that are always present on the skin but that usually are not able to invade the stratified outer protective layer of the skin, may occur in the obstructed, enlarged sebaceous glands; the result is an infected pimple.

Pimples should *never be squeezed,* whether they are red or yellow. Squeezing any kind of infected pimple is apt to force infection back into nearby arteries and veins, resulting in an infection or septicemia in the bloodstream. This may spread rapidly and sometimes is fatal. Touching a red pimple with alcohol 6 to 10 times daily will dehydrate the pimple and frequently dry it up.

Blisters are usually caused by repeated irritation or friction of damp skin. Preventing infection of the blister is most impor-

tant. This can be done by putting a sterile dressing over the blister.

Boils, or furuncles, are caused by staphylococcus infections in a hair follicle. Carbuncles usually are similar to boils but involve several hair follicles. They are apt to occur with the more virulent infectious skin bacteria. Again, these infections should *never be squeezed.* The early use of antibiotics may prevent early infection or prevent its spread. Bacteria have the faculty of becoming resistant to some antibiotics, as the bacteria manufacture enzymes that deactivate the antibiotics. A culture of the bacteria causing the infection should be made and then various antibiotics tested to see which antibiotic is effective. These are called sensitivity tests and may require 48 hours or longer to run. Consequently, during the early phase of an infection and while waiting for the results of the tests, many physicians will prescribe a broad-spectrum antibiotic, that is, an antibiotic known to be effective against many strains of bacteria. Many infections can thus be conquered in an early stage, but in highly resistant infections, sensitivity tests will nearly always be required.

Contact dermatitis is an allergic or irritant reaction of the skin to any substance to which the patient happens to be sensitive. Most contact dermatitis is caused by poison ivy, poison oak, poison sumac, cosmetics, soaps, and other substances. Prevention is important. Napoleon said that every man is a fool or his own physician by the time he reaches 30 years of age. In other words, we all must learn individually by experience what to avoid in our contacts with foods, drinks, and other substances. What is one man's food may be another's poison. A physician's help should be secured if severe or intractable eczema develops, but the primary responsibility for avoiding these contacts obviously rests with each individual.

Hives, or urticarial weals, are itching blotches or patches of swelling that suddenly develop in the skin of allergic people. Various antihistamines, such as diphenhydramine (Benadryl), tripelennamine (Pyribenzamine), or chlorpheniramin (Chlortrimeton) usually provide rapid relief. Again, prevention is better than treatment.

Athlete's foot (epidermophytosis) is a fungus infection between the toes. Blisters and scaling with peeling skin are common. Blisters may be dried up by painting the skin with tolnaftate (Tinactin). Cases are frequently chronic and require a physician's care. Prevention by keeping the skin clean and dry, especially between the toes, is most important.

Birthmarks include port-wine stains, most of which are congenital vascular anomalies. Many people have various sizes of small brown spots known as cafe au lait spots. If these are on the face and are unsightly, they may be covered with cosmetics. Covermark is made specifically for such a purpose.

Moles are the result of growths at the end of sensory nerves. The average person has 20 to 40 moles. Most cause no harm. If a mole begins to grow or becomes tender and inflamed, it should be excised by a surgeon and sent to a pathologist for study, as occasionally moles may rapidly develop into malignant tumors. A wen is a swelling in the skin caused by plugging of an oil gland with resulting accumulation of a "cheesy" material. Removal by minor surgery is indicated, as most of these wens become infected and have a foul odor.

Dandruff is a common scaling of the scalp caused by excessive secretion of oils and peeling of the epithelium of the scalp. Keeping the scalp clean by twice weekly shampooing and the occasional application of alcohol followed by a mild hair tonic will control most dandruff. Selsum, which contains selenium sulfide, is approved by the American Medical Association's Council on Pharmacy and Chemistry for the treatment of dandruff.

Bleaches and permanent waves may dry out the hair but apparently do no other harm unless the person is allergic to the chemicals used.

DENTAL HEALTH

Our teeth are strong but subject to damage; for example, they combine with the jaws to exercise more than 200 pounds of

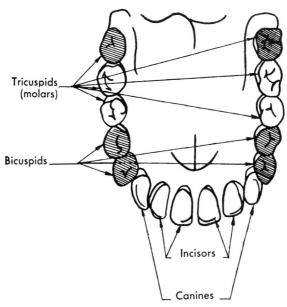

Fig. 3-2. Teeth. The permanent set of teeth includes all of those shown. (Both the upper and lower jaws have the same number and arrangement of teeth.) The deciduous set, or "baby" teeth, lacks the teeth striped in the diagram. (From Anthony, C. P.: Structure and function of the body, ed. 3, St. Louis, 1968, The C. V. Mosby Co.)

pressure in chewing food, yet they are easily subject to chipping and other injury when treated carelessly. They are seen when we smile, so their cosmetic effect can be one of value or detraction, depending on their appearance. Teeth perform a necessary function by chewing up food in preparation for digestion. Many authorities state that 19 out of 20 college students have some kind of dental defect. Guarding and caring properly for one's teeth will pay big dividends in later life. Cervantes, in *Don Quixote*, understood this when he wrote, "Every tooth in a man's head is more valuable to him than diamonds."

Structure and function of the teeth

We speak of teeth by different names, depending on their location in the mouth and their function. The central and lateral incisors are cutting teeth. The cuspid and bicuspid teeth both tear and grind food, whereas the molar teeth are primarily grinding teeth. In childhood there are 20 primary or "baby" teeth.

The incisors first appear from 7 to 9 months of age. The cuspid teeth first appear at 16 to 18 months of age, whereas the molar teeth first appear from 14 to 18 months of age. Figs. 3-2 and 3-3 show the location of primary and permanent teeth. Primary teeth are retained until the incisors of the permanent teeth begin to appear between age 7 to 9 years; the cuspids appear at 10 to 12 years. The first molar erupts at 6 to 7 years, the second molar at 12 to 13

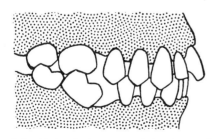

Fig. 3-3. Malocclusion caused by loss of the maxillary (upper) and mandibular (lower) first molars. Note the posterior contact only at isolated points. (From Hirschfeld, L., and Geiger, A.: Minor tooth movement in general practice, ed. 2, St. Louis, 1966, The C. V. Mosby Co.)

years, and the third molar erupts at 17 to 21 years of age.

The teeth are composed of a soft core of connective tissue called the pulp, which is well supplied with nerves, arteries, veins, and lymphatics entering from each root tip. The pulp nourishes the dentin or body of the tooth, which in turn is covered by enamel. The enamel-covered part of the tooth is called the crown and is the only part of the tooth that projects above the gum. Enamel cannot repair itself, so decay of the enamel is permanent once it begins. Cement covers the root and, together with the periodontal membrane, helps anchor the root of the tooth into its bony socket.

It has been proved that teeth are markedly decay resistant where fluorine (about 1 part per million) is found in the drinking water. Most progressive communities now add fluorine routinely to the drinking water. Such a practice could be universal; but a few consistently vocal people have delayed the practice in some communities, and children in these areas are deprived of measures that would help prevent decay of teeth.

Teeth need good alignment, or occlusion. Frequently malocclusion occurs and corrective realignment with braces is necessary. This type of malocclusion occurs most often if the primary teeth have been allowed to decay, causing permanent teeth to fall down and out of their normal alignment in early life. Space maintainers in the mouth will keep neighboring teeth from drifting out of position when primary teeth are lost too early. Some people have a too narrow or too short jaw for proper occlusion. The reduced bony arch in both upper and lower jaws appears to be an evolutionary change in homo sapiens. Teeth are more crowded in modern man than they were in prehistoric man.

Dental caries

Thirty-five percent of the people in this country over the age of 35 have lost all their teeth. Ninety-eight percent of the people have some dental caries (Fig. 3-4). Yet there are people in certain areas, such as the Alaskan Eskimos and people in certain areas

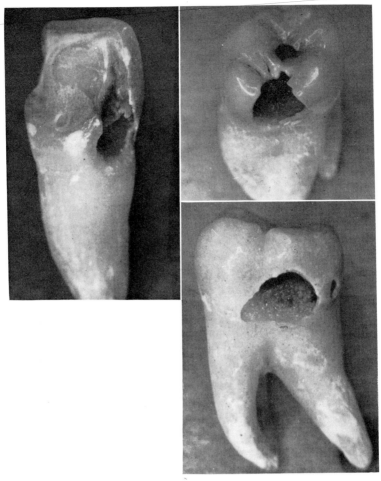

Fig. 3-4. Three examples of caries caused by neglect that commonly result in loss of the tooth because of pulp degeneration. (From Gilmore, H. W.: Textbook of operative dentistry, St. Louis, 1967, The C. V. Mosby Co.)

of Texas and Oklahoma, where dental caries are rare to unknown. Cleansing the teeth and gums by brushing with a stannous fluoride toothpaste at least twice a day and using a water jet to clean particles from beneath the gums, combined with the use of a dental floss to remove particles from between the teeth, will do much to prevent tooth decay and retraction of gums.

A tremendous number of bacteria (*Lactobacillus acidophilus*) are present in the mouth at all times. These form plaques (Fig. 3-5). When sugars or other carbohydrates are metabolized by bacteria in these plaques, acids are formed. These acids can then dissolve the enamel of the tooth and initiate decay. Research indicates that acids form within 5 minutes after sweet foods are eaten, and harmful acid levels build up within 15 minutes. These acids continue to form as long as food is present. Cavities may form underneath the invisible bacterial plaques. It usually takes several days for a plaque to form on a tooth surface. Caries can be prevented if these plaques are not allowed to form. Similar plaques may form between the teeth, so removal of food particles to prevent this is necessary.

Periodontal disease

Periodontal disease (Fig. 3-6), commonly called pyorrhea or gingivitis, begins with a

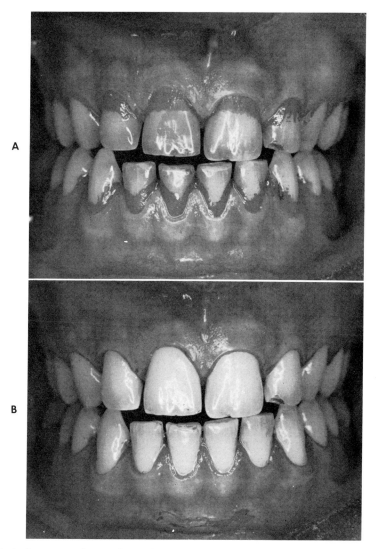

Fig. 3-5. A, Rinsing with 6% basic fuchsin reveals plaque not visible on unstained teeth. **B,** After cleansing teeth, mouth rinsed again with 6% basic fuchsin indicates that plaque has been completely removed. (From Bernier, J. L., and Muhler, J. C.: Improving dental practice through preventive measures, ed. 2, St. Louis, 1970, The C. V. Mosby Co.)

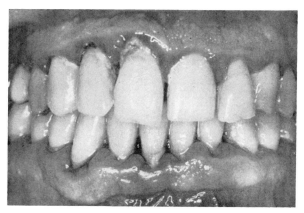

Fig. 3-6. Typical case of periodontitis. (From Grant, D., Stern, I. B., and Everett, F. G.: Orban's periodontics, ed. 3, St. Louis, 1968, The C. V. Mosby Co.)

withdrawing of the gum so that a pocket forms between the gum and tooth, which fills with food particles, bacteria, and later pus. Teeth become loosened and eventually are lost unless proper care is instituted. Again, prevention is better than treatment.

Dental myths

Education has helped to dispel many of the myths about dental care. But many Americans still cling to outmoded or discredited notions. Most of these notions are only silly, but others can be a real threat to a person's dental health. Here, according to the American Dental Association, are the most common fallacies about dental care and the facts behind them.

Fallacy. It is not important to take care of a baby's first teeth, because they are lost anyway. *Fact.* Baby teeth need as much care as permanent teeth, because they not only help maintain the shape of the jaw so the permanent teeth will erupt in the proper position, but are important for chewing, speech, and appearance.

Fallacy. Pregnancy speeds the process of tooth decay. *Fact.* There is no relation between the two. If tooth decay increases during pregnancy, it is probably because of poor mouth hygiene or increased eating of sweets.

Fallacy. Brushing the teeth completely prevents tartar deposits on teeth. *Fact.* Brushing alone cannot prevent the accumulation of tartar deposits, nor can it remove hardened tartar from a tooth. Only a dentist or a dental hygienist using special instruments can remove hardened tartar.

Fallacy. The best times to brush teeth are before breakfast and before going to bed. *Fact.* To be most effective, brushing should be done immediately after eating a meal or even a snack. Bacteria in the mouth quickly turn fermentable carbohydrates, especially sugar, to acid, which attacks the enamel of the teeth. Eventually, these acid attacks result in decay.

Fallacy. Chewing gum helps keep the teeth clean and fight tooth decay. *Fact.* Most chewing gum contains sugar (approximately one-half teaspoon per stick), and

the constant presence of sugar can increase decay.

Fallacy. A toothache does not require the attention of a dentist, since it will often disappear by itself. *Fact.* A toothache is a good warning that something is wrong. Even though the pain may go away for a time, a dentist should be consulted. Toothache may occur because decay has started and is working its way toward the pulp, which contains the nerve. If the pain stops after a few days, it may mean that the pulp and nerve are already destroyed. Pain may also be caused by the pressure of an abscessed tooth. Peridontal disease (affecting the gum or bone surrounding the teeth) may cause pain that is felt as a toothache.

Fallacy. When pain occurs, it is too late to save the tooth. *Fact.* Sometimes this is true, but usually the tooth can be saved by prompt and proper treatment.

Fallacy. Teeth decay because they are soft. *Fact.* There is little difference in the hardness of teeth, and this difference has no bearing on tooth decay. The principal cause of rapidly decaying teeth is improper care. The incorporation of fluorides into the enamel by means of fluoridated water supplies, fluoride treatments, or dietary supplements will also do much to prevent tooth decay.

Fallacy. Large fillings weaken teeth. *Fact.* Unfilled cavities weaken the teeth much more than large fillings do. If a filling is lost, it should be replaced immediately.

Fallacy. Eating foods high in vitamin and mineral content will prevent tooth decay. *Fact.* After all the teeth are formed and calcified, diet has little effect on teeth. However, a balanced diet is needed throughout life for health of all the tissues of the body, including gums and other mouth tissues.

Fallacy. Drinking lots of milk will prevent tooth decay. *Fact.* No amount of milk will prevent tooth decay. Milk, however, is the best dietary source of calcium, a mineral that is essential to the healthy growth of teeth and bones. But once the teeth are fully formed, at about age 13, calcium intake ceases to have any effect.

Fallacy. It is not important to replace a back tooth that has been extracted. *Fact.* If a missing tooth is not replaced with an artificial tooth, the other teeth tend to drift into the empty space. Once they are out of their proper position, there is likely to be too much stress on certain teeth when food is chewed. This causes further displacement of teeth and injury to the jawbone and to the tissues that attach teeth to the jaws. Also, food is more likely to become packed into the spaces between irregular teeth, and this can lead to decay and be a factor in periodontal disease.

Fallacy. Everyone can expect to lose his teeth and to have to wear dentures eventually. *Fact.* Teeth were meant to last a lifetime, and in most cases they will with proper home and professional care.

Fallacy. If you have bad teeth, it is better to have them all taken out and wear dentures instead. *Fact.* In most cases, it is better to keep as many teeth as possible because jawbones shrink after extractions and can become fragile and therefore more easily broken. Your dentist, of course, is the one best qualified to decide when teeth must be removed.*

VISION CONSERVATION

Vision is one of the body's most precious functions. Seventy-five percent of our learning and education is said to occur through visual processes. Together with hearing, good vision is essential for normal function.

Structure and function of the visual apparatus

The eye has been likened to a camera. In the process of seeing, light images pass through the cornea, which must be clear and unscarred. Light then passes through a clear liquid called the aqueous humor, which is between the cornea and lens. The iris forms the pupil and contains radial and circular smooth muscle fibers. The circular

*Adapted from American Dental Association: Folklore and fallacies in dentistry, Chicago, 1969, The Association. Copyright by the American Dental Association. Reprinted by permission.

sphincter muscles of the iris constrict the pupil, whereas the radial sphincter muscles dilate it and thus regulate the intensity of the light images falling on the retina. These light waves pass through the lens, which focuses them on the retina through the clear vitreous humor, which fills the eyeball.

The lens is a jelly-like body enclosed within a capsule, which has a suspensory ligament attaching it to the ciliary muscle. The thickness of the lens can be altered by contraction or relaxation of the ciliary muscle so that rays of light entering from varying distances may be sharply focused on the retina. In the retina are visual receptors called rods that provide for night vision and cones that provide for day and color vision. From the rods and cones visual impulses are carried by the optic nerve to the calcarine fissure of the occipital lobe of the brain where the center for sight is located. About half the sensory fibers of the body are concerned with sight. Each retina contains some 100 rods and 6 to 7 million cones.

Each eye is supplied with pathways from both sides of the brain so that partial vision may be preserved in both eyes with half the brain destroyed. (We are fearfully and wonderfully made.) Fig. 3-9 demonstrates how various lesions affect the vision.

Safeguarding vision

Vision is precious and should be protected by a good eye examination every two years for college students and young adults before the age of 40 and every year after the age of 40. Adult examinations should always include tonometry readings of eyeball pressure to detect early glaucoma, the most common cause of adult blindness in our country today.

Medical care of the eyes should fall only to the most qualified—the ophthalmologist. An ophthalmologist is a doctor of medicine who has spent 3 to 5 years beyond basic medical training in studying disorders and diseases of the eyes. The term oculist is no longer in common usage. An optometrist is not a doctor of medicine, but he has had

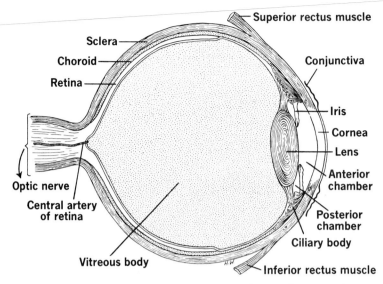

Fig. 3-7. Vertical section of the eye. (From Francis, C. C: Introduction to human anatomy, ed. 5, St. Louis, 1968, The C. V. Mosby Co.)

training in measuring refractive errors and in fitting glasses for these errors. An optician fills eyeglass prescriptions as a druggist fills drug prescriptions. Each of these has a function, but in cases of doubt, an opthalmologist should be consulted, as only he is qualified by training to treat serious disorders, diseases, and infections of the eyes and to operate on the eyes.

The eyelids are nature's way of protecting the eyes from foreign bodies and to diminish excessive light exposure. Man has supplemented nature's protection by inventing shatterproof goggles for modern industrial work where lathes and grinding machinery are used. These machines may flip particles of steel or other substances into the eye, particularly the cornea, giving rise to the phrase frequently used by doctors of a "foreign body in the cornea." Such foreign bodies may produce infections or scarring in the cornea, or both. These injuries can produce blindness, as the scars make the cornea opaque and prevent the passage of light. Three percent of industrial accidents are eye injuries amounting to over 60,000 cases annually. One in twenty cases of blindness now comes from such injuries.

Abnormalities of the visual apparatus and common eye disorders

In nearsightedness, or myopia, objects appear blurred unless they are held close to the eye. This is because the eyeball is usually too long in relation to the lens, and objects viewed at a distance come into a focal point in front of rather than on the retina. When the object is held nearer the eyes, the image moves back onto the retina so that a clear focus is obtained. Glasses with concave lenses shift the focal point in nearsightedness backward onto the retina, and objects held at normal distances are seen clearly. About 5% of children are myopic. In farsightedness, or hyperopia, the eyeball is too short in relation to the lens, and close objects come into a focal point behind rather than on the retina. Convex lenses will correct this disorder.

The lens is very elastic in childhood, but after 40 years of age it becomes firmer and loses some of its ability to alter its curvature. The eyes cannot focus on near objects, and the person needs glasses for reading. This condition is called presbyopia. With bifocals the lower part of the lens is used for close reading, whereas the upper lens has a different focal length and is used to see

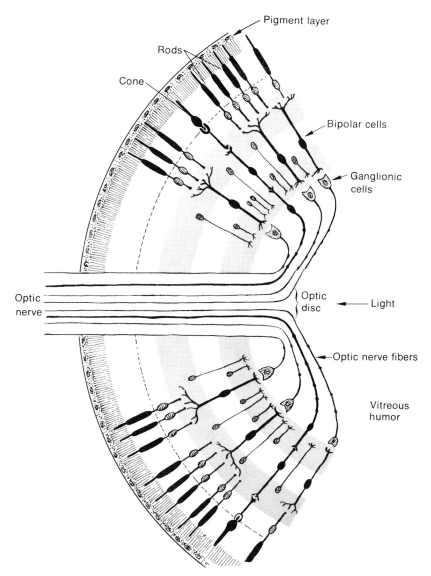

Fig. 3-8. Schematic drawing of a section of a human retina showing principal neuron layers and their connections. (From Tuttle, W. W., and Schottelius, B. A.: Textbook of physiology, ed. 16, St. Louis, 1969, The C. V. Mosby Co.)

objects farther away. Presbyopia is the most common cause of needing glasses.

Astigmatism means "without a point." Irregular curvature of the cornea distorts the light image as it passes through the cornea, and parts of the image formed on the retina are blurred or without a point. Properly fitted glasses, usually given before age 6, can correct this.

At birth the eyes normally do not work together but gradually become coordinated to produce binocular (the two eyes seeing as one) vision by the end of the first year. In some people, muscle imbalance and varying degrees of outward or inward deviation, known as squint or strabismus, may persist. Eye exercises under the direction of an ophthalmologist will benefit some; glasses can correct others; whereas surgery may be required in a few cases of this nature.

Color blindness is transmitted by a sex-linked hereditary factor. It is more common

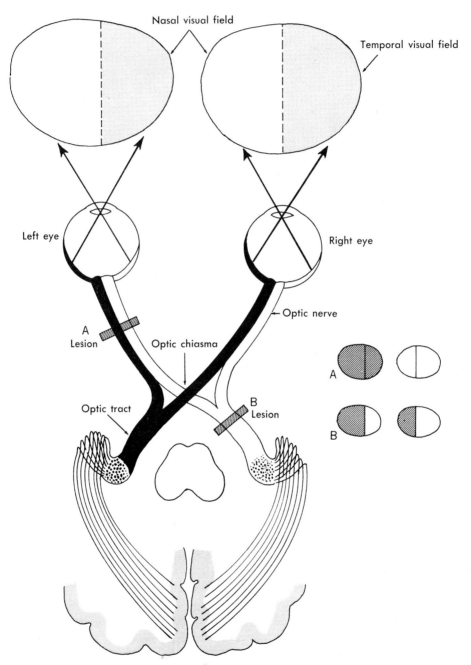

Fig. 3-9. Diagram of the visual pathways. **A,** Left optic nerve destruction causes complete blindness of the same eye. **B,** Right optic tract destruction causes blindness of the nasal visual field of the same eye and of the temporal field of the opposite eye. (From Anthony, C. P.: Textbook of anatomy and physiology, ed. 7, St. Louis, 1967, The C. V. Mosby Co.)

in men than women. An estimated eight million people in the United States are color-blind. The most common type is red-green color blindness. The least common is total color blindness. The color-blind condition is not correctable, but those affected are able to adjust satisfactorily through the detection of subtle differences in their visual images. Chapter 9 offers further information on color blindness as well as other sex-linked characteristics.

Vision should be protected from excessive glare. A pair of Polaroid sunglasses will measurably reduce glare. Television watching for any duration of time is best done about 6 to 10 feet from the screen. The viewing room should not be too dark, since shifting from the screen to the dark room produces strain on the eyes.

Inflammations may involve any part of the eye and are usually named after the part involved. A common inflammation is that of the conjunctiva and is called conjunctivitis. The conjunctiva is a thin, transparent mucous membrane overlying the cornea and the eyelids. Pinkeye is a common form of conjunctivitis. Conjunctivitis can be readily treated by any physician, who will refer the more serious conditions to an ophthalmologist.

Trachoma, a virus-caused infection of the eye producing corneal scarring, is a common form of conjunctivitis found in other parts of the world, although it is uncommon in our country. Tragically, trachoma is still the most common worldwide cause of blindness because of its involvement of the cornea with subsequent scarring.

Glaucoma and cataracts are diseases of later life. Glaucoma is associated with increased pressure in the eyeball caused by improper absorption and circulation of the vitreous humor, the clear liquid that fills the eyeball. Early cases can be detected only by pressure measurements of the eye with a tonometer. This pressure measurement should be a routine part of every adult eye examination. Although this examination is not difficult or painful, it does require skill.

Early glaucoma can be treated by eye drops that constrict the pupil and help circulation and absorption of the vitreous humor, thus controlling the pressure. Occasionally new pathways of absorption must be created by surgery. Two percent of Americans over age 40 are said to have glaucoma. It causes approximately 46,000 cases of blindness in the United States annually.

The causes of cataracts are not definitely known, but it is known that the lens becomes opaque to light because of changes associated with the aging process. Such cases can be readily improved by surgery through removal of the opaque lens and subsequent use of glasses. Cataracts are the most important cause of blindness in the United States.

Two out of every thousand, or about 400,000, people are blind in this country. Half of the cases of blindness can be prevented by early detection, proper diagnosis, and early treatment. Glasses and contact lenses are widely used to correct refractive errors. About 80 million people are estimated to wear glasses, with at least 15 million more needing glasses to improve their vision.

Contact lenses have increased greatly in use with the miniaturization of the lens to a tiny bit of plastic that floats over the cornea on a thin layer of fluid. It has become a common sight at football and basketball games to see all the players suddenly down on their knees looking for a lost contact lens. Contact lenses are used by people who wish, for various reasons, to avoid wearing regular glasses, but they carry the penalty of being irritating to the cornea. The contacting fluid should be clean. The use of saliva with its many bacteria is not recommended as a contact fluid. Probably 10 million people now use contact lenses despite their high cost and their irritating qualities to the cornea.

Corneal transplants to restore vision caused by scarred corneas have become relatively common over the world because of the establishment of eye banks to preserve the donated corneas. Over 60 such eye banks exist in the United States. Probably 35,000 more blind people could regain vision if the corneas were available. The next of kin should remember that donation of the dead person's corneas is a last good deed that person can do for someone else. Many people carry a small card signifying that they have already contacted an eye bank and made arrangements to give their corneas for transplantation. Plastic corneas are in the experimental stage and will probably eventually prove a useful substitute for scarred corneas.

HEARING CONSERVATION

Hearing is, next to sight, one of the most important ways we learn. It is estimated that about one eighth of all our learning reaches us through our ears.

Structure and function of the audio apparatus

The ear is composed of: (1) an outer ear, which receives sound waves; (2) the middle ear, which conveys the sound waves to (3) the inner ear, which contains auditory, or hearing, receptors.

The outer ear, the funnel-shaped appendage that we see, is called the auricle or pinna and includes the external auditory canal, which conveys sound about one and a half inches into the head to the eardrum. This canal is lined with glands, which secrete ear wax or cerumen. This wax protects the eardrum or tympanic membrane from dust and other foreign substances.

The middle ear beyond the eardrum is called the tympanic cavity. It contains three small bones, or ossicles, which help transmit vibrations of sound to the inner ear. These three bones, the hammer (malleus), the anvil (incus), and the stirrup (stapes) are vital to hearing. The hammer is attached to the eardrum; the anvil is suspended by two ligaments to the hammer and the stapes. The stapes fits into the oval window separating the middle and inner ear. Through the lymph of the spiral cochlea, organ of

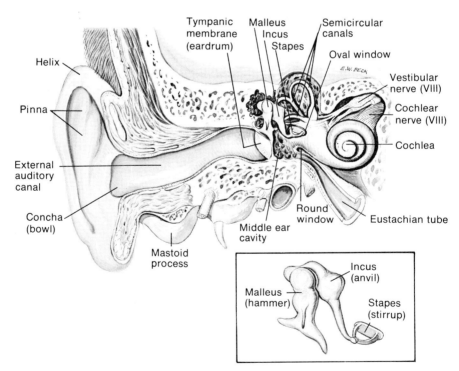

Fig. 3-10. Diagram of the hearing apparatus. (From Tuttle, W. W., and Schottelius, B. A.: Textbook of physiology, ed. 16, St. Louis, 1969, The C. V. Mosby Co.)

Corti sound waves are transmitted to hair cell endings of the auditory nerve and then to the auditory area of the temporal lobes of the brain. The hair cells near the bottom, or entrance, of the cochlea respond to high frequencies; those near the top, or end, of the cochlea respond to low frequencies. The eustachian tubes connect the middle ear with the nasopharynx. These serve to equalize the air pressure on the inner side of the eardrum with the pressure outside the eardrum. If one has a cold or has recently flown at high altitudes, the eustachian tube may become blocked, and the pressure differential on either side of the tympanic membrane may cause pain in the ear with some temporary loss of hearing.

The inner ear also contains, besides the cochlea or hearing portion, a proprioceptor portion concerned with balance and equilibrium. There are three semicircular canals lying in different planes at right angles to each other. These contain lymph, or fluid.

Whenever the head is tipped or moved, this fluid moves about and stimulates nerve endings that float like threads in the lymph. These nerve endings connect with the vestibular nerve. Their stimulation makes us aware of our body position. If this fluid is agitated violently and rapidly, as in riding in a boat on a rough sea, we develop motion sickness. Many drugs are now available that, if taken before the onset of motion sickness, will prevent it.

The saccule and utricle, along with the semicircular canals, make up the labyrinth of the inner ear. The saccule and utricle are proprioceptors that counteract the pull of gravity and tell us which way is up and down. They act through stimulation of minute hair cells, similar to those in the cochlea, as small concretions, sometimes called ear stones, are washed across the tiny hairs. These hairs are extremely sensitive to gravitational pull and act as a righting mechanism to keep us in the upright position.

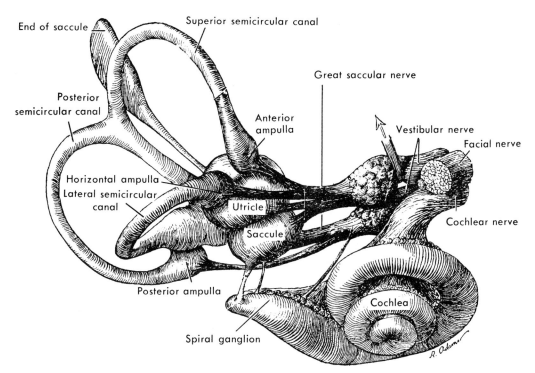

Fig. 3-11. Diagram of inner ear and nerves running from it. (From Mettler, F. A.: Neuroanatomy, ed. 2, St. Louis, 1948, The C. V. Mosby Co. In Turner, C. E.: Personal and community health, ed. 14, St. Louis, 1971, The C. V. Mosby Co.)

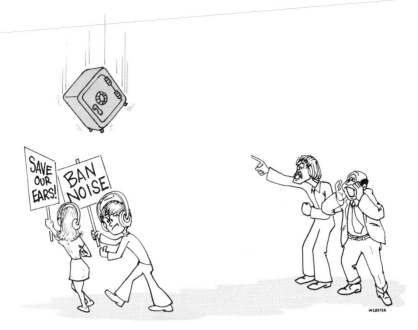

Fig. 3-12. Noise, well described as a pollutant, is a menace to aspects of health other than the sense of hearing. (Courtesy Martin Webster.)

The noise barrage

Noise is unwanted sound, and there is more of that today than we care to listen to. Common noise sources, such as power lawnmowers, kitchen blenders, power tools (especially saws), sink disposals, and vacuum cleaners, generate sounds that could be destructive to the hearing apparatus if sustained for long periods. In most cases, these noise-generating devices are used with relative infrequency.

On the other hand, there is evidence that the general noise background has increased markedly in the past two decades, especially in cities. It has been noted that noise levels in numerous cities have increased 20 decibels since the 1940's. This represents a tenfold increase in the sound pressure present, an increase that cannot be allowed to continue.

Loss of hearing may have a number of causes: birth defects, aging, accidental blows, and exposure to relatively intense noise levels over extended periods of time. There is increasing evidence that large segments of the population have been ad-versely affected by the latter. In this category, at least four types of high-intensity sound levels have been commonplace in the experience of young persons: (1) motorcycle engine noise, (2) gunfire, (3) band practice, and (4) live rock-and-roll music. All of these generate sufficient noise to be harmful to the inner ear structure if one's exposure is extensive. Motorcycles without mufflers generate sound in excess of 100 decibels. Handguns, rifles, and shotguns deliver an instantaneous report that ranges from 140 decibels to more than 160 decibels. Sound levels in band practice rooms exceed 114 decibels. Rock music rises in intensity to levels ranging from 105 decibels to 122 decibels.

Relatively high noise levels coupled with extended exposures damage the hair cells of the cochlea beyond repair. Bent, broken, or missing, they can no longer transmit their message to the brain and constitute a type of nerve damage known as acoustic trauma.

With the advent of mechanization, hearing loss became associated with specific operations notorious for their inherent noise

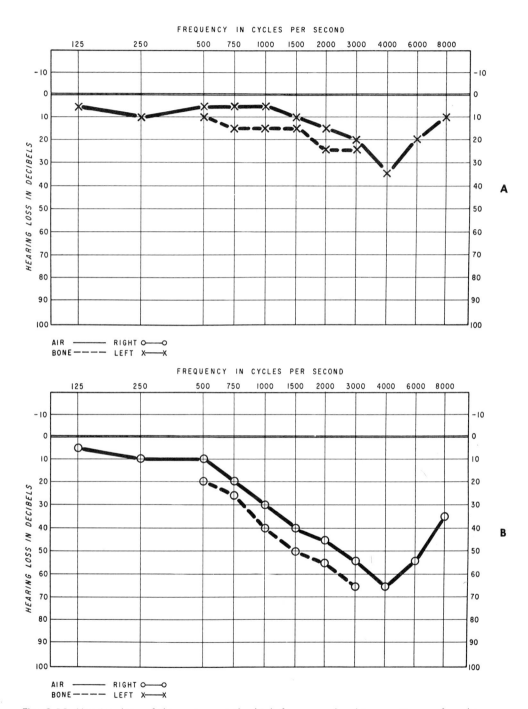

Fig. 3-13. Hearing loss of this nature at the high-frequency level is sometimes referred to as the "boilermaker's notch." (From DeWeese, D. D., and Saunders, W. H.: Textbook of otolaryngology, ed. 3, St. Louis, 1968, The C. V. Mosby Co.)

Table 3-1. Approximate sound pressure levels of familiar environmental sounds

	Decibels	
Jet engine (100 ft.)	140	Pain threshold
	—	Air raid siren
Riveting gun	130	Threshold of feeling (tickle)
	—	
Thunder clap	120	Turbine generators
Modern discotheque	—	
	110	Loud shout (1 ft.)
Power lawnmower	—	Diesel truck (high speed)
New York subway	100	Motorcycle (no muffler)
Jackhammer	—	Electric blender
Shouted speech	90	Speech interference level
	—	City traffic (inside car)
	80	Loud singing (not amplified)
	—	
Noisy restaurant	70	
	—	
	60	Normal speaking level
	—	
	50	Average office
Quiet residence	—	
	40	Quiet office
	—	
	30	Faint whisper

levels. For example, workers in boilermaker and aviation plants slowly but assuredly became deaf.

Initial losses occurred at frequencies of about 4,000 cycles per second (the highest piano note). Although the audiogram was not available when this phenomenon was first identified, a typical audiogram reflecting this loss would have been like that shown in Fig. 3-13. Note that little or no loss has occurred above this frequency; but, more important, little loss has occurred below this frequency. Otologists refer to this form of acoustic trauma as the "boilermaker's notch."

At this stage neither the person affected nor his associates were aware of this loss. The speech range predominantly includes frequencies between 500 and 2,000 cycles per second; Fig. 3-13, **A** shows an average loss of about 4 decibels in these frequencies. Continued exposure, however, caused further damage in the 4,000 cycles per second range, and more important, also affected hearing at lower frequencies. The notch be-

came deeper and wider as reflected in the audiogram of Fig. 3-13, **B,** with decided hearing loss in the speech range. It was now apparent to anyone conversing with a person so affected that he had difficulty in hearing them unless the ordinary speech level was replaced by moderate shouting.

David Lipscomb, Professor of Audiology and Speech Pathology at The University of Tennessee, has been prominent in pointing out the noise-producing problems in our present society and in suggesting appropriate preventive measures. In a January 1970 speech he identified ten areas of concern.

1. *Discotheques.* These establishments must be required to reduce the intensity of the sound environment to a much more acceptable level—e.g. 90 dB as measured on the "A" scale of a sound level meter. Enforcement of this code could likely be effected by agencies which issue cabaret licenses, food and drink certificates, or some such established regulatory board. I have been told by the musicians that they do not wish to play loudly, but that they cannot find a job if they do not. Cabaret owners have told me that they can't see how the patrons can stand the noise, but, they groan "If we regulate the musicians, we can't get

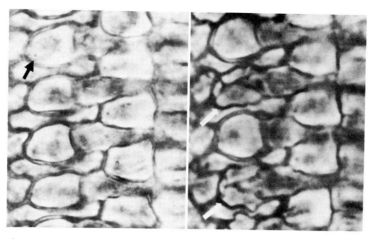

Fig. 3-14. Composite photograph showing the cell structure of a guinea pig cochlea. **Left,** normal outer hair cells. **Right,** two white arrows point to cells damaged by high-intensity noise stimulation (a total of 88 hours of rock music spread over 27 different periods covering a 56-day time span). (From Lipscomb, D. M.: Ear damage from exposure to rock and roll music, Arch. Otolaryng. **90**:29-39, November 1969.)

them back for a return engagement." It appears that both sides are pointing a finger at the other, thus, there is need for legislation which will attenuate the excessive sound present in these establishments.

2. *Traffic noise.* The state of California Assembly recently passed a bill (#2254) which establishes the maximum allowable sound produced by a moving vehicle as a function of its speed. The New York legislature (Bill #3974) has provided for the regulation of horns and other warning devices stating that horns, for example, should have two volume levels, one for use in congested areas and the higher volume allowable on the open highway. Some cities have enacted vehicle codes which prohibit the use of automobile horns altogether.

3. *Provision for adequate mufflers on moving vehicles.* Quite related to the previous suggestion is an appeal for reduction of engine noise through the use of an effective muffler (e.g. N. Y. Bill S. 4167—an act for prohibiting operation in large cities of motorcycles with inadequate noise muffling devices).

4. *Industrial noise.* In 1969 the revision of the Walsh-Healy Government Contracts Act initiated federal regulation of noise levels present in the plant environment of nearly all suppliers to the U. S. Government. These same regulations should be incorporated into state law so as to protect not only the workers in plants with government contracts, but all workers throughout the state.

5. *Aircraft noise.* The state of California has created an advisory committee for the Public Utilities Board in order to suggest airport noise standards (Bill #645). The bill provides that two of the advisory board members be representative of homeowners concerned with aircraft noise. It is important to establish basic criteria for airport noise as soon as possible before the further expansion of existing facilities precludes such regulation.

With the future addition of super-sonic transports, some states have begun to anticipate the sonic boom problem (e.g. California Senate resolution No. 7, dated June 9, 1969, urged the President and his staff to forestall overland flights at super-sonic speeds).

6. *Ear protection in recreational shooting.* The singlemost destructive sound has been found to be impulse (impact) noise. This is sound which reaches peak intensity in a very brief time span (e.g. the crack of a rifle). It is suggested that legislation be introduced to protect the sports shooter by requiring firing ranges to provide and enforce the use of good quality ear muffs for all persons on the firing line. Further, protection should also be extended to the employees of such facilities.

7. *Neighborhood industrial noise.* Many cities have codes which are designed to limit the intensity of sound produced by a manufacturing plant. This sound is measured at the boundary limits of the industry and must not exceed a prescribed level.

8. *Building codes.* There is a great deal which needs to be accomplished in the realm of multiple dwelling noise, including: regulating the noise of machinery such as air conditioners, etc. (N. Y. Bill S. 3035–A. 4771), construction standards (N. Y. Bill S. 3049–A. 4770), noise from construction activity (N. Y. Bill S. 3033-A. 4769),

and regulation of the amount of noise which is generated within the building (N. Y. Bill S. 3566–A. 5406). In this time of high-rise apartment living, it is vastly important that the acoustic environment be given equally as much consideration as the interior design and decor to the residence.

9. *Construction noise.* Construction machinery is among the most noisy of all sound generating devices. Much of this sound can be reduced with the implementation of efficient mufflers, proper maintenance to reduce the squeaks and squeals which result from metal rubbing against metal, and better design. Further reduction of the irritating quality of construction noise can be introduced by regulating the work hours for construction equipment which exceeds a pre-determined sound level (e.g. N. Y. Bill S. 3566–A. 5406 which delimits the permissible work hours of construction conducted near multiple-dwellings).

10. *Environmental quality control.* In 1969 California amended the government code relating to environmental quality control to include noise as one of the factors depreciating the quality of the environment. This is a necessary addition to our state and local codes which define boards, committees, consultants, etc., for the purpose of preserving the environment.

I realize this list will never be complete, but it constitutes a beginning. The representatives in our state legislature who are now fervently attempting to conduct the business of our state government are urged to lend an ear (no pun intended) to these suggestions, make appropriate additions, and design appropriate, meaningful, worthwhile and enforceable legislation directed at the noise problem. I am confident that I speak for the rest of the persons in the hearing health community when I say that we stand ready and willing to assist in every way we can.*

In our relationship to others and to our environment the influence of noise is no small deterrent to personal health. The problem promises to become more acute until and unless we are able to control it through collective and individual efforts.

Common auditory disorders

Wax in the ear canals is a common cause of deafness. Hard wax may be softened by hydrogen peroxide dropped into the ears. Care should be used in removing wax. In difficult cases it is wise to remember the advice, "do not put anything smaller than your elbow" into the ear canal, and instead, to seek the help of a physician.

Ear canal infections are painful. Staphylococci are apt to cause a boil in the canal, whereas streptococci produce cellulitis of the tissue. Both are painful. Canal infections either by gram-negative bacteria or fungi are not so painful but are more persistent and tend to be chronic. Aid and advice should be secured from a physician in the persistent cases. Swimming for long hours daily may keep the ear canal and eardrum soggy. This wet condition makes an ideal climate for infections that thrive in damp and wet skin areas. Alcohol dropped in the ear canals daily after prolonged swimming helps dry the ear canal and eardrum and can prevent many infections from developing in the ear canal.

Middle ear infections (otitis media) may be acute or chronic. Pus may accumuulate, and the pressure can rupture the eardrum. Rupture is usually accompanied by pain and fever. Acute infections of the middle ear may travel to the mastoid. Chronic infections of the middle ear may lead to permanent loss of hearing when the vibrating bones (malleus, incus, and stapes) become glued together with scar tissue. In long-continued chronic otitis media, the infection may occasionally invade channels to the brain and cause a temporal lobe abscess of the brain. The early and wide use of broad-spectrum antibiotics has sharply reduced these complications.

Audiology centers have been established over the country and are aiding persons with hearing difficulties in prevention, diagnosis, and treatment of hearing losses. The American Hearing Society has local chapters in nearly all major cities where information may be secured for help. Many hearing problems of children could have been prevented or greatly reduced by early diagnosis. Prevention and early diagnosis with corrective measures supplied early are the keys to better hearing and a reduction in other disabilities that hearing losses may produce, particularly in children.

---

*Lipscomb, D. M.: Excerpt from speech presented to the Knoxville, Tennessee, Civitan Club, January 23, 1970.

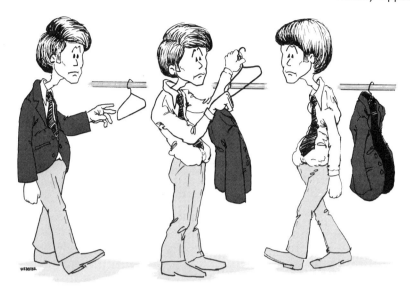

Fig. 3-15. "A picture is worth . . ." (Courtesy Martin Webster.)

Deafness may be caused by nerve failure or interference with the auditory nerve, so-called nerve deafness. Nerve deafness is readily diagnosed and differentiated from middle ear deafness by those trained and qualified in audiology.

POSTURE AND APPEARANCE

The alert, erect, healthy, graceful person radiates a feeling of poise, optimism, and self-confidence. When being interviewed for a position in competition with others, the person with good posture often gains an edge over those who lack it.

The mechanics of posture, carriage, and bearing of the body

The old Army adage, "Suck in your gut and throw out your chest," has much to recommend it. "Stand tall" is another bit of good postural advice. If we add to that, "Keep your head back and chin up," we immediately describe the ideal comfortable position of posture for most people. Good mechanical posture will make the body a more efficient and effective machine. How can you tell if your posture is good or bad? A commonly used test of posture is to stand with your back against a wall with your weight resting evenly on the balls of your feet. Your shoulder blades and buttocks should touch the wall. If only your back or midthoracic region touches, your spine is bent or flexed too much. Standing up straight with the head back aligns the ear, shoulder, hip joint, kneecap, and the instep in the ideal postural position.

To align the body and carry it gracefully yet efficiently, we use the bones and muscles of the body as levels and weights. Approximately 200 bones are divided into long, flat, short, and irregular bones. Muscles are of three types. Cardiac muscle, the muscle of the heart, differs from other muscle in that it normally has a "beat" of its own. That is the reason a heart continues to beat when it is transplanted. Smooth muscle is the automatic muscle of the blood vessels and intestines. Striated muscle is the regular muscle of the extremities. We are concerned in posture with striated or skeletal muscle, so called because it is attached to the skeleton. Over 600 muscles help to maintain our position and balance. Each muscle has "sensors" constantly feeding information to our computer, the brain, via the nerves and spinal cord. Muscles may become tired or abnormally stretched with poor posture and so weaken our body or even disable it, as happens in low back pain. In 80% of such cases the cause is bad posture and muscle deficiency.

The foundation of the body's weight bearing and carriage is the feet. Each foot has 26 bones, 117 ligaments, and 19 muscles with 2 arches. One arch is a longitudinal arch from toe to heel. The other is a transverse arch across the top of the foot's width. A weak longitudinal arch, causing flat feet, shifts the body's weight to the inside of the foot, throwing the ankle and leg out of line and so causing foot pain. High heels may cause transverse arch troubles by shifting weight from the heel and outer arch directly to the transverse arch.

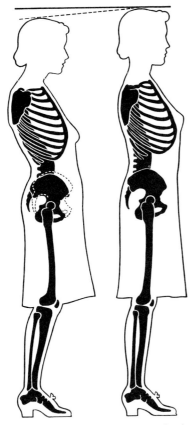

Fig. 3-16. Standing posture. **Left,** bad; **right,** good. In good posture head is straight above chest, hips, and feet; chest is up and forward, abdomen in, or flat, and usual back curves are not exaggerated. In poor posture head is forward, chest flat, abdomen relaxed, and back curves are exaggerated. (Courtesy Samuel Higby Camp Institute for Better Posture.)

Deviations in posture

Man's upright position has mechanical disadvantages outweighed by increased speed and versatility of movement. The lower spine of some people develops an abnormal swayback appearance, caused by poor muscle tone, which physicians call lordosis. Some older people tend to get stooped in the upper thoracic region. This condition is called kyphosis. A lateral curvature of the spine is termed scoliosis. All of these deviations of the spine may be associated either with poor muscle development or muscle strain and may produce pain. A physician's help, usually that of an orthopedist, in strengthening and overcoming the muscle defect producing such conditions, should be sought. Inadequate development of muscles and sagging between the chest and pelvis because of disregard for posture or appearance produce many postural defects.

Maintaining good posture

Maintaining good posture is largely a matter of constant attention to many small details of our body's carriage plus the development of the right muscles. Developing good habits of sitting and lifting will prevent many muscle strains. There are three common exercises to help strengthen muscles and improve posture:

1. To strengthen neck muscles, stand straight with the hands clasped behind the head. Force your head back against the pressure of your hands, keeping the chin in.
2. To strengthen abdominal muscles, lie flat on the floor with your hands behind your head. Keep the legs stiff and straight. Slowly raise the heels 10 inches off the floor. Then weave the legs side to side while keeping them stiff and straight. Do this at least 10 times initially and increase the number of times gradually to 30 times daily. A variation of this is to hook the feet under a sofa while lying flat and then lift the head and trunk off the floor to the upright position 10 times.

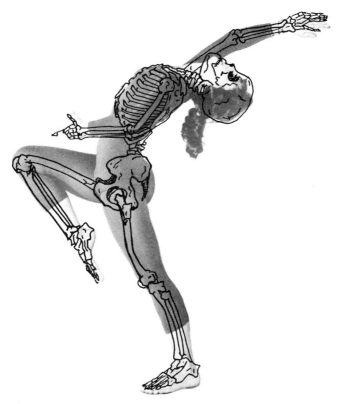

Fig. 3-17. Satisfactory posture is a combination of heredity and conscious effort over time. The grace of an attractive dancer reflects good musculature and adequate skeletal alignment from head to toe. (Drawing courtesy Lois Wallace.)

3. To strengthen the low back muscles, sit on the edge of a chair with your legs spread wide apart. Slowly flex forward and touch the floor, then slowly return to the erect position. Do this a minimum of 10 times daily and gradually increase to 30 times daily.

Isometric exercises, in which little or no movement of the skeleton is involved but which are merely active contractions of the muscles, have become popular for building up a muscular appearance. Other exercises such as those pictured in Fig. 3-19 are helpful in keeping one's body carriage graceful and the muscles in efficient tone. Persistent difficulties need the aid of a physician, usually an orthopedist, but there is much each of us can do to prevent minor, nagging postural deviations. Physical fitness, an extension of the primary postural concerns, is discussed in the next chapter.

A HAPPY APPEARANCE

We would not debate the importance to total health of clear, vibrant skin, well-positioned, lustrous teeth, normal vision and hearing, and esthetic posture. But probably no single feature will add more enjoyment to your own zestful living than a smile. A smile lightens up the atmosphere of daily living like a bright light on a dark night. A smile adds immeasurable zest and attractiveness to its wearer. Wear a smile in your everyday activities and you will generate about you an atmosphere of gracious friendliness that will cause people to seek you out "just because you make them feel good." A smile will soften the sharpest words of criticism and censure. A smile will open doors of friendship and business to you that will go far beyond your training and talent. Laughter and a smile are the oil of life that ease the daily friction of living.

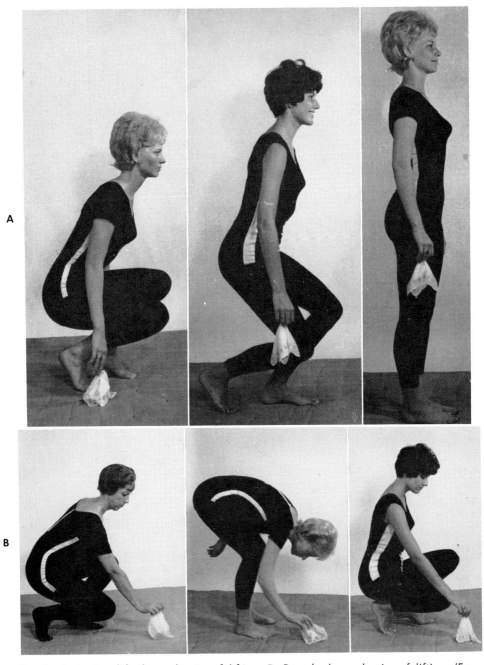

Fig. 3-18. A, Good body mechanics of lifting. **B,** Poor body mechanics of lifting. (From Barney, V. S., Hirst, C. C., and Jensen, C. R.: Conditioning exercises, ed. 2, St. Louis, 1969, The C. V. Mosby Co.)

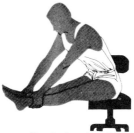

Exercise for waist and abdomen. Sitting with legs together straight out, bend forward and grasp the legs just below the knees. Press down with the hands, at the same time press up against the hands with both legs.

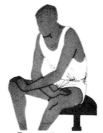

Exercise for chest and legs. Placing the feet about four inches apart, bend forward and place hands against inside of opposite knees. Attempt to press knees together while at the same time holding them apart with the hands.

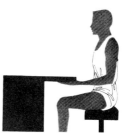

Exercise for the upper arms. Sit straight, grasp the underside of a heavy desk or table with palms up, forearms parallel to desk. Push up as hard as possible.

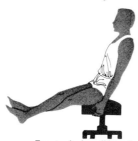

Exercise for legs. While sitting forward on the edge of the chair, lean back; hold legs straight out. Hook one foot over the other and hold tightly. Rest feet on floor; keep legs straight; then try to pull the feet apart.

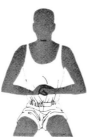

Exercise for arms, chest, and shoulders. Sit straight with chest out and arms held across chest; place one fist inside the other. Press together using all the strength of the arms and shoulders.

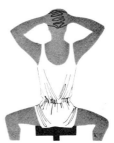

Exercise for the neck. Sitting straight, clasp the hands behind the neck holding elbows forward. Pull forward with the hands and at the same time press the head backwards.

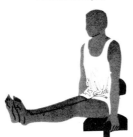

Exercise for shoulders, arms, abdomen. Keeping the back straight, lean forward and place the hands palms down against the side of the chair. Hold legs straight out, attempt to raise body about one inch off the chair.

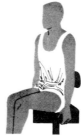

Exercise for arms and shoulders. Sit straight, grasp the sides of the chair tightly with both hands and pull up as hard as possible.

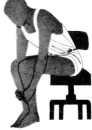

Exercise for the back. Keep back straight and lean forward until you can grasp your legs or braces of chair. Pull straight up using back muscles only.

Fig. 3-19. Selected exercises for postural improvement.

Laugh, or smile, and the world smiles with you; weep, or frown, and you do so alone.

What is real? It is how you feel when all is right with you and your world. It can be quite unrelated to the actual state of your physical health. This feeling of "rightness" is often difficult to achieve, but certainly a smile helps you along the way. A smile will create, inside you, a greater feeling of joyful, zestful living; for as a man thinks in his heart, so is he. Above all our assets in a personal health inventory, we place first a smile.

CHAPTER 4

Point counterpoint: food and activity

How we live is determined by a myriad of choices that we make continuously. We have already seen, in Chapters 2 and 3, that the consequences of these choices are apparent in many aspects of health. The consequences are particularly and perhaps more rapidly apparent when we consider nutrition and activity.

NUTRITION

"Socrates said, 'Bad men live that they may eat and drink, whereas good men eat and drink that they may live.' " (Plutarch)

It is important to make an early distinction between nutrition and food. *The American College Dictionary* describes nutrition as "the process by which the food material taken into an organism is converted into living tissue, etc." and food as "what is eaten or taken into the body for nourishment." At first glance, if there is a difference in these two definitions, it is slight. Nutrition appears to be more scientific with the reference to conversion, whereas food is given the less technical status of simply providing nourishment.

Implied in these two definitions, however, is a difference that is most important. On the one hand, the definition of nutrition implies no possibility of choice. For example, the energy needs of our body are met by carbohydrates, proteins (both yielding about 4 calories per gram), and fats (9 calories per gram) at a constant, never changing rate, whatever their food source. On the other hand, the definition of food does imply the possibility of choice, and the decisions we make regarding food are deter-

mined by our responses to the environment. Last night you overate at sorority rush. This morning you had an English exam, but rose late so that you only had time for a glass of milk (not bad, but not good either) before class. Your brother was married last Saturday, and what a feast they threw—every delicacy imaginable and no end to the liquid refreshments. After all, marriage is a time for celebration, and what better way than with food! But the question is whether your choice of food provided you with the nutrition you need.

Daily dietary needs

The basal metabolic rate. If a person remained in bed, ate nothing, maintained a normal temperature, and was relaxed and motionless but wakeful, the energy consumed to remain alive would be his basal metabolic rate. For young men this is about 1,600 calories per day; for young women it is about 5% less, or 1,520 calories. From many determinations of basal metabolic rates in different people, tables are available giving the average basal metabolic rate for any age, sex, and given body area (usually inferred from height and weight). An individual's basal metabolic rate, determined either by measuring total body heat given off or by measuring the rate of oxygen consumption, is recorded as a percentage greater or lesser than the average found in these tables. Like the heartbeat, some variation (up to $\pm 10\%$) from the average is of no health consequence. Basal metabolic rate is reasonably constant once full growth has been achieved, up to the third decade of life.

Each decade thereafter, there is an approximate 2% decline.

Recommended dietary allowances. In the United States the accepted standard for nutrient intake is that of the Food and Nutrition Board of the National Research Council. These standards are presented as the recommended daily dietary allowances and represent the opinion of nutrition experts relating to daily intake levels that will not only protect against deficiency but allow for a relatively wide margin of safety. Recommendations are made only for nutrients for which the information available permits an estimate of human requirement. Allowances are made for variations in dietary requirements that relate to age, sex, and activity, and also to needs associated with pregnancy and lactation. The most recent revision (1968) of the "Recommended Daily Dietary Allowances" is reproduced in Table 4-1.

Energy. A physicist would define energy as the property of a system that diminishes, when the system does work on any other system, by an amount equal to the work done. The unit of measure used to describe energy is the calorie; a kilocalorie is the amount of heat required to raise 1 kilogram (2.2 pounds) of water 1 degree centigrade. As used in nutrition studies, this unit is the large calorie, and once was designated with a large "C." The small calorie, which will not be referred to again, is one-thousandth (1/1,000) of a kilocalorie.

Life itself requires energy as indicated in the discussion of the basal metabolic rate. Increased activity requires increased energy. Sedentary existence requires approximately 2,500 calories daily: 1,600 for basal needs; 200 for food digestion; and 700 for the additional muscular activity, including increased heart rate. Increasing caloric needs, beginning with basal needs are seen in Table 4-2.

Physical laws apply to nutrition. If the calories taken in equal the calories burned, body weight will remain constant as long as total water content remains constant. When calorie intake exceeds energy requirements,

there is a weight gain. Thus an excess of 20 calories per day, if maintained, would result in the gain of nearly 2 pounds in a year (4,218 calories equal 1 pound of fat). Altough this sounds insignificant, the consequences are of serious medical concern when viewed over two or more decades. When calorie intake is less than energy requirements, there is a weight loss. First carbohydrates, including stored glycogen, then stored fats, and ultimately, as in extreme starvation, enzymes and structural proteins are metabolized to provide energy. More on overweight and underweight is included later in this chapter.

It is important that the total number of calories consumed in the diet coincide with the level of activity. Unfortunately, when it does not, today's youth are inclined to solve the dilemma by reducing their activity. There is mounting evidence that this imbalance contributes to obesity, degenerative arterial disease, diabetes mellitus, and many other complications. There is little doubt that a higher level of individual health would be reached if the population were more active and increased its calorie intake accordingly.

Carbohydrates. All carbohydrates contain carbon, hydrogen, and oxygen, with hydrogen and oxygen always present in a 2 : 1 ratio. Carbohydrates are found in foods in three forms: as monosaccharides (a single six-carbon chain as in glucose, $C_6H_{12}O_6$); as disaccharides (two six-carbon chains joined together as in sucrose, $C_{12}H_{22}O_{11}$); and as polysaccharides (many six-carbon chains joined together as in starch $[C_6H_{10}O_5]_x$, where x represents the unknown but very large number of single sugars that make up the starch molecule).

About 47% of the caloric intake in the American diet is made up of carbohydrates. They represent the most inexpensive and therefore the most important source of food energy. Because they are inexpensive, it is not uncommon for the average diet in developing countries to derive more than 80% of its energy source from carbohydrates. In the United States during the last 60 years

Table 4-1. Recommended daily dietary allowances[1] (revised 1968)

	Age[2] years from up to	Weight (Kg)	Weight (lbs)	Height (cm)	Height (in)	K (calories)	Protein (gm)	Vitamin A activity (I.U.)	Vitamin D (I.U.)	Vitamin E activity (I.U.)
Infants	0-1/6	4	9	55	22	kg X 120	kg X 2.2[3]	1500	400	5
	1/6-1/2	7	15	63	25	kg X 110	kg X 2.0[3]	1500	400	5
	1/2-1	9	20	72	28	kg X 100	kg X 1.8[3]	1500	400	5
Children	1-2	12	26	81	32	1100	25	2000	400	10
	2-3	14	31	91	36	1250	25	2000	400	10
	3-4	16	35	100	39	1400	30	2500	400	10
	4-6	19	42	110	43	1600	30	2500	400	10
	6-8	23	51	121	48	2000	35	3500	400	15
	8-10	28	62	131	52	2200	40	3500	400	15
Males	10-12	35	77	140	55	2500	45	4500	400	20
	12-14	43	95	151	59	2700	50	5000	400	20
	14-18	59	130	170	67	3000	60	5000	400	25
	18-22	67	147	175	69	2800	60	5000	400	30
	22-35	70	154	175	69	2800	65	5000	—	30
	35-55	70	154	173	68	2600	65	5000	—	30
	55-75+	70	154	171	67	2400	65	5000	—	30
Females	10-12	35	77	142	56	2250	50	4500	400	20
	12-14	44	97	154	61	2300	50	5000	400	20
	14-16	52	114	157	62	2400	55	5000	400	25
	16-18	54	119	160	63	2300	55	5000	400	25
	18-22	58	128	163	64	2000	55	5000	400	25
	22-35	58	128	163	64	2000	55	5000	—	25
	35-55	58	128	160	63	1850	55	5000	—	25
	55-75+	58	128	157	62	1700	55	5000	—	25
Pregnancy						+200	65	6000	400	30
Lactation						+1000	75	8000	400	30

From Food and Nutrition Board, National Research Council.

[1]The allowance levels are intended to cover individual variations among most normal persons as they live in the United States other nutrients for which human requirements have been less well defined.

[2]Entries on lines for age range 22-35 years represent the reference man and woman at age 22. All other entries represent allo

[3]Assumes protein equivalent to human milk. For proteins not 100 percent utilized factors should be increased proportionately.

[4]The folacin allowances refer to dietary sources as determined by *Lactobacillus casei* assay. Pure forms of folacin may be effec

[5]Niacin equivalents include dietary sources of the vitamin itself plus 1 mg equivalent for each 60 mg of dietary tryptophan.

there has been a reduction in the consumption of cereals and potatoes (polysaccharides) and an increase in the consumption of refined sugars and syrups (monosaccharides and disaccharides). There is good evidence that this shift has resulted in increased dental caries, particularly for diets high in sucrose. More recent investigations suggest a relationship between high carbohydrate diets (with a high ratio between simple as compared with complex sugars) and heart disease.

Water soluble vitamins							Minerals				
Ascorbic acid (mg)	Folacin[4] (mg)	Niacin (mg equiv[5])	Ribo-flavin (mg)	Thiamine (mg)	Vitamin B6 (mg)	Vitamin B12 (μg)	Calcium (gm)	Phos-phorus (gm)	Iodine (μg)	Iron (mg)	Mag-nesium (mg)
35	0.05	5	0.4	0.2	0.2	1.0	0.4	0.2	25	6	40
35	0.05	7	0.5	0.4	0.3	1.5	0.5	0.4	40	10	60
35	0.1	8	0.6	0.5	0.4	2.0	0.6	0.5	45	15	70
40	0.1	8	0.6	0.6	0.5	2.0	0.7	0.7	55	15	100
40	0.2	8	0.7	0.6	0.6	2.5	0.8	0.8	60	15	150
40	0.2	9	0.8	0.7	0.7	3	0.8	0.8	70	10	200
40	0.2	11	0.9	0.8	0.9	4	0.8	0.8	80	10	200
40	0.2	13	1.1	1.0	1.0	4	0.9	0.9	100	10	250
40	0.3	15	1.2	1.1	1.2	5	1.0	1.0	110	10	250
40	0.4	17	1.3	1.3	1.4	5	1.2	1.2	125	10	300
45	0.4	18	1.4	1.4	1.6	5	1.4	1.4	135	18	350
55	0.4	20	1.5	1.5	1.8	5	1.4	1.4	150	18	400
60	0.4	18	1.6	1.4	2.0	5	0.8	0.8	140	10	400
60	0.4	18	1.7	1.4	2.0	5	0.8	0.8	140	10	350
60	0.4	17	1.7	1.3	2.0	5	0.8	0.8	125	10	350
60	0.4	14	1.7	1.2	2.0	6	0.8	0.8	110	10	350
40	0.4	15	1.3	1.1	1.4	5	1.2	1.2	110	18	300
45	0.4	15	1.4	1.2	1.6	5	1.3	1.3	115	18	350
50	0.4	16	1.4	1.2	1.8	5	1.3	1.3	120	18	350
50	0.4	15	1.5	1.2	2.0	5	1.3	1.3	115	18	350
55	0.4	13	1.5	1.0	2.0	5	0.8	0.8	100	18	350
55	0.4	13	1.5	1.0	2.0	5	0.8	0.8	100	18	300
55	0.4	12	1.5	0.9	2.0	5	0.8	0.8	90	18	300
55	0.4	10	1.5	0.9	2.0	6	0.8	0.8	80	10	300
60	0.8	15	1.8	+0.1	2.5	8	+0.4	+0.4	125	18	450
60	0.5	20	2.0	+0.5	2.5	6	+0.5	+0.5	150	18	450

under usual environmental stresses. The recommended allowances can be attained with a variety of common foods, providing

wances for the mid-point of the specified age range.

tive in doses less than 1/4 of the RDA.

All carbohydrates are reduced to mono-saccharides in the stomach or small intestine before being absorbed into the bloodstream. Once in the bloodstream, some carbohydrate is used immediately as an energy source. Normally the glucose level is be-tween 80 to 120 mg. per 100 ml. of blood. Brain cells, because of their inability to store sufficient quantities of glucose and their limited ability to use fats or amino acids as energy sources, are the first to suffer when the glucose level falls below

Table 4-2. Examples of energy expenditures in calories per minute

Activity	Man (154 lbs.)	Woman (128 lbs.)
Sleeping and reclining	1.1	1.0
Sitting	1.5	1.1
Standing	2.5	1.5
Walking	3.0	2.5
Running	9.4	8.0

this. Thus, the depression that many college students experience is often caused by faulty and irregular eating patterns and the resulting widely fluctuating levels of blood glucose. Weakness, trembling, and fainting are further signs of low blood glucose, and in the extreme, unconsciousness, convulsions, and death will result if the blood glucose level does not rise.

Carbohydrates above immediate needs are stored either in the liver or muscle cells as glycogen or, if in excess beyond the need for glycogen, are transformed to fat for storage.

A factor controlling the blood glucose level is insulin, produced by the islet cells of the pancreas. Normally when the blood glucose level approaches 140 mg. per 100 ml. of blood, sufficient insulin is produced to utilize glucose or convert it to the more stable compounds for storage. Insufficient insulin allows the glucose level to rise above 140 mg. per 100 ml. of blood, and glucose may appear in the urine (glycosuria). This is a feature of diabetes mellitus, sometimes called "sugar diabetes."

A daily minimum requirement for carbohydrate is difficult to determine and is virtually unnecessary in the American diet. At least 100 grams per day are desirable to avoid ketosis (incomplete combustion of fatty acids) and the excessive use of protein as an energy source. The latter is of special concern when full growth has not yet been attained.

Fats. The same elements found in carbohydrates are also present in fats; namely, carbon, hydrogen, and oxygen. However,

there is more carbon and less oxygen, and there is a much greater concentration of energy than in carbohydrates (9 calories per gram of fats compared with 4 calories per gram of carbohydrates).

The American diet includes about 41% calories from fat. Although the proportion of animal fats has decreased and that from vegetable sources has increased in recent years, animal sources are still high when compared with typical diets found in most other countries. In the presence of fats other foods are more palatable, and the satiation level is higher. In addition, fats serve to provide a protective cushion around vital organs, to facilitate digestion, to retain body heat, and as carriers for fat-soluble vitamins.

Each fat molecule is composed of one molecule of glycerol and three molecules of fatty acid. All fats contain glycerol, but differ in the kinds of fatty acids present. Certain of the latter are termed essential— linoleic, linolenic, and arachidonic—in that their lack will result in impaired growth and reproduction, dermatitis, and reduced efficiency of energy utilization.

Fatty acids are either saturated or unsaturated. Those that are saturated contain as much hydrogen as their carbon atoms are capable of holding. Unsaturated fatty acids contain one or more double bonds between certain carbon atoms and so could hold more hydrogen atoms. The saturated fats have been linked to high cholesterol levels in the blood and heart disease, but a definite relationship between cholesterol and heart disease has not been demonstrated. Although high-risk persons (those prone to heart disease) exhibit high cholesterol and triglyceride levels (the latter may be related to high simple-sugar consumption), they also demonstrate other characteristics (reduced physical activity, higher smoking levels, different body characteristics, etc.) that set them apart from so-called low-risk persons.

Our supply of fat is derived from three sources: animals and dairy products, most of which are saturated, and plant oils that are partially unsaturated. Plant oils come from nuts and seeds. Peanut oil, margarine, and olive oil are common examples. Margarine is a hydrogenated vegetable oil with nutritive values equivalent to creamery butter when fortified. A consequence of hydrogenation, of course, as when a liquid cooking oil is transformed into a shortening, is to make a fatty acid more saturated than it was previously through the addition of hydrogen in place of some of the double bonds between carbon atoms.

Proteins. Proteins, the so-called building blocks of the human body, are chemically unique in that each protein molecule combines, as one small part of its long chain, a carboxyl group (COOH) at one end and an amino group (NH_2) at the other end to form an amino acid. Each protein is the consequence of hundreds of amino acids joined head to tail in a complex chain. The prime element in protein, not seen in our discussion of carbohydrates or fats, is nitrogen. It is interesting that life as we know it has been ruled unlikely on Mars because of its apparent absence of nitrogen. It may be, however, that more sensitive instrumentation and eventual on-site investigation will reveal nitrogen on Mars or other planets.

Some 25 amino acids have been identified, and at least another 10 are suspected to exist. These combine in an almost unlimited variety to form the largest, most complex molecules so far identified. An example is hemoglobin, the oxygen-carrying molecule found in the blood. Its complexity is seen in its formula: $C_{3032}H_{4816}O_{872}H_{780}S_8$-$Fe_4$. The body is able to synthesize all but eight of the amino acids at a sufficient rate to meet its basic needs. These eight, called essential, must be provided by dietary protein. They are isoleucine, leucine, lysine, methionine, phenylalanine, threonine, tryptophan, and valine. A ninth amino acid, histidine, is essential to infants. All of these must be present simultaneously for the necessary protein synthesis to be accomplished.

The American diet is rich in protein. Foods such as milk, meat, eggs, fish. cheese, and nuts are excellent sources. These, in combination with protein from plant sources, can reduce cost while maintaining nutritional adequacy. Yet protein deficiency does exist among small segments of the population who are ignorant of nutrition science, or have insufficient money to purchase the necessary protein. Pregnant women and the elderly are especially likely to be victims. Marginal protein deficiency among children in depressed communities may be more prevalent than realized. The first symptoms of protein deficiency are a decreased muscle mass, followed by swelling of the legs because of accumulation of fluids.

In many developing countries extreme protein deficiency has long been a serious problem. Protein foods from animal sources are expensive, and overpopulated, agriculturally inefficient countries cannot afford the time or the luxury of letting animals graze on land that must be cultivated for plants. Consequently, kwashiorkor, which means "disease of the firstborn" (because the first child usually developed it when removed from his mother's breast at 9 to 12 months of age to make room for the second), has plagued sections of Asia, Africa, and South America for centuries. It is characterized by apathy, edema, diarrhea, skin lesions, hair discoloration, protruding abdomen, and anorexia. The focus of the world's food problems is found in the lack of adequate protein; and until a means to produce inexpensive, palatable protein-rich foods is discovered, the problems will become even more acute.

Vitamins. Chemically, there is very little difference between the essential amino and fatty acids and the host of substances known as vitamins. All are simple organic substances, essential for life, and cannot be synthesized by man rapidly enough to meet his needs. Since amino and fatty acids are needed in much greater quantities, however, the term "vitamin" is reserved only for those substances required in minute quantities. So small is their requirement, for example, that although all vitamins could be

Table 4-3. Fat-soluble vitamins

Vitamin	Important functions	Effect of deficiency	Best sources	Stability in foods
Vitamin A	Integrity of mucosal epithelium Production of visual purple Normal growth Health of the skin	Dry and scaling skin Faulty bone and tooth development Night blindness Xerophthalmia and other epithelial tissue disorders	Fish liver oils Milk (whole) Butter and fortified margarine Vegetables (the dark green and deep yellows)	Soluble in fat but not in water Stable to heat Destroyed by oxidation, drying, thawing, and light
Vitamin D	Absorption and metabolism of calcium and phosphorus Normal development of bones and teeth	Rickets (in children) Osteomalacia (in adults) Convulsions Dental decay	Fish liver oils Milk (fortified) Exposure to sunlight	Soluble in fat but not in water Stable to heat and oxidation
Vitamin E	Normal reproduction Antioxidant of carotene and vitamin A in intestine Fertility in male rats Normal fat deposition	Humans: mild anemia, hemolysis of red cells Animals: muscular dystrophy, male sterility, resorption of fetus in females	Wheat germ oil Corn and cotton seed oils Milk Butter Eggs Liver	Soluble in fat but not in water Stable to heat Not affected by acid Oxidized by alkali, rancid fats, iron salts, and light
Vitamin K	Production of prothrombin Normal liver function	Prolonged clotting time Intestinal disease (obstruction, colitis, diarrhea, sprue)	Synthesis in intestine Liver Green leafy vegetables	Soluble in fat but not in water Stable to heat Unstable to alkalis and light

a source of energy, their potential for this purpose is minute.

Vitamins do not become a part of the body as do proteins, fats, and minerals. Instead, they serve as catalysts to accelerate various chemical reactions within the body. They serve primarily to convert food substances into the forms necessary for utilization. For example, vitamin D is needed for the normal absorption and utilization of both calcium and phosphorus.

When vitamins were first discovered early in the twentieth century, the number of different vitamins was unknown. It seemed easier then to assign the next letter of the alphabet to each new vitamin as it was described. Complications soon developed as more than a dozen variations of the original vitamin B were uncovered. Today nearly 30 different vitamins are known to exist, in-

cluding biotin, cobalamin, choline, folacin, inositol pantothenic acid, para-aminobenzoic acid, and pyridoxine. Although the practice of letter identification remains for those first so described, most are referred to now by their chemical name.

It is accepted practice to divide vitamins into those that are fat soluble (A, D, E, K) and those that are water soluble (most others). Tables 4-3 and 4-4 summarize information about the major vitamins classified in each of these two categories.

Minerals. At least 17 minerals contribute to important health functions of the body. The major minerals in terms of quantity found in the body are calcium, phosphorus, potassium, sulfur, sodium, chlorine, and magnesium. Minerals referred to as micronutrients or trace elements, because the body's need for these is much smaller, include iron, manganese, copper, iodine, cobalt, fluorine, zinc, chromium, molydenum, and selenium. Although the need for iron, iodine, and fluorine is small, they are usually considered separate from the other micronutrients because of their established importance. Minerals make up about 4% of total body weight, of which calcium and phosphorus account for three fourths, or 3% of total body weight. We are bombarded by advertising about iron-deficiency anemia, yet iron represents less than 0.005% of body weight, whereas calcium represents between 1.5 and 2.2%. Adults are usually more deficient in calcium than in iron. If a diet contains adequate amounts of minerals for which recommended levels have been set (see Table 4-1), the biologic requirements for the others will more than likely be met also, with the possible exception of fluorine. Information about selected minerals is summarized in Table 4-5.

Water. The body is 50% to 75% water by weight. All chemical reactions take place in its presence, and a 10% loss will result in serious health impairment. Any deficit or excess of more than a few percent that lasts beyond a few days (even as few as three) is incompatible with health.

Adults require 6 to 8 cups of water daily to offset losses. Average water losses occur in the feces (5% of total), urine (55% of total), and via the lungs and sweat glands (40% of total). In addition, physical activity, environmental and body temperature, humidity, and the movement of the surrounding air will add to the water intake needs.

Hemorrhaging, diarrhea, fever, and burns are conditions that result in excessive water loss. Any person even mildly ill should pay close attention to his liquid intake. To "force fluids" may not be easy, but it is a dire necessity during any illness, and recovery will be quicker if the normal water balance is maintained.

It is possible for a positive water balance to be maintained under certain conditions. Excessive water retention by cells is called edema. In its extreme form a finger pressed into the skin will leave a depression that fills slowly like water filling a hole dug at the beach. Disturbances of protein nutrition and circulatory and renal complications may result in edematous conditions.

Food in America today

Your daily food plan. Without the application of sound nutritional knowledge the average young adult's diet would be inadequate. This is unquestionably the case for many beginning college students who are free, often for the first time in their lives, to choose their complete diet. If you are selecting your own diet and you permit hunger and instinct to be your guide, the chances are good that some needs are not being met and that others, for example energy needs, may be met to excess. Yet it is less difficult in America today to obtain the nutrients needed for satisfactory growth and development than in most other countries of the world. At least it is less difficult if attention is given to certain basic facts.

In 1957 the United States Department of Agriculture revised its earlier listing of the "basic 7" food groups to include only a "basic 4." These have served with some minor adjustments since that time as the foundation guide for a balanced diet. The "basic 4" includes the following:

Milk group: some milk daily
Children under 9	2 to 3 cups
Children, 9-12	3 or more cups
Teen-agers	4 or more cups
Adults	2 or more cups
Pregnant women	3 or more cups
Nursing mothers	4 or more cups

    Cheese and ice cream can replace part of the milk requirement.
Meat group: two or more servings
    Beef, veal, pork, lamb, poultry, fish, and eggs, with mushrooms and nuts as substitutes
Vegetable-fruit group: four or more servings
    A dark green or deep yellow vegetable (important for vitamin A) at least every other day
    A citrus fruit or other fruit or vegetable (important for ascorbic acid) daily
    Other fruits and vegetables, including potatoes
Bread-cereals group: four or more servings
    Whole grain, enriched, restored

Table 4-4. Water-soluble vitamins

Vitamin	Important functions	Effect of deficiency	Best sources	Stability in foods
Thiamin (B₁)	Utilization of carbohydrates Normal growth Appetite Digestion Normal nerve functioning	Loss of appetite Indigestion Constipation Beriberi Fatigue Irritability Cardiac lesion	Liver, kidney, heart Whole-grain cereals and bread (enriched) Soybeans Peanuts Milk Pork and beef	Destroyed by heat in alkaline solution Stable in acid solution Highly soluble in water, not in fat Not affected by drying
Riboflavin (B₂ or G)	Utilization of carbohydrates Health of skin, eyes, mouth Normal growth Vigor	Loss of appetite and weight Cheilosis (cracking at corners of mouth) Vascularization of cornea Photophobia (intolerance of light) and blurred vision General weakness	Milk Meats Liver, kidney, heart Eggs Green leafy vegetables Dried yeast Possible synthesis in intestine	Stable to heat and oxidation Sensitive to light and alkali Mediumly soluble in water, not in fat
Ascorbic acid (C)	Integrity of intercellular substances through formation of collagens Metabolism of amino acids Absorption of iron Normal bone and tooth development Transforms folic acid to biologically active folenic acid	Irritability Mucosal hemorrhaging, including bleeding gums Edema Scurvy	All citrus fruits Cabbage Dark green leafy vegetables Potatoes Cantaloupe	Destroyed by drying, storage, and exposure to air Neutralized by alkali Highly soluble in water, not in fat
Niacin (nicotinic acid)	Health of skin Normal growth Normal nervous system functioning Carbohydrate metabolism	Pellagra (dermatitis, diarrhea, dementia, death)	Meats Liver, kidney Milk Green leafy vegetables Salmon Yeast	Stable to heat, oxidation, and light Stable to acid and alkali Slightly soluble in water, not in fat
Folacin	Carbohydrate metabolism Regeneration of blood cells Protein metabolism	Megaloblastic anemia Inflammation of tongue (glossitis) Diarrhea Malabsorption Sprue	Liver, kidney Yeast Green leafy vegetables Beef Wheat cereals	Oxidized by acid and sunlight Slightly soluble in water, not in fat
Pyridoxine (B₆)	Carbohydrate, fat, and protein metabolism, but especially protein and amino acid metabolism	Depression Nausea and vomiting Conjunctivitis Dermatitis	Peanuts Corn Liver, kidney Wheat germ Soybeans	Destroyed by heat and ultraviolet light Mediumly soluble in water, not in fat

Table 4-4. Water-soluble vitamins—cont'd

Vitamin	Important functions	Effect of deficiency	Best sources	Stability in foods
Cobalamin (B$_{12}$)	Protein metabolism Nucleic acid and nucleoprotein synthesis Maturation of all cells Carbohydrate metabolism Nervous system and intestinal tract functioning	Retardation of growth Pernicious anemia Sore tongue Amenorrhea	Liver, kidney Milk Cheese Eggs Most meats	Stable to heat in fluids Neutralized by strong acid and alkaline solutions and by light Slightly soluble in water, not in fat

Milk is the leading source of calcium, riboflavin (B$_2$), and high-quality protein, and provides many other vitamins, minerals, carbohydrates, and fats. In addition, vitamin A, thiamine (B$_1$), and niacin are present in smaller quantities. Vitamin D is normally found in whole milk only in small quantities, but a quart of irradiated or fortified milk contains sufficient vitamin D to provide the recommended daily allowance. Fig. 4-2 shows the contributions of two cups of milk or its equivalent to the recommended daily allowance for the average adult.

The foods of the meat group contribute nearly 50% of the body's protein plus considerable iron, thiamine, riboflavin, and niacin. Other minerals and vitamins and variable quantities of fat are contained in the food of this group. The essential amino acids can come only from the meats (containing high-quality protein) of this group and from milk and certain vegetable com-

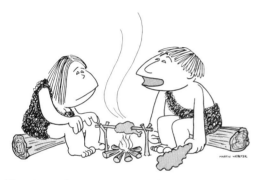

Fig. 4-1. "Sometimes I wonder whether we're getting a good balance of the basic 4 food groups." (Courtesy Martin Webster.)

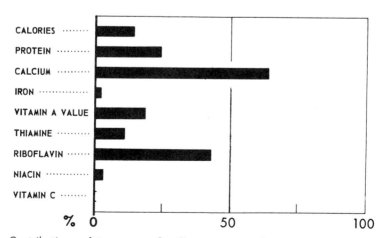

Fig. 4-2. Contributions of two cups of milk or its equivalent to the recommended daily allowance for the average adult. (From Agricultural Research Service, U. S. Department of Agriculture.)

Table 4-5. Minerals

Mineral	Important functions	Effect of deficiency	Best sources
Calcium	Bone and tooth formation Muscle contraction Clotting of blood Irritability of nerves Contraction of muscles Iron utilization	Retardation of growth Rickets Malformed teeth Osteomalacia (bone soften- ing in adults) Blood clotting slowed	Milk, cheese Oysters, salmon Green leafy vegeta- bles
Phosphorus	Bone and tooth formation Fat and carbohydrate metab- olism Neutrality of blood Fatty acid transport	Retardation of growth Rickets Malformed teeth Lack of vigor and endurance	Milk, cheese, eggs Nuts, legumes Whole-grain cereals Fish
Potassium	Normal heart rhythm Irritability of nerves and muscles Intracellular fluid balance Cellular enzyme function	Deficiency complicates many pathologic conditions Diabetic acidosis Muscle weakness Nausea Excess harmful to heart	Meats Fish Fruits Cereals
Sulfur	Contributes to formation of hair, nails, insulin, cartilage, melanin	Dermatitis Poor development of hair and nails	Found in combina- tion with all pro- tein foods
Sodium	Extracellular fluid balance (complements potassium's role in intracellular balance)	Weakness Nerve disorders Loss of weight Disturbed digestion "Salt hunger"	Salt Baking soda and powder Milk Eggs
Chlorine	Osmotic pressure pH of body Formation of gastric juice Metabolic processes Muscular action	"Salt hunger" Loss of weight Disturbances of digestion Incomplete water retention	Salt Meat Milk Eggs
Magnesium	Formation of bones and teeth Enzyme activator in carbo- hydrate metabolism Irritability of nerves and muscles	Convulsions Retarded growth Disgestive disturbances Accelerated heart beat Vasodilation	Meat, milk Fruits Vegetables
Iron	Formation of hemoglobin, red blood corpuscles, respiratory enzymes Normal epithelial tissue	Anemia Lowered vitality Pale complexion Retarded development Reduced hemoglobin level	Enriched cereals Asparagus Prunes Raisins Eggs Liver, kidney
Iodine	Normal development of thyroid gland Formation of thyroid Regulation of basal metabolic rate	Goiter Hypothyroidism Retardation of physical, sex- ual, and mental develop- ment (cretinism)	Broccoli Cod liver oil Iodized salt Seafood

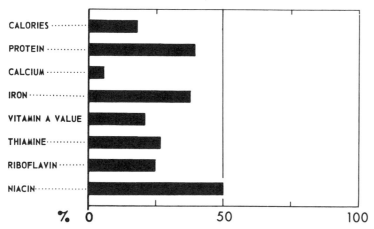

Fig. 4-3. Contributions of two servings from the meat group to the recommended daily allowance for the average adult. (From Agricultural Research Service, U. S. Department of Agriculture.)

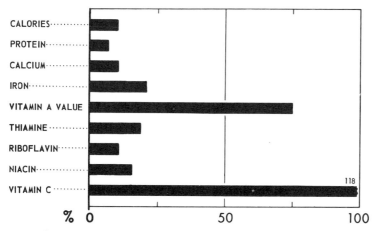

Fig. 4-4. Contributions of four servings from the vegetable-fruit group to the recommended daily allowance for the average adult. (From Agricultural Research Service, U. S. Department of Agriculture.)

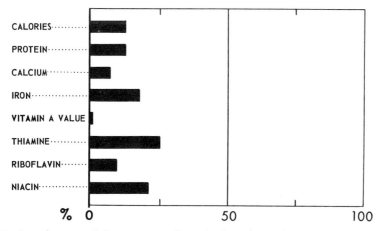

Fig. 4-5. Contributions of four servings from the bread-cereal group to the recommended daily allowance for the average adult. (From Agricultural Research Service, U. S. Department of Agriculture.)

binations. Although dry beans, peas, and nuts serve as alternatives, these contain protein of lower quality. Fig. 4-3 represents the contributions of two servings from the meat group to the recommended daily allowance for the average adult.

Foods from the vegetable-fruit group are valuable because of the vitamins and minerals they contain, as well as for the interest they add to meals and for the roughage they provide. Vitamins A and C are particularly well represented, but many other nutrients are included in significant quantities. Fig. 4-4 summarizes the major contributions of this group to the daily diet.

Breads and cereals *comprised of whole grains, enriched, or restored,* contain significant amounts of thiamine, protein, iron, and niacin as well as several other nutrients in lesser quantities. This group is more important, however, because the cost per serving is somewhat less than that for the other three groups. Thus, many contributions to the nutritional smorgasbord are made inexpensively. Included in this group are bread, cooked cereals, ready-to-eat cereals, cornmeal, crackers, flour, grits, macaroni, noodles, rice, rolled oats, and spaghetti. The amount of calcium provided depends on the quantity of milk, milk solids, and yeast foods found in the bread. Iron, thiamine, riboflavin, and niacin are standard supplements to most cereal foods. Unenriched, refined breads and cereals offer variety to the daily diet. Fig. 4-5 summarizes the major contributions of the bread-cereal group.

Selection of a variety of foods as outlined in the "basic 4" provide most of the nutrients for an adequate diet. The servings indicated provide most, but not all, of the nutrients needed by the young adult. Fig. 4-6 shows the contributions of the four groups combined compared with the recommended daily allowance shown as 100%. The margin of difference up to the minimum recommended allowance, shown in precise quantity in Table 4-1, may be achieved through larger helpings of the same foods and with other foods between or during meals to provide sufficient energy and maintain desirable weight.

This presentation of the "basic 4" has been straightforward, and it seems that individual adherence to the varieties and amounts indicated should be all that is basically necessary to know about nutrition. Unfortunately, it is not. There are a number of other factors that contribute to make wise food selection difficult.

Social and emotional factors. Would you enjoy a meal that included rattlesnake, eel, snails, beetles, grasshoppers, or ants? Most, if not all, of these are foreign to the

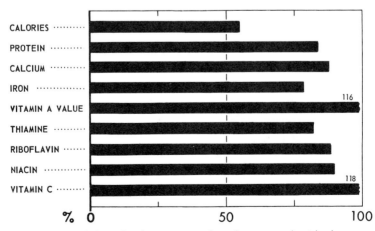

Fig. 4-6. Contributions of four food groups combined compared with the recommended daily allowance (shown as 100%) for the average adult. (From Agricultural Research Service, U. S. Department of Agriculture.)

American diet, and chances are you would find them quite unpalatable—if you knew what you were eating in advance. Yet these foods are delicacies in other cultures.

But, let's not be quite so extreme. Could you enjoy bread or biscuits made from fish flour, a product containing almost the protein equivalent of fresh beef steak? Fish flour is made from so-called trash fish, which is of low fillet quality, in a complicated process that refines the entire fish, including head, fins, and intestines. A number of firms in this country would like to produce fish flour, but so far the Food and Drug Administration has declared it "esthetically undesirable" and has refused to issue a license. Consequently, it cannot be sold in this country, and sales to foreign countries are slow: "If it's not good enough for you, it's not good enough for us!" The chances that you would consume fish flour, given a thorough knowledge of the refinement process, are 50/50. Certainly they are much better than that you would eat grasshoppers or ants. This is because the choices you make in food selection, and all your food habits, are inexorably entwined in all the other aspects of our culture. Hopefully you are the master of these habits, but the task is difficult at best. Many factors influence our choice.

From birth to death major events in our life take place in the presence of food. Fathers announce a new son or daughter with special sweets. The new grandmother welcomes her daughter and grandchild home from the hospital with a special meal. Birthdays and graduations are events that call for dinner out or a traditional feast at home. Marriage, wedding anniversaries, and family reunions are centered around expensive and expansive banquets. Even death, sad for some, joyful for others, is steeped in the tradition of food.

Religion, whether Buddhism, Christianity, Hinduism, Islam, Judaism, or any other, uses or denies food in primary ways. For example: the Buddhist monk may not eat after midday, although he is allowed to drink tea and coconut milk; the Last Supper is reenacted in every Christian church several times each year; most Hindus are strict vegetarians, since all animals contain a part of Brahman, the Universal Spirit, and are sacred; among Islamic traditions no animal food except fish and locusts is considered lawful unless, at the instant of slaughter, the person killing the animal repeats, "In the name of God, God is great"; and in the Jewish religion the influence of food is most evident during the eight-day Festival of Pesach (Passover) when only specially prepared (Kosher) foods may be used. In earlier times the rain dance, harvest feast, and animal (and human) sacrifice tied food and religion together. Today, tradition continues with the saying of grace at mealtime and the line in the Lord's Prayer that asks, "Give us this day our daily bread."

Thousands of people earn their livelihood in the growing, preparing, distributing, cooking, serving, tasting, removing, and destroying of food. The farmer, milkman, cook, waiter, brewmaster, busboy, and sanitation worker are easily identified in their working garb. The best chefs bring handsome salaries. Annually, more than a few housewives earn sizeable prizes for new recipes. Every state fair must have its home-canning contest to honor food skills now nearly obsolete.

There are many ways in which food may be used as reward, punishment, or a form of bribery. Dessert may be forthcoming if "you clean your plate," or withheld if you don't. An approved act may bring candy; an unapproved act may bring banishment to the bedroom without dinner. Success on a midterm exam or a 3.5 grade point average for the whole freshman year may warrant the best meal in town; conversely, failure at these tasks may result in self-imposed withdrawal from food. Job success and a salary increase may lead to a dinner for two. Under the influence of such conditioning there is little wonder that we like and dislike foods because of events, some remembered, but many long since forgotten.

Certainly food serves to relieve the stresses in life—an argument with a friend, boredom, loneliness, the loss of a job, new people in a strange place, adjustment to college, and countless other situations. For the baby, milk means security, an association that may last a lifetime. In World War II milk was seldom available to the soldier overseas. Many craved it, because its attainment was synonymous with returning home; to confirm this the Red Cross met incoming troops with a glass of milk for everyone. Conversely, many adults abhor milk because it conjures experiences of being treated like a baby that they would sooner forget.

In most of these situations the meaning of food may be only vaguely related to the specific nutrients it provides for the body. There is no doubt that food has a psychologic as well as physiologic base. Both, and probably to an equal extent, determine the physical person we become through the food we eat. Of course, problems can result from such a basis for choice.

Overweight. Despite, but more likely because of, our affluence a number of serious nutritional problems prevail today. Without question, the primary nutritional problem in America is overweight. One adult in every five is overweight, and increasing numbers of adolescents and young adults are

heavier than they should be. There is little real difference between overweight and obesity, except in the case of a well-conditioned athlete where muscle mass and retained water will create a temporary pseudo-overweight condition. Unless you are this well-conditioned athlete, you are overweight if you are 10% above normal and obese if you are 20% or more above normal. The former is only a step on the road to the latter if food habits don't change and medical counseling is not sought.

There is a better way to tell if you are overweight than simply to look at yourself in the mirror. Do you feel bloated? Does your abdomen protrude beyond your chest? When you pinch a roll of flesh over the rib cage or on the back, fleshy side of the upper arm, is there more than an inch between your fingers? Finally, how do you compare with normal men and women your same age as seen in Table 4-6? More important, if your present food habits continue (and activity and basal metabolic rate decrease), what will you weigh at 30, at 40, and beyond?

The rapidly maturing adolescent and the young adult should apply the height-weight tables to themselves with extreme caution.

Table 4-6. Height and weight charts*

Men (ages 25 and over)				Women (ages 25 and over)			
Height in shoes (1″ heels)	Weight in pounds (in indoor clothing) Small frame	Medium frame	Large frame	Height in shoes (2″ heels)	Weight in pounds (in indoor clothing) Small frame	Medium frame	Large frame
5′ 2″	112-120	118-129	126-141	4′10″	92- 98	96-107	104-119
3″	115-123	121-133	129-144	11″	94-101	98-110	106-122
4″	118-126	124-136	132-148	5′ 0″	96-104	101-113	109-125
5″	121-129	127-139	135-152	1″	99-107	104-116	112-128
6″	124-133	130-143	138-156	2″	102-110	107-119	115-131
7″	128-137	134-147	142-161	3″	105-113	110-122	118-134
8″	132-141	138-152	147-166	4″	108-116	113-126	121-138
9″	136-145	142-156	151-170	5″	111-119	116-130	125-142
10″	140-150	146-160	155-174	6″	114-123	120-135	129-146
11″	144-154	150-165	159-179	7″	118-127	124-139	133-150
6′ 0″	148-158	154-170	164-184	8″	122-131	128-143	137-154
1″	152-162	158-175	168-189	9″	126-135	132-147	141-158
2″	156-167	162-180	173-194	10″	130-140	136-151	145-163
3″	160-171	167-185	178-199	11″	134-144	140-155	149-168
4″	164-175	172-190	182-204	6′ 0″	138-148	144-159	153-173

*For girls between 18 and 25, subtract 1 pound for each year under 25. From Metropolitan Life Insurance Co.

Because of differences in rate of vertical growth, in muscular development, and in speeds of sexual maturation, the 12 to 20 year old introduces variables not present in the younger child or in the adult. Also, as pointed out above, the 6-foot, 225-pound tackle who is overweight according to the tables is not fat by the standard criteria. His extra weight is caused by his well-developed, heavier-than-average muscles and above-average retention of water.

In a physiologic sense, the cause of overweight is simply stated: more calories are taken in than are burned. But we now know that there are many factors that combine to cause overweight.

The interaction of heredity and environment is difficult to analyze. A child with two parents of normal weight has less than a 10% chance of becoming overweight himself. With one obese parent his chances increase to 40%, and with two obese parents, there is an 80% chance that he will also be obese. There is increasing evidence to support belief in the existence of a recessive "obese" gene. As has been shown with mice, a thin male and a thin female, both carrying the recessive "obese" gene, will produce fat, lethargic, contented offspring. These offspring are decidedly less active than thin mice; and when fasted, they still carry more fat than their normal counterpart while their muscles waste away as they lose protein.

The research of Jean Mayer at Harvard has shown that overweight adolescents are less active than those not overweight. There is a decided passivity that characterizes the overweight person. Although some believe that this passivity is an expression of dependency on the person's families, present prior to the onset of obesity and continuing through its development, Mayer believes it is an effect of social pressure on the obese person. He states that the obese person: (1) accepts in part the disapproving attitudes regarding himself held by other members of the community, and (2) suspects isolation from and rejection by his peers and compensates by withdrawing himself. Con-

sequently, his inactivity becomes even more pronounced.

Our mode of living is not likely to provide incentive or necessity for physical activity. Electric can openers open the breakfast orange juice. Mechanized transportation is taken even for short distances (climb those stairs instead of taking that elevator). A remote-control device tunes the television set. The electric toothbrush is becoming more popular.

Leisure time, ever on the increase, should reduce obesity but doesn't. Americans should exercise during their free time; instead they converse and consume. Our football stadiums remind us of Rome shortly before its decline. If there is a difference, it's in the fact that our gladiators are better paid, and the carnage isn't quite as great. But Americans are as great spectators as were the Romans, and obesity is one most definite consequence.

Finally, we are reminded by a myriad of skillful advertising techniques of the gastronomic delights that are within our reach. Food preservation, packaging, and distribution have made gourmet foods available to everyone—a fact that television, radio, billboards, and even skywriters seldom let us forget. There is considerable irony that eating has become a popular indoor and outdoor leisure activity.

What is the great problem about obesity? The reasons are most compelling. Many studies, including the classic longevity study conducted in Framingham, Massachusetts, from 1950 to 1960 with follow-up studies still continuing, have directly associated obesity with heart disease, high blood pressure, diabetes, gallbladder disease, and arthritis. It interferes with the proper functioning of the heart and lungs and overburdens the bones and joints. The brain is dulled, since normal oxygen uptake into the lungs is impaired. The fat person has more accidents and illnesses than the nonfat person, and his recovery is slower and more difficult. The daily limitations cannot be overlooked: fat people get in and out of cars with embarrassed difficulty; normal school, work, and recreational activities take place at a reduced pace and with reduced efficiency.

Mortality statistics are awesome in themselves, and obesity is a primary villain. The death rate for obese men ages 24 to 74 because of coronary heart disease* is greater than 40% above the expected rate. Other mortality figures are equally awesome: cerebral hemorrhage, 60% above; chronic nephritis, 90% above; cancer of the liver and gallbladder, 70%; and diabetes, nearly 300% above. When other factors are also involved, such as high blood pressure, high blood cholesterol, and a familial history for obesity, mortality rises even more sharply.

Quite obviously, obesity is a disease of complex etiology that not only has serious social and emotional ramifications but also initiates and contributes to a large number of earlier deaths. Unfortunately, the problem is so complex that there is no quick remedy for the afflicted. Four points may serve as guides, however:

If you are within your normal weight range now, work to remain there. Eat adequately and sensibly, and develop activity patterns that become habitual. Understand that your basal metabolic rate will gradually drop off after age 30 (you have no control of this), and in all likelihood so will your activity (this you can control if you wish to). Consequently, caloric intake must be reduced over time in order to hold your weight at its present level.

If you are overweight now, make a serious effort to cut down (not out) on the quantity of food you eat. The necessary diet for you may be nothing more than an overall reduction.

Establish a routine of regular activity. Do this at the same time each day, and try not to deviate. Concentrate now on learning several individual sports skills that will carry over to the middle and later years. Swimming, horseback riding, tennis, squash,

handball, canoeing, sailing, waterskiing, skating, and golf are all excellent.

When the problem is acute, see a physician or competent diet counselor. If you try each new diet fad that appears in the popular literature, you will be practicing what Mayer has called the "rhythm method of girth control," and the results could be even more severe than if you lived with your obesity. Similarly, don't brood over your problem and suddenly motivate yourself into a spasm of extreme activity. Even jogging without gradual prior conditioning can be dangerous. Skilled medical and dieting advice should be your first step toward correcting the problem of obesity.

Underweight. Less than normal weight is of concern to many young adults. The underlying cause may be more serious than the manifest sign of underweight itself: a perceived but undiagnosed illness, such as hyperthyroidism or diabetes; a less than adequate diet because of poverty, overpopulation, war, or famine. In our society and among your age group the cause more likely is overactivity, irregular hours, inadequate sleep, and poor eating habits—in short, the social merry-go-round. If you find yourself going in circles with a resultant weight loss, we hope you will step back occasionally to appraise your goals and the most appropriate means to achieve them.

It is well to keep in mind that a constant weight throughout life that is slightly below average appears to contribute significantly to a continuing level of good health.

Dental caries. Dental caries are a rampant disease in America today, with the 15 to 35 age group especially affected. The loss of teeth after 35 is usually caused by gingivitis and more extreme gum disorders. Caries, the actual destruction of tooth enamel, are caused by the action of simple carbohydrates, particularly sticky candies, in the presence of oral bacteria (p. 60). At the start of this century, sugars and sweets represented about 20% of the total carbohydrate in the food supply, with the flour-cereal products constituting about 56%. At the start of the eighth decade of the twentieth

---

*From Mayer, J.: Overweight: causes, cost, and control, Englewood Cliffs, N. J., 1968, Prentice-Hall, Inc., p. 103.

century 36% was furnished by simple and refined sugars, while only 37% came from the flour-cereal products. The shift to the simpler carbohydrates over the last 10 years may account for some of the observed increase in blood lipids, especially cholesterol and the triglycerides. There is little doubt that this shift accounts for the increase in dental caries. Skipping the candies and other refined sweets and shifting to fruits and raw vegetables for between-meal snacks will reduce dental caries. The esthetic value, but more important the functional value, of being able to masticate food into the later years with your own teeth instead of with dentures is well worth the controlled discretion in food choices that you need to make now.

Subclinical deficiencies. Even though we are a well-fed nation, certain segments of our population exist on diets that are nutritionally marginal. Children in ghettos and depressed rural communities and the elderly are particularly affected. Marginal nutrition manifests itself in a number of subclinical deficiencies: retarded growth and development among the young, lowered resistance to infection, slow convalescence from injury and illness, inefficient and confused mental processes, lost time from school and work, depression, and unhappiness. Because of the vagueness of the symptoms, the victims of subclinical deficiencies often fall prey to falsely advertised food supplements and nutrition quacks.

Food fallacies. As knowledge of the science of nutrition has increased, the chasm between what we know and ignorance has become wider and wider. The bridge across this chasm is education, and although those who teach nutrition—physicians, nurses, dentists, nutritionists, dietitions, teachers— perform well, they are unable to reach all people as effectively as they might. Consequently, folklore and fallacies about food are perpetuated, and charlatans abound.

Fallacies about food combinations are common. Fruit and milk is considered bad because the acid curdles the milk—even though all milk is curdled by stomach acids.

Milk and fish is another bad combination; and, according to the "Hayites," meat and potatoes form an evil combination. Still other combinations that are presumed to cause disease are: milk with oysters or cucumbers, and carbohydrates with proteins.

Equally ridiculous are the misconceptions, old and new, that somehow remain with us: no food should be retained in the bowel more than 24 hours after eating; animal secretions (milk being the prime example) cause cancer if consumed beyond weaning; all food must be chewed 30 to 70 times; cooked foods are "dead" foods and are to be avoided; any one of the five wonder foods—skimmed milk, brewer's yeast, wheat germ, yogurt, and blackstrap molasses— eaten daily will add 5 youthful years to life. Other bits of nutrition nonsense are probably familiar to you: fish is brain food; oysters make you potent; vitamin C prevents colds (Linus Pauling's discourse on vitamin C in *Vitamin C and the Common Cold* notwithstanding); water at meals is bad; meat causes cancer.

Many fallacies and misconceptions are perpetuated through ignorance. They need little help to continue them through the years. In addition, a persistent campaign is being carried on to undermine public confidence in the nutritional value of staple foods. Four major themes constitute the attack:

All diseases are caused by a faulty diet. According to this myth, it is almost impossible to obtain a completely adequate diet. No matter how carefully food is purchased at retail stores, some nutrients will be missing, which can be supplied only by the addition of a certain food supplement. The suggested supplement contains a long list of ingredients, many known, but others not yet known to food scientists, that possess secret health benefits.

Soil depletion causes malnutrition. Advocates of this myth contend that our soil has been depleted by continual cropping, is now impoverished, and foods grown on it are inferior. Chemical fertilizers are attacked also because they "poison" the land and the food grown on it. Although it is true that farmed-out soil will yield stunted crops, what does grow contains as much food value as food grown on rich soil. The one disease associated with a deficiency in the soil is goiter, caused by the lack of iodine. Iodized salt has provided the solution to this problem.

Overprocessing destroys food values. This myth states that food is processed to death. Although some vitamins and minerals are lost in commercial and home preparation of food, more than at any previous time the techniques of harvesting, canning, freezing, packaging, distributing, and final cooking and serving have been perfected to retain or restore nutritional values at peak levels. Examples of this are the additions to flour, bread, milk, and margarine that supply the known dietary requirements of important nutrients. The success of this effort is witnessed by the disappearance from the American scene of both rickets and pellagra, diseases that once were prevalent.

Subclinical deficiencies abound. This myth is a good example of a half truth that has been magnified in importance at the expense of other truths. To say that a condition is subclinical means that it is not possible to obtain any observable evidence of a deficiency, but a deficiency is proposed as a theoretical explanation of the symptoms. Some may be very real, as discussed earlier. Others, however, are not. "Do you have a tired, run-down feeling when you want to do things?" is the familiar pitch. Most people do at one time or another, and some are eager to take the proffered supplement that promises to relieve their symptoms. Hadacol, so popular in the 1950's, was one of these; many others are on the market today. You should distrust any suggestion of self-medication with vitamins and minerals to cure diseases of the nerves, bones, blood, liver, kidneys, heart, or any other organ.

The nutritional con-man. A quack or charlatan is a pretender. There are many who play the field of nutrition. They exploit the fears, hopes, apprehensions, and pride that reside in all people. Those who can't or won't be critical of the claims, those who fear the truth, those who are gullible—all these and others become their victims.

The successful author, Upton Sinclair, was one of these. He was an advocate of fasting. His book, *The Fasting Cure,* published in 1911, describes how prolonged fasting will combat asthma, Bright's disease, cancer, the common cold, liver disorders, syphilis, tuberculosis, and even locomotorataxia—the consequence of a destroyed nerve. Horace Fletcher was the promoter of the chewing theory referred to earlier. He flourished in the early years of this century, but there are still masticating advocates today. Jerome I. Rodale was and still is a raw food fanatic, and Daniel C. Munro argued for the high protein diet, since "Methuselah lived 969 years because he ate mostly meat." Gayelord Hauser's pitch was for the five wonder foods (p. 97), which are only available in concentrated form through natural-food stores at high prices. Their limited virtues, however, the best scientific, nutritional, and medical opinion tells us, can be obtained from ordinary foods at far less cost.

The methods the nutritional con-men use are very little different today from those of the frontier medicine man. Through health-food lectures, they claim, directly or by inference, that the products they are advocating will prevent or cure specific ailments. Some meetings often rise to the emotional level of a revival, while others are carried off with a scientific and medical aplomb that would do credit to a Schweitzer. A second approach is by door-to-door selling, while still a third is through pseudoscientific books and journals. Rodale, for example, once had three monthly magazines going at the same time. All presented a case for the prevention of disease through organic farming, and throughout each, sunflower seeds were heralded as the great forgotten food.

Legal constraint. A number of agencies try to protect the public in specific ways. The Food and Drug Administration enforces regulations pertaining to the labeling of a product. Major legislation that gives the

FDA regulatory power includes the following:

1. Federal Food and Drug Act of 1906 —made illegal the adulteration of food transported across state lines for sale.

2. Federal Food Drug and Cosmetic Act of 1938—regulated imports and exports as well as interstate commerce. This legislation also made truthful labeling mandatory.

3. Amendments to the 1938 law include the Miller Pesticide Amendment of 1954, which set standards for safe levels of pesticide residue permitted to remain on fruits and vegetables; the Food Additives Amendment of 1958, which required the food processor to show that all food additives were safe before they could be sold to the public; and the Color Additive Amendment of 1960, which forbade the use of any food coloring known to be or suspected of being carcinogenic to man or animal.

4. The 1969 Meat Packing Control Act was passed as a direct result of the pressure that Ralph Nader and his "Raiders" (young law students working in Washington investigating various government agencies) brought to bear on an important segment of the food industry on behalf of the consumers. Nader's efforts are exemplary of what can be done to correct ecologic trends that will most assuredly be deleterious to total health if allowed to continue.

The Federal Trade Commission is empowered to take action against false and misleading advertising, and the United States Post Office prosecutes those who receive money for misrepresented products sold through the mails.

It's your choice. The fact is that under normal circumstances no one is force-fed— at least not after the first few years of his life; and certainly you're on your own now. What goes in your mouth you put there. We hope it does you as much good as it gives you enjoyment. If it does, your nutritional status is most likely quite satisfactory.

EXERCISE

Perhaps no subject related to health has been before the American public to a greater extent in recent years than that of exercise and physical fitness. The barrage of information and conversation about physical fitness falls into a consistent pattern of concern for both lay and professional persons alike. What is it? Why should I get any? How much is enough? How do I get it? These are the questions that are being asked and that will be answered here, within the limitations of space.

What is physical fitness?

Physical fitness is an inseparable part of total fitness for effective living. In a special report on fitness and exercise, total fitness has been described as follows:

Fitness involves interrelationships between intellectual and emotional as well as physical factors. Good health, a basic component of fitness, implies in addition to freedom from disease, sufficient strength, agility, and endurance to meet the demands of daily living and sufficient reserves to withstand ordinary stresses. Adequate nutrition and exercise, sufficient rest and relaxation, suitable work, and appropriate medical and dental care are important in maintaining fitness.[*]

Captured in this more inclusive definition is the concept of physical fitness that permeates most of the literature: that is, "sufficient strength, agility, and endurance to meet the demands of daily living and sufficient reserves to withstand ordinary stresses."

We believe that you'll accept this definition of physical fitness. The difficulty lies in its utilization. What exactly are the "demands of daily living"? On the one hand we advocate exercise and fitness, and on the other we extend the philosophy of "why walk when you can ride" to every aspect of existence possible. It's unfashionable to exercise. You feel different if you do, because few others are; and besides it's hard work and no fun. At least that's the unfortunate image that exercise conveys to most Americans. If Americans could be physically fit without working at it, we'd be the most physically fit nation in the world. We try with passive exercise machines, bed vibrators and the like, but there seems to be

---

[*]Special report: exercise and fitness, J.A.M.A. **188**:433, 1964.

no short cut. Because there isn't, because fitness requires energy, we rationalize that the results are not really worth the effort; and so we find ourselves among the most unfit nations—our Olympic athletes notwithstanding.

But, happily, there's a positive side to the activity question, at least among today's youth. It's also fashionable to be slim, firm, vital, and exuberant. The price for these is activity, and many are paying it willingly. Whether enough are doing so for it to make a significant difference in the general level of physical fitness is currently in debate.

Why physical fitness?

Sustained activity continued to the point where the heart rate is demonstrably increased, and repeated at regular intervals, will effect certain physiologic changes. Obviously, these changes take place in both men and women and are important, healthwise, to both sexes. First, the efficiency of the heart is increased. Its strength is increased, and as a consequence it is able to pump more blood with each beat. As this happens, the number of beats necessary to supply blood to all parts of the body is fewer, and so the heart slows down. Fewer beats per minute, perhaps 20 fewer beats, means the heart has a longer rest period between each beat under conditions of normal activity. When demand suddenly increases, your heart doesn't beat as fast to supply the needed oxygen when you are fit to meet the challenge as it would if you weren't.

Second, regular sustained activity increases the number and size of the blood vessels carrying oxygenated blood to all portions of the body. Among the several advantages of this change is the clear fact that recovery following a heart attack is better in the conditioned person: the conditioned heart with its increased number and size of blood vessels is able quickly to establish an alternate supply route to the injured muscle or muscles.

Third, lung capacity and efficiency is increased. All activity requires oxygen. If we breathe in 21% oxygen with each inspiration but expire 18%, we are not very efficient. This is the case among those who are unfit. Contrary to popular attitude, there is an end to the supply of oxygen—at the site

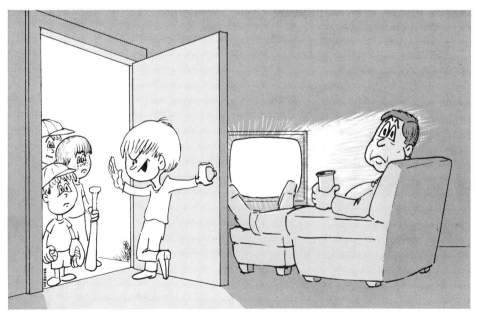

Fig. 4-7. "Naw, I'm gonna grow up and be a spectator, like my dad." (Courtesy Martin Webster.)

where it's needed, the individual cell. If you can use 25% of the inspired oxygen instead of only 10%, cellular activity will be more efficient, and so will you. Regular sustained activity enables you to transport nearly twice as much oxygen in your blood as you otherwise would.

Fourth, muscle tone is improved—"fat becomes muscle"—and the body is generally toughened up. A concomitant is an average reduction in blood pressure during rest, although this benefit is a consequence of the first three advantages as well. The esthetic contributions of supple skin and good muscle tone to general appearance are appreciated most in their absence, and there is much appreciation, but more envy, for these by the average American today.

Fifth, there is increasing evidence that the fit person, the person who exercises regularly, is less susceptible to the ravages of many diseases than the unfit. True, we know of persons who have succumbed to a heart attack while exercising, and exercise by implication becomes the scapegoat. This may be true in a certain percentage of cases. But many people die each year of heart attacks, over 700,000 in 1971, and the statistical chances that some of these would occur while the victims were exercising are good. But the evidence clearly tells us that those who have a regular regimen of physical activity are less likely to suffer the consequences of heart and blood vessel disorders, respiratory ailments, diabetes, ulcers, arthritis, and other chronic illnesses and diseases. Even those with physical problems fare better on an exercise program under the guidance of a physician.

It has been said that although we may be in the Golden Age of Medicine, we are in the Dark Age of Prevention. We can design and install artificial heart valves and with limited success even give a person someone else's heart, but we fail to convince people what they must do to prevent the debilitating condition in the first place.

Finally, regular sustained activity develops a feeling of well-being that can only be appreciated by those who have experienced it. Although this is difficult to document scientifically, the claims of thousands bear it out. The routine of daily life is fatiguing. Most people believe that fatigue is relieved by rest, and so they sit—and eat. Their symptoms, muscle soreness, low back pain, aching feet, get worse rather than better, and the logical answer for them is more rest. Instead, more activity than normal, rather than less, is the answer. With conditioning you learn to relax and are better able to deal with the stresses of daily life. Surprisingly, those in condition report that the sense of body awareness, of pleasurable fatigue that they experience, gives them a feeling of confidence that results in improved performance both on the job, with the family, and in all other aspects of life.

But until you've been there, until you've experienced what Kenneth Cooper in his book *Aerobics* has called "the training effect," you cannot appreciate the euphoria we are describing. Someone once said that a fetus, if given the choice, would not choose to be born, because existence for it, without knowledge of life outside the womb, must seem perfect. Yet once born and able to experience the joys and the sorrows of life, few would wish to return to the womb. The fetus is comparable to the unfit person. Most persons, once they have achieved a satisfactory level of conditioning, will not voluntarily permit themselves to return to the rolls of the unfit.

How much activity is enough?

"Okay," you say, "I'm motivated; now how much is enough? I can't spend all my time exercising. How do I know if I'm in condition, and how do I maintain it?" A fair question. Fortunately there are better answers today than there were even a few years ago.

At the outset, as with the relationship between energy needs and activity, there is a similar relationship between oxygen needs and activity. We have seen that regular sustained activity improves the body's efficiency to transport and utilize oxygen. You might conclude then that a task performed today in 15 minutes and performed tomorrow in 14 minutes means there has been an improvement in conditioning. This is not necessarily true. There are two aspects we need to consider: the relationship between the anaerobic and aerobic oxygen supply, and the motivation during activity.

Anaerobic and aerobic metabolism. Most Americans perform an inordinate amount of anaerobic activity: that is, activity of short duration that causes shortness of breath, increased heartbeat, tightened chest, and subsequent reduced activity until recovery. Running to catch the 8:19, shoveling snow, and those infrequent two steps at a time to the third floor all qualify. These activities are performed in the absence of adequate oxygen, and an oxygen debt is created rapidly. The small amounts of oxygen available at the cells are quickly depleted, and

without replenishment the person must slow down and maybe even sit down until he "can catch his wind." Athletes experience "second wind," the adjustment of the body to a new and greater level of oxygen demand than normal. The man who gets his exercise only by running for that train never reaches this state, and he may well be doing himself real harm by his infrequent, strenuous activity.

To demonstrate anaerobic activity on the other end of the continuum, the conditioned athlete will perform "wind sprints" and interval training as part of his conditioning program. For example, distance swimmers will devote some time to interval swimming: a warm-up period, then five 100-yard sprints in 1 minute 15 seconds with 30 seconds between, then four 200-yard swims in 2 minutes 45 seconds with 30 seconds

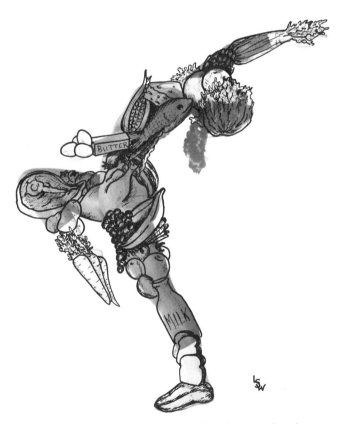

Fig. 4-8. We are what we eat is made clear in this abstract of a dancer in classic pose. Regular activity and good nutrition will allow this girl to maintain her figure throughout her full life span. (Drawing courtesy Lois Wallace.)

between, and so on through the planned program. The heart and lungs cannot supply the necessary oxygen if this activity is extreme, and the athlete must rest for a short time. Gradually, however, he does this more quickly and efficiently, and he conditions himself to move from anaerobic into aerobic energy utilization with a minimum of stress and discomfort.

Young adults are most usually able to weather all anaerobic activity, whatever their condition. Their blood vessels, particularly in the heart, but throughout the entire body, have a resiliency that allows them to dilate sufficiently to carry the required oxygen. This fact creates the delusion that they have excellent health, and in the short run of a few years they do. Youth are blessed with resilient and unobstructed blood vessels, with freely moving joints, and with lungs not yet affected seriously by extrinsic factors such as air pollution and smoking. But changes take place early in life, as autopsies on soldiers killed during the Korean War revealed. The American diet is conducive to the early development of atherosclerosis, the narrowing and stiffening of arteries caused by deposits of cholesterol. We once thought this was a condition of middle and late life; it is clear, however, that atherosclerosis begins in the twenties. When this degenerative disease is complicated by heavy smoking, reduced activity, and the stresses of new job and family responsibilities, to be over 30 may in fact mean that life—effective, productive, enjoyable life—is over.

In nearly 50% of all heart attacks that prove fatal, no clot or other obstruction is found. There is necrosis—dead tissue—and much scarring of the heart muscle tissue, but no clot, which once was thought to be the triggering event to the attack itself. Research around the world has shown evidence of other causes of death from heart attacks. Emotional stress and smoking cause the adrenals to pump increased adrenaline into the bloodstream. This increases cellular activity and elevates the demand for oxygen in the heart. Unless oxygen can be delivered, symptoms ranging from mild discomfort to

those of a severe heart attack will transpire. The attack is caused by lack of oxygen in the heart as often as by a clot.

The Swedish scientist, Ulf von Euler, has contributed technical evidence to indicate that another substance besides adrenaline is active. This is noradrenalin, produced by fibers of the sympathetic nervous system located within the heart muscle tissue. Normally, both adrenaline and noradrenalin help to regulate blood flow within the heart and throughout the body. Under stress, noradrenalin is pumped directly into the heart muscle and, along with adrenaline coming from the adrenals, serves to accelerate the heartbeat and increase the heart's blood-pumping action. Such action is good if the amount of oxygen supplied by the coronary blood vessels is equal to the amount used by the heart. Usually it is. The heart vessels dilate; they carry more blood and oxygen to the heart muscles, and the important oxygen demand is met. But atherosclerotic vessels victimized by inactivity, smoking, and emotional stress finally are unable to meet the challenge. When this happens, an oxygen deficit can occur, and the heart will suffer injury in direct proportion to the amount of oxygen it needs.

We've included the extreme consequences of anaerobic activity because they are most relevant to the general level of physical fitness today. Also, they underscore dramatically the need for each person to achieve and maintain a condition in which oxygen requirements are met to their aerobic maximum: that is, activity in the presence of a steadily replenishing supply of oxygen.

A most significant study designed to establish, in the wide area of normal health, meaningful categories of physical fitness according to aerobic capacity is that by Bruno Balke.* In working with several hundred Federal Aviation Agency workers he was able to demonstrate that within the range

*Balke, Bruno: A simple field test for the assessment of physical fitness, CARI, Report 63-6, Oklahoma City, Civil Aeromedical Research Institute, Federal Aviation Agency.

of aerobic work, a nearly linear relationship exists between running speed and oxygen requirements per unit of body mass. This was accomplished by comparing the maximum oxygen intake attainable—determined in a standardized treadmill test—with the oxygen requirements estimated for average velocities achieved in best-effort runs over various distances. Balke showed that performances in runs of 12 to 20 minutes duration, expressed in amounts of required oxygen, closely matched the objectively measured aerobic capacity. Using his findings, Balke established a field test of a 15-minute run over a known distance at best individual effort for the assessment of physical fitness. From the accurate distance and time measurements, the average velocity in meters per minute was determined and converted into the physiologically meaningful value of equivalent oxygen requirement. Balke concluded that when the performance is a "best effort," this value represents very closely the aerobic work capacity and provides an objective rating of physical fitness.

Note that Balke talks about "best effort." If there is any medical concern, such a field test should be performed only on the advice of a physician. Once this fact is established, the next consideration is of the fact that "best effort" requires considerable motivation. At your age it isn't likely that there is a serious physical problem that would prevent your participation in such a field test; the issue of motivation may be something else.

Dr. Balke showed the relationship between aerobic and anaerobic oxidation over the 15-minute period (Fig. 4-9). From these data it is clear that a very short strenuous effort, for example, running 100 yards in 10 seconds, is accomplished almost completely anaerobically. As the task is extended, however, anaerobic activity diminishes and aerobic activity increases. The curve is almost flat beyond 10 minutes and is virtually so at 15. Consequently, Balke arrived at a field test of 15 minutes as the time necessary to assess a person's available functional reserves, or his physical fitness. In less technical phraseology, the distance you can run and/or walk in 15 minutes reflects your state of physical fitness.

The theoretical findings of the Balke research fall short in their practical applications for the average person, who wants to

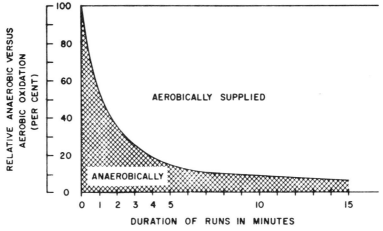

Fig. 4-9. The relative role of anaerobic and aerobic oxidation for supplying the total amounts of oxygen required during best-effort runs at defined time intervals. (From Balke, Bruno: A simple field test for the assessment of physical fitness, Report 63-6, Civil Aeromedical Research Institute, Federal Aviation Agency, Oklahoma City, Okla.)

know how much activity of what nature is needed to put him in shape and keep him there. One of the most recent practical programs designed to do this is found in *Aerobics* by Kenneth Cooper. Cooper studied under Balke and undoubtedly was inspired by him.

Dr. Cooper has developed, as he puts it, a pharmacopeia, a catalog of activity described in measurable amount so that anyone can select any activity and know exactly how much participation in it is necessary to produce a beneficial effect. His program is based on the principle that any exercise must be strenuous enough to produce a sustained heart rate of 150 beats per minute or more and that under this condition the training-effect benefits begin about five minutes after the activity commences and continue for the duration of the activity. If you compare this principle with the Balke curve, you will see the great proportion of aerobic oxidation at five minutes as compared with anaerobic oxidation. Balke's "best effort" would be equivalent to 150 heartbeats per minute.

Using this principle, Dr. Cooper has developed a system that translates the amount of oxygen required by various activities into points. Some activities are more strenuous and so receive more points; those less strenuous receive fewer points. For example, if you cycled two miles in 7 minutes 45 seconds or less five times in one week, you would receive 10 points. This would not signify physical fitness by either the Balke or the Cooper criteria but nonetheless is a starting point. On the other extreme, you are in excellent physical shape if you are able to swim 1,000 yards in 20 minutes 30 seconds four times in a week. This goal receives 34 points. According to *Aerobics,* an exercise regimen that produces 30 points per week, distributed among any combination of activities that appeal to the performer and spread over a minimum of three sessions during the week, will maintain physical fitness.

The beauty of the point system is that the energy expenditure of most activities is translated into points even for the shortest

distances. For example, to walk a mile in 14.5 to 12.0 minutes is worth 2 points. If you did this 15 times a week, you would have your 30 points.

Motivation. Early in his presentation of *Aerobics,* Dr. Cooper is quick to identify the bane of all exercise programs ever developed—motivation.

> If you've got the proper motivation, if you're truly concerned about getting your body into condition and keeping it there, I can give you a program of exercise that will match whatever motivation you bring to it.*

Any activity necessarily involves movement. Movement is work, to do work requires effort, and effort requires motivation. The motivation you possess is equal to the level of physical fitness you wish to achieve and maintain, no more no less.

Your self-concept is mirrored in your physical appearance and condition. What you perceive this to be will determine the effort you expend now and in the future. Certainly *Aerobics* or a similar program offers a handy guideline for you to follow. Whether you do or not is a function of your motivation.

Selecting the appropriate activity

Which activities do you prefer? *Aerobics* recommends running, swimming, and cycling as the best exercises, followed by walking, stationary running, handball, basketball, and squash. Isometrics, weight lifting, and calisthenics, though good to a point, do not serve as conditioners. They do not improve aerobic performance, the penultimate criterion of physical fitness. Sports like golf, tennis, volleyball, and others fall somewhere between the best activities and the worst.

A small booklet by Arthur H. Steinhaus, which is dated but still excellent, includes the recommendations seen in Table 4-7. If you are concerned with your level of physical fitness but to a less precise degree than you will achieve following *Aerobics,* the information included in Table 4-7 is quite satisfactory for your needs.

---

*Cooper, Kenneth H.: Aerobics, New York, 1968, M. Evans and Co., Inc., p. 5.

Table 4-7. Rating of sports

Sport	Endur-ance	Agility	Strength			Age range recommended
			Leg	Abdo-men	Arm and shoulder	
Archery	L*	L	L	M*	H*	All ages
Badminton						
singles-doubles	H—M	H	H	M	M	Singles under 50
Basketball	H	H	H	L	L	Under 30
Baseball (hard)	M	H	H	M	M	Under 45
Bicycling	M	L	H	L	L	All ages
Bowling	L	L	M	L	M	All ages
Boxing	H	H	H	H	H	Not recommended*
Canoeing and rowing						
recreational	M	L	M	M	H	All ages
competitive	H	L	H	M	H	Under 30
Field hockey	H	H	H	M	M	Under 30
Football	H	H	H	H	H	Under 30
Golf	L	L	M	L	L	All ages
Handball						
singles-doubles	H—M	H	H	M	H	Singles under 45
Heavy apparatus						
tumbling	L	H	H—M	H	H	Under 45
Hiking	M	L	H	L	L	All ages
Horseshoes	L	L	L	L	M	All ages
Judo	H	H	H	H	H	Under 30
Lifesaving	H	M	H	H	H	Under 45
Skating						
speed	H	M	H	M	L	Under 45
figure	M	H	H	L	L	All ages
Skiing	H	H	H	M	M	Under 45
Soccer	H	H	H	M	L	Under 45
Softball	L	H	M	M	M	Under 50
Swimming						
recreational	M	L	M	L	M	All ages
competitive	H	M	H	M	H	Under 30
Table tennis	L	M	M	L	L	All ages
Tennis						
singles-doubles	H—M	H	H	M	M	Singles under 45
Touch football	H	H	H	M	M	Under 30
Track						
distance	H	L	H	M	M	Under 45
jumps	L	H	H	H	M	Under 45
sprints	M	M	H	M	M	Under 45
weights	L	M	H	M	H	Under 45
Volleyball	L	M	M	L	M	All ages
Wrestling	H	H	H	H	H	Under 30

From Steinhaus, Arthur H.: How to keep fit and like it, ed. 2, Chicago, 1952, The Dartnell Corp., p. 70. Reprinted by permission of the Dartnell Corporation.

*H—high, M—medium, L—low, referring to contribution to physical fitness.

Exercise—a woman's right and need

A myth exists that women should not exercise, but if they do certainly they should stop before they begin to perspire; to sweat is "unladylike." This attitude toward activity by women is widespread and unfortunate. It deprives many females of wholesome enjoy-ment and improved health. Fortunately, influential sports groups and respected researchers are providing clear evidence to support the case for increased female participation in sports and physical activity.

Why is it that so many American women complain of fatigue, vaguely defined backaches, and menstrual discomforts? Is it a woman's lot to suffer from these "female complaints," or can something be done to reduce or eliminate them? A study by Gendel and Weinhold supports the notion that these complaints stem from a simple lack of exercise.*

The authors studied 67 college freshmen women ranging in age from 17 to 25. Of this number, 55 were single, 12 were married. All were normal, healthy young women but not particularly athletic. Nearly all of them complained of menstrual discomforts. After carefully examining the medical and fitness records of these girls, the authors concluded that physical fitness was the most important factor in the amount of sickness each girl reported.

Of the test group, 21 were classified as more physically fit and 46 as less. In comparing these two groups the authors state that:

> The more physically fit group had less of all the common complaints—menstrual discomfort, backache, digestive disorders, fatigue, colds, and allergies.
> The married girls experienced fewer menstrual pains but more chronic backaches, reported less abdominal strength and muscle tone.

The authors also believe that American women as a group are not fit enough to bear children without these telltale signs of strain.

> Pregnancy and delivery epitomize all the elements of the most strenuous work-capacity tests that can be given. In general, girls and women are not prepared for this task. . . . If this much chronic symptomatology exists at a time when physical activity for most women is decreasing, the pool of women whose future pregnancies could precipitate further disability is startling.

Swimming, hiking, biking, dancing, even jogging are activities that women can do and find enjoyable. If no medical reason exists to advise otherwise, all young women should participate regularly in strenuous activity. Standards of performance for women, such as those in the Royal Canadian Air Force exercise program (XBX), *Aerobics,* and the physical fitness standards for women of the American Association for Health, Physical Education, and Recreation are available. The rewards are irrefutable and happily enticing —an improved state of physical fitness with fewer "female complaints" and an improved figure with more male compliments.

RELAXATION AND SLEEP

The best insurance for satisfactory relaxation and uninterrupted sleep is careful adherence to the key recommendations included in the discussion of nutrition and exercise. Nonetheless, a few additional remarks are appropriate.

Our wakeful existence is increasingly complex. You are faced with more problems today than you were a year ago. The challenge of college has created many problems for you. All these problems demand attention. Some you can solve immediately; others you have to work at piecemeal over time before they can be worked through to a satisfactory conclusion. It is natural that you should become tense and perhaps even lose some of your poise under the pressures. The key is to recognize when the tensions and conflicts become too severe and to reduce them through controlled relaxation. If you don't, the consequences may be severe. Worry, inefficiency, irritability, and anxiety may be the first signs that something is wrong. If you permit the tensions to continue without relief, nervous disorders, loss in weight, sleeplessness, and more serious illness may be the consequences.

Let's start with the premise that pressure is part of our way of life. How we control it—not how it controls us—is the key to our being able to live successfully with it. Fundamental to coping with pressure is your ability to relax. You must be able to let go, forget your concerns, and orient your mind and body to other tasks, even for a short time. The following points show how this can be done.

Organize your life. What are the things that are important to you? What are your goals, in the short run—today, tomorrow—

---

*Gendel, E. S., and Weinhold, C. R.: Fitness and fatigue in the female: the relationship of strenuous activity to medical disability and chronic complaints in young women, presented at Denver, Colorado, February 1970.

and in the long run—this year, next year, professionally, in your lifetime? Once you identify these, establish priorities; learn to break each task into its parts, take each part and work it through, then leave it and go on to the next. Some tasks can only be done with intermittent attention over longer periods of time. Identify these, work at them for awhile, drop them for awhile—a day, week, or maybe even a year—but always come back to them until they are accomplished. Someone once said the way to eat an elephant is to take a bite and start chewing. Writing a book is much the same. So is anything worth doing.

If you are organized, you will be able to see progress and feel successful. As you do, your periods of relaxation, both short periods and those of longer duration, from several hours to several days, will take care of themselves.

To relax for short periods is vital. President Johnson rested for 20 minutes following lunch. It was one of his solutions to pressure-filled days. If possible, rest in dim light and with your eyes closed. Eyestrain is accumulative and contributes to tension. Be sure your clothes fit comfortably, especially the shoes. As you work, check your muscular state. Are your hands clenched, brows furrowed, jaws tense, teeth grinding? Check for these tensing characteristics occasionally, and consciously strive to eliminate them.

Reduce or eliminate as much extraneous noise as you are able. Loud radios and record players should be lowered to pleasurable sound levels or turned off. Music is soothing when you are working at rote tasks but may interfere with creative effort. The research of Dr. David Lipscomb at The University of Tennessee has shown (p. 72) that our modern rock music at the volumes it is played and listened to actually destroys hearing. We know that noise is a serious health problem today, and you must control the noise in your life if you are to learn how to relax.

Participate in regular strenuous activity. We've already explained the necessity of exercise. Note of it is made here to under-score the relationship of exercise to relaxation. The feeling of well-being that we discussed earlier is a pleasurable product of exercise that is most relaxing.

Learn to "vacation." We place quotes around vacation because we don't mean it in the typical sense—that is, a two-week sojourn across the country, or fishing in the mountains—although this may well be the most relaxing thing for you. By vacation we mean a change from your normal routine. The desk worker might have a glorious vacation building an extra bedroom onto his house; the carpenter might have equal fun and relaxation reading some texts on geology if he happens also to be a "rock hound." Anything that is a change of pace, that is different from your normal routine, and that you enjoy doing will contribute to relaxation. Discover them now and use them continually.

The ultimate in relaxation of course is sleep. You require between 8 and 10 hours of sleep in each 24, and the odds are good that you get this, although irregularly.

Sleep, a phenomenon not completely understood, is a condition characterized by periodic loss of consciousness and reduced cortical and physical activities. Physiologically, in sleep the metabolic rate drops 10% to 15% below the normal basal level; systolic blood pressure falls 10 to 30 mm. of mercury; the heart slows by 10 to 30 beats per minute; respiration slows and is irregular; body temperature drops and is lowest in the middle hours of sleep; and the muscles relax. Sleep is deepest in the second and third hour and then gradually becomes less deep until complete wakefulness is again achieved.

It is not uncommon for the young adult to abuse the need for sleep. At one extreme he will go long periods without adequate sleep, and at the other he will force sleep and/or bed rest far beyond his normal requirements. The appropriate balance of course is to get enough sleep to meet the recovery needs (and growing needs where these still remain) of the body, but not to use sleep as an escape mechanism from the challenging tasks of conscious life.

Worry, tension, anxiety, and fear are the great enemies of sleep and the most common causes of insomnia. Not to be able to sleep when you know you need to is discouraging. If the problem persists, it may become harmful. In addition to the need for adequate nutrition and exercise there are a number of specific aids to sleep that you may wish to follow.

Regular sleep habits are important. We are creatures of habit, and recovery during sleep is most complete when we regularly go to bed and get up again at nearly the same times.

A quiet activity, such as reading, just before sleep will serve as a relaxant.

A small quantity of food prior to retiring aids sleep. This should be solid food, since liquids will cause bladder distention and wakefulness earlier than desired.

If you bathe before bed, the water should be warm but not hot. For most persons, hot water will dilate peripheral blood vessels, thus increasing the blood flow to all parts of the body. The effect is stimulatory and is not conducive to sleep.

Bedroom temperature should be 55 to 60 degrees. A colder temperature requires more blankets, and their weight will be discomforting.

FATIGUE

To be tired or fatigued as a consequence of daily activities is normal. How we respond to fatigue, both physical and mental, will contribute significantly to our total health status.

Physical fatigue

Most likely you would describe fatigue as a feeling of tiredness or weariness resulting from continued activity. A physiologist might describe it as a disturbed balance between wear and repair. In either case the result is the same: in fatigue our ability to respond to stimuli is reduced or lost. Local manifestations of physical fatigue include tiredness in the active muscles, a general state of bodily tiredness, or a feeling of sleepiness. Also, there may be a feeling of tenseness and obscure pain in the back of the head, pain and soreness in the muscles, and stiffness in the joints.

Fatigue results from (1) a depletion of the most efficient energy source, carbohydrate, or (2) the buildup of metabolic wastes that hinder continued activity, or (3) a serious alteration in homeostasis, the body's normal physiochemical balance. Fatigue caused by carbohydrate depletion is best demonstrated by the "midmorning slump." This phenomenon is accentuated by a deficient or absent breakfast and obviously results in reduced performance. Fatigue caused by the buildup of metabolic wastes occurs during periods of extended activity, as for example the 100-yard dash. If you run that distance as fast as possible, you cannot run much further at the same speed until you have rested. The waste products of activity, lactic acid, carbon dioxide, and certain acid phosphates, are not removed rapidly enough; and their increased presence in the muscles serves to depress and inhibit further muscle contraction. Fatigue caused by disruption in homeostasis occurs, for example, when there is abnormal loss of body salts, as with profuse sweating. Persons living in tropical countries or working in high temperatures for extended periods must increase their salt intake accordingly to offset the possibility of this form of fatigue.

The interrelatedness of fatigue and physical fitness is clear. If three men of the same age and build run to exhaustion, the distance each travels will be directly related to his physical state at the outset. Our discussion of phyical fitness has explained this relationship. The point to be made here is that fatigue limits performance, not only in the athletic sense. Your ability to stay at any task to its completion will depend on your carbohydrate reserves and on your ability to deliver oxygen to and remove waste products from the active cells, whether muscle, brain, or other.

Mental fatigue

The college population more than any other group is acutely aware of the phenomenon of mental fatigue. In mental fatigue there is an inability to fix attention, memory is impaired, new ideas are not clearly understood, and reasoning is difficult and slow. As with strenuous physical activity, continued mental work without interruption, rest, or change will result in fatigue. Serious, conscientious college students will attest to this fact, and many potential students fail because they are unable to cope with it. Your coping process may be aided by the following points.

Recognize that learning is difficult. New ideas must be studied, thought through, and assimilated gradually into your intellectual base. You may need to read material two and three times before it is clearly understood. This very process is fatiguing. It is one price we pay, over and over, for the privilege of learning.

Adjust the subjects studied to your attention span. Apply yourself to one endeavor for a while, and when your powers of concentration wane, shift to something else. If a task is especially difficult, leave it for a while, then return to it. Surprisingly, it will often become easier.

Alternate physical activity and quiet study periods. A short walk, when studying seems to drag, will prove beneficial, and even more strenuous activities such as running or swimming might be preferred. If your studying is goal-oriented in the short run, for example, a paper that is due or a chapter that must be read, be careful not to overtire yourself and force the need for more complete relaxation than studying will allow.

Serious concerns in fatigue

Fatigue caused by prolonged homeostatic imbalance is of serious concern. When fatigue persists day after day and is not relieved by the normal sleep pattern (a condition referred to as chronic fatigue), there is very likely an underlying cause.

Poor nutrition is the most common cause of chronic fatigue. Earlier sections of the chapter have covered this subject. Young adults in college could probably trace many study and work difficulties that they blame on fatigue to poor nutrition. When lack of nutrition is severe enough, there may be a problem of malnourishment. Fad diets used indiscriminately may result in nutritional imbalances that become manifest as chronic fatigue.

Certain circulatory disturbances, such as heart disease or anemia, may interfere with the supply of oxygen and energy materials to the cells.

Respiratory disturbances may interfere with the adequate delivery of oxygen and energy to the cells.

Endocrine disturbances, such as diabetes, hyperinsulinism (the excessive production of insulin), and menopause, may lead to chronic fatigue.

Emotional conflicts, frustration, worry, and boredom if persistent may lead to chronic fatigue.

Continued sense-centered fatigue may engender a more generalized chronic fatigue state. Those who work in noise-producing circumstances—the foundry worker, the rock-and-roll drummer, the jet plane maintenance man—are susceptible victims of chronic fatigue. Continual visual fatigue may have a similar effect.

POINT COUNTERPOINT

It is impossible to separate nutrition from activity in any consideration of personal health; the former is an energy source, the latter is an energy consumer. In a world that grows smaller by the day, that threatens to be overpopulated by any standard by the year 2000, that is struggling to supply enough food for those here now (and obviously not succeeding), and that is destroying or polluting both farmlands and oceans at an alarming rate, catastrophic nutritional problems well may befall large portions of the earth in the not too distant future. Organized, cooperative activity on a worldwide scale is necessary if we are to deter such a tragedy.

CHAPTER 5

Safety in a dynamic environment

Each year a tremendous amount of money and human effort are expended on co-ordinated programs geared to the reduction of accidents and disasters in all phases of human existence. Industry, educational institutions, safety organizations, the press, and radio and television all conduct concentrated programs that seek to create a safer environment.

In recent years accidents have consistently been ranked fourth among the leading causes of death; accident mortality is exceeded only by the major illnesses of heart disease, cancer, and stroke. Nonetheless, although accidents rank high, accident mortality has actually declined over the past 20 years. But this decline has been more than offset by the facts that people are living longer and that mortality from other conditions has fallen more rapidly than those from accidents.

No matter how good a safety program is, it has to contend with the attitudes of the individual specifically and the public in general. The individual or the public will judge a program, a service, or a product on its ability to do a job better or to make life simpler or more convenient. The typical college student will not judge safety success. He or she simply assumes it. Herein lies much of the controversy over the importance of meaningful programs. It goes without emphasizing too much, that the college student assumes himself or herself to be potentially the self-styled safety expert in terms of cause, effort, and solution.

There is clear evidence that in industry where its importance is recognized, safe behavior can be and is effectively reinforced. This is caused in part by the relative ease of isolating the safety problem and determining the causative factors. Additionally, where controls and enforcement are necessary, they are readily implemented.

THE PROBLEMS

Of all the causes of death of man, those resulting from accidents, homicide, and suicide appear to be the most unwarranted. This section of the chapter is devoted to a review of the problems that a safe mode of living would eliminate or at least reduce.

Tables 5-1 through 5-3 point out the relative severity of accidents as a cause of death. Death statistics often are considered important data for indicating America's level of health and safety. In the second or two it will take you to read this sentence, someplace in America someone will be seriously injured. Every five or six minutes, someone in the United States is killed as a result of an accident. Approximately 11,000,000 disabling injuries are sustained each year. The total cost of all accidents in which deaths and injuries occur is estimated at about 23 billion dollars each year. In recent years, accidents have caused the death of over 100,000 persons annually.

The accident problems in this country present a rather grim picture. You may even be tempted to blot it out of your mind. Statistics of death are indeed boring. However, even you may at one time become vulnerable to or involved in an accident. Because accidents do affect you, you need to know how you can become involved and

Table 5-1. Deaths for all ages, United States, 1970

Cause	Number of deaths			Death rates*		
	Total	Male	Female	Total	Male	Female
All causes	1,930,082	1,087,220	842,862	966	1,115	824
Heart disease	744,658	425,796	318,862	373	437	312
Cancer	318,547	173,694	144,853	159	178	142
Stroke (cerebrovascular disease)	211,390	96,701	114,689	106	99	112
Accidents	114,864	79,424	35,440	57	81	35
Motor vehicle	54,862	39,788	15,074	27	41	15
Pneumonia	66,430	37,285	29,145	33	38	28
Diabetes mellitus	38,352	15,781	22,571	19	16	22
Arteriosclerosis	33,568	14,645	18,923	17	15	18

Data from Accident facts, 1971, National Safety Council.
*Deaths per 100,000 population.

Table 5-2. Deaths for children ages 1 to 14, United States, 1970

Cause	Number of deaths			Death rates*		
	Total	Male	Female	Total	Male	Female
All causes	30,580	18,129	12,451	54.4	63.3	45.1
Accidents	13,112	8,574	4,538	23.3	30.0	16.4
Motor vehicle	5,773	3,641	2,132	10.3	12.7	7.7
Cancer	3,760	2,095	1,665	6.7	7.3	6.0
Congenital anomalies	2,442	1,301	1,141	4.3	4.5	4.1
Pneumonia	2,062	1,081	981	3.7	3.8	3.6
Heart disease	651	341	310	1.2	1.2	1.1
Homicide	514	287	227	0.9	1.0	0.8
Stroke (cerebrovascular disease)	403	210	193	0.7	0.7	0.7

Data from Accident facts, 1971, National Safety Council.
*Deaths per 100,000 population.

Table 5-3. Deaths for youths ages 15 to 24, United States, 1970

Cause	Number of deaths			Death rates*		
	Total	Male	Female	Total	Male	Female
All causes	41,140	29,953	11,187	124.4	183.5	66.8
Accidents	23,012	18,480	4,532	69.6	113.2	27.1
Motor vehicle	16,543	12,911	3,632	50.0	79.1	21.7
Homicide	3,357	2,688	669	10.1	16.5	4.0
Cancer	2,731	1,637	1,094	8.3	10.0	6.5
Suicide	2,357	1,789	568	7.1	11.0	3.4
Heart disease	946	545	401	2.9	3.3	2.4
Pneumonia	851	492	359	2.6	3.0	2.1

Data from Accident facts, 1971, National Safety Council.
*Deaths per 100,000 population.

what you can do to prevent the involvement.

The four major causes of accidental death among the various age groups, according to rank order are:

1-4 years	*5-14 years*
1. Motor vehicle	1. Motor vehicle
2. Fires, burns	2. Drowning
3. Drowning	3. Fires, burns
4. Poison	4. Others

15-24 years	*25-44 years*
1. Motor vehicle	1. Motor vehicle
2. Drowning	2. Drowning
3. Firearms	3. Falls
4. Poison	4. Fires, burns

45-64 years	*65-74 years*
1. Motor vehicle	1. Motor vehicle
2. Falls	2. Falls
3. Fires, burns	3. Fires, burns
4. Drowning	4. Drowning

75 years and over	*All ages*
1. Falls	1. Motor vehicle
2. Motor vehicle	2. Falls
3. Fires, burns	3. Drowning
4. Ingestion of food, objects	4. Fires, burns

The principal classes of accidents and the number of deaths and disabling injuries within each class for 1970 were as follows:

Class	Deaths	*Disabling injuries*
Motor vehicle	54,800	2,000,000
Public nonwork	51,300	1,900,000
Work	3,300	100,000
Home	200	20,000
Work	14,200	2,200,000
Non–motor vehicle	10,900	2,100,000
Motor vehicle	3,300	100,000
Home	26,500	4,200,000
Non–motor vehicle	26,300	4,000,000
Motor vehicle	200	20,000
Public	22,000	2,700,000

Data from Accident facts, 1971, National Safety Council.

THE ANATOMY OF A HAZARDOUS EVENT

The records on safety reveal that the human behavior component is the most obscure and unpredictable factor in hazard-ous events. Accidents don't just happen, they are caused. They are caused mostly by inadequacies in attitude, knowledge, skills, and judgment. They are also caused by defective agents, environmental factors, "acts of God," and a host of other things.

An accident is commonly defined as that occurrence in a sequence of events that usually produces unintended injury, death, or property damage. The sequence of an accidental death or injury may be described as follows:

1. Lack of knowledge and skill
2. Poor attitudes
3. Unsafe act
4. The accident
5. Results

Lack of knowledge and skill

Far too many people possess inadequate or incomplete knowledge and skills to cope with the many complexities of today's potential hazards. It normally follows that the more one knows about and is expertly capable of safe behavior the more one is likely to avoid hazardous events. If you drive, do you know how to respond correctly in the more common emergency situations? Do you know how to enter and exit limited-access highways? What do you know about the possible fire hazards in your home? Many hazardous events may be attributed to ignorance and lack of skill, as well as to lack of the necessary physical and emotional capabilities.

Poor attitudes

From a personal standpoint, a safe mode of living is realized when you put safety knowledge and skill to work. Safe habits and skills are responses to the stimuli of good attitudes. It is a basic fact that almost every single emotion of which the human body is capable can be expressed in feelings, actions, and reactions to a potentially hazardous event. The attitudes of any person vary according to his knowledge, skills, environmental experiences since birth, ignorance of safe practice, and many other factors. Some of the compensating mental and emotional mechanisms discussed in Chapter 2 may also be operative here.

What makes one who knows what is safe execute an unsafe act? The two attitudes that follow cast some light on this perplexing question.

Predestination. Under the influence of this belief, the person assumes that if death, damage, or injury occurs it is caused by Divine determination. It is generally felt that a power greater than the self sits in judgment of the events to which one is exposed. The attitude may be, "If it is to happen, it will, so let it be."

Invincibility. The person believes that it is impossible for him to be injured or killed as a result of an accident. The attitude portrayed here is one that asserts, "It always happens to someone else, not me."

Most of your attitudes concerning a safe mode of living develop basically the same way as any other attitude. They were not present when you were born but have developed to be a crucial influence in your current behavior. Do you do some of the following?

1. Correct unsafe conditions and agents when you first observe them
2. Refrain from taking unnecessary risks
3. Increase the time necessary to do a thing to make the experience safer
4. Set a precept and example for safe acts
5. Refuse to engage in a potentially hazardous experience of which you have no knowledge, skills, or abilities

Unsafe act

An unsafe act may be defined as a deviation from a normal, prudent, or accepted procedure. It is an unnecessary vulnerability to a hazard that minimizes the safe state, although not all unsafe acts produce accidents. Some unsafe acts are:

1. Driving an automobile 70 MPH in a 30 MPH speed zone
2. Smoking in bed while drowsy or sleepy
3. Allowing charcoal to accumulate in enclosed places

4. Mowing a yard without checking for hazardous objects in the yard
5. Using a defective ladder
6. Placing space rugs on a slippery floor
7. Using improperly grounded equipment in a home laundry
8. Riding in an automobile without using safety belts
9. Overloading an electric circuit in the home
10. Failing to install or have installed lightning arrestors for the television antenna

The accident

This is the event that may occur as a result of an unsafe act if conditions are conducive to its occurring. Using the unsafe acts cited above, we can project each to the advent of the accident that might occur.

1. The automobile crashes.
2. The burning cigarette of the sleeping person ignites a fire.
3. A spontaneous combustion occurs.
4. A piece of glass is thrown from the mower and strikes a passerby.
5. The ladder breaks, and the person falls.
6. A fall is sustained.
7. The person is electrically shocked.
8. The person is ejected from the automobile in a collision.
9. A fire occurs in the home.
10. The television set is struck by a bolt of lightning.

Results

The kind and degree of damage sustained in an accident is quite variable. A fall may result in nothing more than personal embarrassment or may lead to death. The fire caused by smoking in bed could result in the burning of only the bedclothing, or it could result in the death of the imprudent smoker and also completely destroy the house.

Even if an accident occurs, all is not hopeless. When experiencing an accident, one may do much to prevent or reduce the severity of the results. Falling is one case in point. In many cases, one who has developed the skill of falling will have better success in falling "safely" than one who has not. Other sections of this chapter are devoted to preventive and corrective factors.

TRAFFIC SAFETY

The motor vehicle has taken a toll of lives over twice that caused by all the wars in American history: over a million during a period of 67 years. More than 55,000 persons are killed each year. More than 2 million persons are injured, and the costs annually exceed 10 billion dollars. From 1900 through 1970, motor vehicle deaths in America totalled more than 1,800,000. The deaths of American military personnel in all wars through 1970 totalled 1,470,673. Among passengers in the different types of vehicles, the following death rates were reported for 1970:

Kind of transportation	Death rate per 100,000,000 passenger miles
Passenger automobiles and taxis	2.10
Scheduled airliner	0.00
Buses	0.19
Railroad passenger trains	0.09

As a young adult, if you should die today chances are you would most likely die from an accident. The same holds for your being seriously injured. If you should die from an accident, the greatest chances are that you will die from a traffic-related accident. Again, the same holds for your being seriously injured. Considering these morbid factors, you must understand the significance of the basic factors of traffic safety as they relate to your safe mode of living.

Traffic safety is best understood in terms of its basic components: traffic education, traffic engineering, and traffic enforcement. All too often persons who have an interest in traffic safety will take a position of declaring the all-importance of one of these three basic E's. Some traffic educators assert that education is the panacea to all traffic safety problems; some traffic engineers assert

that traffic engineering is the panacea; whereas many traffic enforcement officers assert that traffic enforcement is the panacea. Obviously, each has an important role to play in the ultimate realization of traffic safety.

Traffic safety education may be learned in many forms, both formal and informal. As a young adult, your traffic education may have been as sophisticated as a comprehensive driver and traffic safety education course or as informal as learning to drive by yourself. The most commonly offered formal education is high school driver and traffic safety education. Other courses are offered through the National Safety Council's defensive driving course, by colleges and universities, by traffic courts, and by other private and public agencies.

High school driver education

High school driver and traffic safety education is a course of instruction designed to develop the knowledge, skills, and attitudes necessary for safe and enjoyable driving. The minimum requirements for such a course should be 30 hours of classroom instruction and 6 hours of behind-the-wheel instruction. Many of you may have had this course, or you may yet take it in college. In recent years much attention has been devoted to increasing the amount of class time for a more comprehensive education. The laboratory or behind-the-wheel phase of the course has been implemented by adding simulation instruction and multiple-car driving range experiences. In simulation, the student drives a simulated (mock) automobile in response to situations developed on film and projected onto a large screen. In multiple-car range instruction, one instructor teaches six or more students at the same time. Each student drives an automobile in response to the directions of the instructor who communicates with them either by a power megaphone or a radio communication system.

In recent years many states have made instruction mandatory for every teen-ager who seeks to be licensed before age 18, and require that the course be given for credit no later than the sophomore year, that it be taught by certified instructors, and that it be available to all pupils in the state whether attending private or public schools. At the end of 1970 thirty-one states had such a law in force. There is much that you can and must do to support comprehensive driver education courses in your college and in high schools throughout the country.

Driver and traffic safety education in high schools is an important course. Its worth has been verified, as seen in the following statements.

With very few exceptions, comparison of driver education students with other students has revealed that those who have taken driver education have fewer accidents.

Whatever the correlation between driver education and accident experience, it is a fact that many of America's automobile insurance companies give up to 15% premium discount for drivers under age 21 who have successfully completed a driver education course.

One large insurance company reported that its figures substantiate the often heard axiom that trained drivers have half as many accidents as untrained drivers.

Another large insurance company asserted that its automobile loss experience was 20% better for male teen-age drivers who had had driver education than for the untrained teen-age drivers. The results were reflected in the reduced premium rates granted by the company.

College and university programs

Colleges and universities are mainly concerned with the preparation of specialists who would teach not only the teen-age drivers but also with the preparation of teachers of teachers. Only in recent years has much attention been given to the role that higher education plays in driver and traffic safety education. Comprehensive programs of all types exist at all levels—junior college through graduate school. Most of the programs that currently exist devote large amounts of time to driver and traffic safety education. If you haven't quite made up your mind about a career, you might consider the great demand for good safety specialists.

Colleges and universities also serve as state safety centers that do research and perform many traffic safety services. A few of the institutions that have outstanding centers are Cornell University, University of California at Los Angeles, Michigan State University, University of Michigan, Ohio State University, Pennsylvania State University, and Central Missouri State College.

Commercial driving schools

Commercial driving schools exist in every major city. They range in size and comprehensiveness from the one-man operation to the large company. Most of these schools teach only the operative, or manipulative, skills of driving. The majority of the people who attend these schools failed to learn to drive at an early age.

Engineering

Education for traffic safety is supported by traffic engineering. The streets and highways are designed, constructed, and signed by traffic engineers. These professionals use much expertise in deciding the design of the roadway, intersections, medians, and roadsides. They determine safe speed limits and the proper traffic signs for various driving conditions. The role of the traffic engineer is an essential one that people should strive to understand.

Enforcement

Traffic laws and regulations are basically sound. They serve as the basis for driver conduct on the streets and highways. The majority of these laws should be self-enforcing. Many man-made traffic laws are based on the natural laws of physics; one example is the safe speed limits set on curves. Law enforcement officers and the traffic courts perform important enforcement responsibilities, but your objective, as related to your driving, should be self-enforcement.

Recommendations for better traffic safety

You should work to see that the following things are done in your state.

1. State inspection should be required of all cars twice a year to make sure vital parts are in safe working order.
2. Uniform motor vehicle laws should be passed in all states so that rules of the road, signs, and signals are the same throughout the country.
3. The minimum age limit should be raised to 18 for all new drivers, except for youths of 17 who successfully pass a certified high school driver education course.
4. More realistic speed limits, now often too low, should be set, but tougher enforcement and penalties against speeders should be imposed.
5. Adequately staffed traffic engineering units in all states and large cities should be set up to improve traffic safety conditions on the roads.
6. The level of alcohol a driver must consume before he is legally presumed to be drunk should be lowered, and severe penalties should be given for those who drive while drunk.
7. Requirements to get a driver's license, including a medical examination, should be stiffened, and all drivers should be reexamined periodically.

The above recommendations are in harmony with the brief discussion of law and order near the end of this chapter. You may not agree with some of the above, but you are obligated to assist in finding a solution to the greatest safety problem of all young Americans. Alternate recommendations, if appropriate, are always in order.

RECREATIONAL SAFETY

The amount of leisure time available to people is continually increasing. The 40-hour, 5-day week is standard. Even the 35-hour or 30-hour week is not unusual. The ultimate potential of leisure time and recreation is incomprehensible. Recreation is probably the fastest-booming business in America. Americans are currently spending about 150 billion dollars a year on recreation, and it is anticipated that this amount will increase to 250 billion dollars by the middle of the 1970's. The range of activities is virtually impossible to define.

In recent years, the problems related to off-the-job activities have attracted the attention of industry. As shown earlier in this chapter, work deaths and injuries were the lowest of the four major classes of accidents. Many of the deaths and injuries in the other classes might technically be attributed to some recreational endeavor. A leisurely Sunday driver forgets about the normal flow of traffic and precipitates a collision. A weekend do-it-yourself enthusiast loses a finger while using a power saw to build a bookcase. A once-in-a-lifetime hunter kills a friend while deer hunting. All you need do is recall the many cases you know of or have read of during the last few months in order to appreciate the significance of recreational safety.

Hunting

Approximately 20 million Americans go hunting each year, and each year several hundred of these die from accidental gunshot wounds. The weapons used are of many types. The National Rifle Association recommends the following essentials for safe hunting and handling of firearms.

1. The first rule of gun safety is to treat each gun as if it were loaded.
2. Guns carried into camp or home, or when otherwise not in use, must always be unloaded, and taken down or have the actions open.
3. Always be sure the barrel and action are clear of obstructions and that you only have ammunition of the proper size for the gun. Remove oil and grease from the chamber before firing.
4. Always carry your gun so that you can control the direction of the muzzle, even if you trip and fall.
5. Be sure of your target before you pull the trigger; know the identifying

features of the game you intend to hunt.

6. Never point a gun at anything you do not want to shoot; avoid all horseplay while handling a gun.
7. Unload all unattended guns, and store guns and ammunition separately, beyond the reach of children and careless adults.
8. Never climb a tree or fence or jump a ditch with a loaded gun; never pull a gun toward you by the muzzle.
9. Never shoot a bullet at a flat, hard surface (for example, a smooth body of water); when at target practice, be sure your backstop is adequate.
10. Avoid alcoholic drinks before or during shooting.

The safe use of firearms is not the only factor in safe hunting. Many more hunters are killed and injured in accidents that don't involve firearms. Overexertion, falls, drowning, and excessive exposure are other important considerations. Remember that most good hunting sites are remote to medical facilities.

All of the accidental deaths and injuries caused by firearms do not occur in the field; more occur in the home. In 1970, 1,200 deaths by firearms occurred in the home, whereas fewer than 800 occurred while hunting.

Water safety

Water is the focal point of outdoor recreation. People want water to sit by, to swim in, to dive under, to ski across, to fish in, and to drive their boats over. Although water provides these many pleasurable experiences, it unfortunately takes approximately 7,000 lives each year. Of this total, about 1,500 are of college age. This age group has the poorest water safety record of all age groups. Some general water safety tips are presented below.

Swimming:
1. Refrain from swimming alone; swim under supervision, or use the buddy system where possible.
2. Start each swimming season slowly if you do not swim all year.

3. Refrain from swimming when you are tired or immediately after a meal.
4. Always be familiar with the water you swim in; look for pollution, undertow, cross currents, depth, and debris.
5. Know how to administer artificial respiration.

Boating:
1. Know and observe nautical rules. Stop to help others if necessary.
2. Don't overload the boat.
3. Always have a companion with you.
4. For trips, a "travel plan" should be filed with a responsible authority.
5. Don't take a boat out if you or a partner can't handle it.

Water skiing:
1. Wear a life jacket.
2. Make sure there are two persons in the boat, one to drive and one to watch.
3. Make sure the tow is taut before signaling a start.
4. Refrain from skiing at night or in shallow water.
5. When tired, stop skiing.
6. Be sure that all participants know the basic water skiing signals.
7. Skiers should avoid showing off, for this is the major cause of water skiing accidents.

Hiking and camping

Many Americans in search of the return to nature go hiking or camping. Unfortunately, a few end up lost or are responsible for forest fires or other similar catastrophic events. Some of the recommended safety precautions are cited below.

1. Hiking and camping generally require a special type of dress. Consider the general ruggedness of the activity, and dress accordingly.
2. If you are not an experienced hiker or camper, make sure that at least one in your party is experienced.
3. Know the procedures for caring for a camp fire.
4. Exercise the proper care in the use of camp equipment and tools.
5. Make sure that you have reasonable

knowledge and skill for dealing with poisonous plants and snakes.

6. Remember that the compass is an essential piece of equipment. Know how to use it.
7. Whether you are camping or hiking, make sure that someone knows of your destination.
8. If by chance you become lost, do the following:
   a. Stop, rest, and think; it is better to wait than wander.
   b. Note distinctive landmarks.
   c. Find or build shelter.
   d. Build a fire if it is cold or getting dark.
   e. Give a single periodic yell or other signal.
   f. Shoot three blasts from a pistol or gun if you have one.
   g. Travel in a single and logical direction.
   h. If available, follow a stream; it usually leads to a habitated area.

HOME SAFETY

About half of the fatal accidents or injuries that occur in the home strike persons over 65, and one-sixth of them happen to children under 5. Among the causes of home accidents, physical handicap or frailty and poor judgment are high on the list, although

Table 5-4. Products involved in home accidents

Product	Percent
Knives	12.5
Chairs, tables, cabinets	9.0
Cooking ranges, ovens	8.5
Tools	7.5
Furniture, misc.	7.0
Pots, pans	6.0
Minor appliances	6.0
Bottles, cans, jars	4.8
Utensils, pointed objects	4.5
Razors	4.3
Toys	3.5
Bicycles	3.3
Other	23.1

Data from Accident facts, 1969, National Safety Council.

emotional and psychologic factors are also operative. Five major factors associated with accidents around the home are:

1. Poor lighting
2. Failure to repair or replace defective equipment
3. A person too young or too old doing chores beyond his physical ability
4. Too much of a sense of security as related to one's home
5. Crowded or disorganized home

The principal cause of home deaths in each age group is as follows:

Age	Type of accident	Death rate per 100,000 population
Under 1 year	Mechanical suffocation	15.2
1 to 4 years	Fires, burns	4.5
5 to 14 years	Fires, burns	1.4
15 to 24 years	Poisoning by solids and liquids	2.2
25 to 44 years	Poisoning by solids and liquids	1.7
45 to 64 years	Fires, burns	3.6
65 to 74 years	Falls	13.2
75 years and over	Falls	80.3

Table 5-4 identifies the products instrumental in home accidents. Most of the injuries involving these products are minor, usually requiring only first aid.

Falls

More than 40% of all accidental home deaths and serious injuries are the result of falls. The National Safety Council reported that 9,600 persons died in 1970 as a result of falls. This figure includes deaths from falls from one level to another, that is, stairs, ladder, and roof, and on the same level, that is, floor, ground, and sidewalk.

Stairs are most frequently involved. This is especially true of dimly lit second-story or basement stairs. The stairs should be uncluttered and have handrails high enough so that one may grasp them without stooping. They should be of a nonslip texture. It is recommended that in all cases, the bottom stairs should contrast, in color, the surface floor below. Other general safety factors are:

1. A sturdy stepladder is safer than a chair or box.
2. Space rugs should be anchored to prevent slides and falls.
3. Surfaces should be kept free of grease, ice, mud, and other substances that may contribute to a fall.
4. The shower or tub bottom should be covered with a rubber mat if the bottom is of a slippery texture.

Fires and burns

In rank, fires and burns are next to falls among the common causes of home injuries and accidental deaths. Over 5,600 persons died in 1970 as a result of fires and burns. The causes of home fires are listed below.

Cause of fire	Percent
Smoking and matches	19.1
Heating and cooking equipment	15.2
Electrical	14.3
Rubbish	8.8
Lightning	6.6
Chimneys and flues	5.5
Flammable fluids	4.7
Children and matches	4.0
Spontaneous combustion	3.8
Exposure	3.1
Sparks on roof	2.3
Hot ashes and coals	2.1
Candles and open flames	1.9
Combustibles near heater	1.5
Pyromanic actions	1.1
Other causes	6.0

It is estimated that each year about one million people are victims of burns requiring medical attention; over 60,000 are hospitalized. The great majority of those so affected are the very old or the very young who cannot help themselves in emergencies. Fires are easily prevented if you understand the extent of the dangers and take simple precautions. Some of the basic precautions are:

1. Buy materials made of flame-resistant fibers. Among these are chemically treated cottons, modacrylic fibers, high-temperature nylon, blends of flame-resistant and flammable fabrics, material made of glass fibers, and wools that do not ignite easily.

2. Keep heating units clean, and have them inspected. Check all heating units before winter. Use protective screens for fireplaces and for gas and electric heaters.

3. Don't overload circuits. Have adequate wiring, particularly for heavy-duty appliances, and have it checked by a certified inspector. Keep wiring and cords in good condition.

4. Keep matches away from children; don't smoke when you are sleepy, or while using hair spray or nail polish. Provide enough ashtrays, and check them for smoldering cigarettes or cigars before emptying.

5. Handle explosive vapor carefully, and dispose of trash and rubbish safely. Store all flammable material away from the furnace and other sources of heat; keep oily mops and rags in closed containers; keep flammable liquids away from the living area. Burn leaves in a special container if your community permits this type of disposal under its air pollution code.

Suffocation

Accidents that smother the victim have preventable causes. The major means of suffocation are mechanical or by an ingested object. Of the 2,300 deaths reported for 1970, 900 were of children under 4 years of age. Some of the major causes are ingestion or inhalation of objects or food, bedclothes, thin plastic materials, and cave-ins and mechanical strangulation.

Home security

A break-in can jeopardize the personal safety of your family as well as your property, and it is usually a nerve-racking experience. It is essential that you and your family adopt some family security guidelines and see that they are adhered to. Guidelines to ensure the security of your living quarters include the following:

1. Make sure the locks on your doors are of top quality and used consistently. Keep your doors locked day and night.

2. Be careful with your keys. If you move, have new lock cylinders in-

stalled, have the keys changed. Don't leave house keys on a car-key chain. They could be duplicated while left at a parking lot.

3. Don't open your door at every knock or ring. First, find out who's there. If it's necessary to open the door a little, keep the chain guard on. Instruct babysitters to do the same.

4. From dusk until bedtime leave one or more houselights and yard lights on, whether the family is home or not.

5. Don't brag about family collections, valuables, or new acquisitions. Someone with "instant collecting" habits may get the word.

6. Consider installing a burglar alarm system in a new home that you may purchase.

7. Get a dog, large or small. It's his bark, not necessarily his bite, that discourages possible intruders.

8. When you're out of town for a few days, don't let stacked-up papers, milk deliveries, closed blinds, or the unattended yard or walks advertise your absence. Ask a neighbor to care for such things for you. If you have a light timer that turns a light on after dark, then off in the morning, tell the neighbors what hours it's set for.

9. If a prowler gets into the house, don't interfere with his getting out, laden or empty-handed. Never risk your life to save possessions. If you return and find a room ransacked, don't investigate the rest of the house. Call the police from a neighbor's house.

CIVIL DEFENSE EMERGENCIES AND DISASTERS

The area of safety that is designed for protection against the effects of major disasters is civil defense. Fires, hurricanes, tornadoes, wars, earthquakes, riots, and floods have confronted man throughout his history. Whether these disasters strike you individually or in a group, they can be modified or controlled by positive action. The American settlers who constructed a palisade and a block house to stop hostile bullets and arrows, and perhaps a levee to check a flood, were practicing civil defense. When they guarded against enemy attack and criminal acts, fought fire, and organized their villages and towns with local governments to provide the necessary survival services, they were developing civil defense as an essential guardian of life and as an essential part of government and of the community. The concept of civil defense is basic to our existence.

Earthquakes, potential riots, tornadoes, and other disasters are still with us. They affect us in some manner whether we experience them directly or indirectly. Local government, with the legal and material support of the state and the nation, has the responsibility of alleviating suffering; of saving lives; and of giving aid to people in disasters, whether man-made or of natural cause.

Warfare

Americans can no longer turn a deaf ear to the threat of outside aggression, for even little countries whose names may be difficult to pronounce are beginning to show military might. Singly, most do not pose a significant threat. Collectively and politically, they do pose a threat. Americans and Russians no longer hold exclusive expertise in the development of nuclear capability.

It is important to remember that a foreign bomb has never been dropped on America's mainland during a war. Our safe mode of living, in the military sense, has not been directly affected during the twentieth century. During most of the principal wars in which Americans have been involved, almost 50% of the casualties occurred in wars fought in other countries. Table 5-5 summarizes the total American casualties in the principal wars.

Nuclear arms were not used in any of the wars listed. If relative calm on the international scene cannot be maintained, the threat of major confrontations will grow. Although the concept of civil defense is not new, its form must ever change to meet

Table 5-5. U. S. military casualties in principal wars

War	Total deaths
Revolutionary War (1775-83)	4,435
War of 1812 (1812-15)	2,260
Mexican War (1846-48)	13,283
Civil War (1861-65)	
Union forces	364,511
Confederate forces	133,821
Spanish-American War (1898)	2,446
World War I (1917-18)	116,708
World War II (1941-45)	407,316
Korean War (1950-53)	54,246
Vietnam War (1961-)	53,316

Data from Accident facts, 1971, National Safety Council.

the challenges. As more nations become overpopulated, poorer, and stifled by the lack of food and space, they look for assistance from the richer and more powerful nations. On the other hand, some look for more land or smaller countries to conquer. The relevance of nuclear arms to these possibilities should be obvious.

Many wars throughout history have been fought because of ideological differences. During the latter part of the twentieth century, however, more threats of war may develop because of extreme pressure of one or more severe ecologic conditions. These conditions may cause some nations to seek homeostasis and identification in the changing world structure through military means.

Nuclear attack

Weapons. The arsenal of weaponry is unlimited. The weapons may be dropped from airplanes, sea-to-surface missiles shot from submarines, intercontinental ballistic missiles, air-to-surface missiles, and many other types. Where each weapon bursts, the fireball—with cloud, light, heat, blast, and

shock—would be accompanied by effects any person could well visualize. Depending on the intensity of the blast, on the distance from ground zero (ground zero is the exact point at which the weapon hits), and possibly on some protective features of intervening terrain, varying amounts of personal and property losses would occur within a radius of several miles. A nuclear explosion that releases the same amount of energy as approximately 1 million tons of TNT is termed a 1-megaton burst. A 5-megaton burst would cause total destruction from ground zero up to 3 miles, severe damage from 3 to 5 miles, moderate damage from 5 to 7 miles, and light damage from 7 to 9 miles.

Fallout. In nuclear warfare, radioactive fallout is the major threat to most people, rather than the threat of a direct hit. The areas of most severe fallout are near the explosion and downwind. Depending on the bomb yield, wind, weather, and other factors, the area of severe fallout may extend for several miles upwind and 300 or more miles downwind. The intensity of fallout is not necessarily uniform throughout the local fallout area, and a lighter fallout might extend outward from ground zero.

Radiation. Radiation is emitted from fallout particles. The air through which fallout passes and the surfaces on which it settles do not themselves become radioactive. It is the radiation originating from these particles that constitutes the major danger to living things. Of the three types of radiation, gamma radiation is the most hazardous of the fallout materials. Beta and alpha radiation are not major hazards and are fairly easy to defend against. However, protection from gamma rays requires considerable amounts of very dense materials or a great distance between people and the source of radiation in order to prevent radiation damage. Such protection can be provided, using facilities that exist, with necessary improvements, and by making judicious plans and preparation.

Radioactive decomposition. Time is on your side in relation to survival. The image of a world permanently contaminated and unable to support human life is a very dramatic setting for fiction, but it isn't true in terms of nuclear science. The radioactive isotopes, formed as a result of detonation of a nuclear weapon and carried by the wind as fallout, lose their capacity for radiation at a rapid rate. This phenomenon is called radioactive decay. Research has shown that the rate of radioactive decay of the fallout from the explosion of a nuclear weapon can be estimated by the "7-to-10 rule." For each multiple of 7 in terms of time, the radiation rate dwindles to one-tenth of its former intensity. For example, if radioactive survey meters showed 100 roentgens per hour (100 r/hr) at peak radiation about 1 hour after the nuclear explosion, 7 hours later the same meters would register approximately 10 r/hr, and about 50 hours later 1 r/hr.

Exposure. Radiation illness may be mild or severe, depending on exposure. Fortunately it is not contagious. Both the intensity of the radiation and the period of exposure are factors in determining its effects. Beta burns can result under certain conditions from significant amounts of fallout remaining in direct contact with the skin, but either shielding body surfaces from the particles or removing fallout particles before damage occurs is a fairly simple preventive measure. Gamma radiation, however, affects people who are some distance from the fallout itself. The severity of its effects on persons exposed to a given dose varies greatly. A summary of the estimated short-term effects on human beings of external gamma-ray exposures of less than 4 days is shown in Table 5-6.

Shielding. Gamma radiation has the ability to penetrate mass, but this of course is limited by the density of the mass. The more dense the mass, the less the penetration. A basic protective feature, then, is to interpose a substance between the radioactive fallout and the people.

The basic objective of civil defense is to identify for Americans the places they may go to be protected from fallout and to make

Table 5-6. Short-term dose of gamma-ray exposure and visible effect—four days or less

Short-term dose	Visible effect
50 r	No visible effects
75-100 r	Brief periods of nausea on day of exposure in about 10% of the group
200 r	Some of the symptoms of radiation sickness in as many as 50% of this group. (Although only 5% to 10% may require medical attention, no deaths are expected.)
450 r	Serious radiation sickness in most members of the group followed by death of about 50% within 2 or 4 weeks
600 r	Serious radiation sickness in all members of the group followed by death of almost all members within 1 to 3 weeks

Data from A realistic appraisal to civil defense, 1966, U. S. Office of Civil Defense.

those places available and ready to support life until local conditions permit emergence from shelter. The thickness and density of the shielding substance are the prime factors.

In addition to time and shielding from radiation, a third factor is distance from the existing fallout, as in being well within the interior of a building or in underground shelter.

Nuclear warfare may never occur in this country, but it is quite reasonable to conclude that preparedness is a major deterrent. When the threat of war is remote, there is a tendency for citizens to be little concerned about preparedness. Conversely, when the threat becomes more immediate, citizens tend to clamor for the establishment of surer means to deal with the threat. Civil defense against possible outside aggressors is not a popular subject. It is an expensive proposition that is approached in various ways by different states and communities. You should carry your share of the civil defense burden. You must become as informed as possible of the programs in your city and state. If your city does not have a viable program, then you are obligated to work for the development of a good program.

Natural disasters

Natural disasters are those caused by uncontrollable forces of nature. It is generally impossible to determine exclusively when these disasters will occur. The United States Weather Bureau is responsible for forecasting the occurrence of storms and other disasters, including hurricanes; but these forecasts cannot pinpoint the exact time a storm will occur at a given location.

Nature is often mutable, especially in certain geographic areas of this country. When the unpredictable acts of nature occur in heavily populated areas, widespread damage, great inconvenience, and frequently loss of life occur. Previous knowledge of possible disasters will enable you to take needed precautions that will reduce damage, even if the storm or impending disaster cannot be deterred. Parts of the Southeast and the Midwest are vulnerable to tornadoes; parts of the Gulf states are suscep-

tible to hurricanes; and parts of the West, California in particular, are exposed to the possibility of earthquakes. Add to the above, landslides, floods, snowdrifts, and other natural disasters, and you should readily recognize the potential gravity of the threats to your safe mode of living.

Hurricane Camille, which occurred in 1969, was the second strongest hurricane ever to hit the United States. It literally shattered portions of south Mississippi and Louisiana. More than 300 persons were killed as a result of the hurricane and subsequent floods. Thousands were left homeless. Businesses and recreation areas were destroyed. Not only were the physical factors of property damage involved but also health factors, such as the purity of drinking water, diseases, and other things that contribute to the safe and healthful mode of living.

Many natural disasters of significance have occurred in America. A list of the major natural disasters in which more than 200 lives were lost is shown in Table 5-7.

Table 5-7. Major natural disasters—200 or more lives lost

Type	Places	Year	Deaths
Flood	Johnston, Pennsylvania	1889	2,209
	Galveston, Texas	1900	6,000
	Ohio and Indiana	1913	732
	Texas	1921	215
	St. Francis, California	1928	450
	Ohio and Mississippi River Valleys	1937	360
Hurricane	Texas	1915	375
	Louisiana	1915	500
	Texas	1919	287
	Florida, Alabama, and Mississippi	1926	243
	Florida	1928	1,833
	Florida	1933	409
	New England states	1938	657
	Louisiana and Texas	1957	395
	Mississippi and Louisiana	1969	300
Tornado	Illinois	1925	606
	Mississippi, Alabama, and Georgia	1936	402
	Arkansas, Tennessee, Missouri, Mississippi, and Alabama	1952	229
	Indiana, Ohio, Michigan, Illinois, and Wisconsin	1965	272
Earthquake	San Francisco	1906	452

Data from Accident facts, 1971, National Safety Council.

Tornadoes. The tornado is nature's most vicious storm. It is a funnel-shaped cloud with upward spiraling winds of great velocity. The cause is attributed to the colliding of hot and cold masses that create a tremendous difference in pressure between the inside and the outside of the funnel. As the spiraling winds within the funnel increase in velocity, the pressure outside decreases. When the funnel passes over a building, there is less pressure on the outside than on the inside, and it actually causes the building to explode.

Tornadoes are usually more prevalent in the spring and early summer. The pathway of tornadoes is most generally from southwest to northeast at about 25 to 40 miles per hour. The diameter of a tornado is small, but its length may extend for one-fourth mile. A tornado is very erratic in that sometimes it touches the ground, but then its base may rise several hundred feet in the air for a period of time only to suddenly strike the ground again. Some reasonable safety measures to take when a tornado strikes are:

1. Take cover in a shelter, ditch, or basement. The southwest corner of any structure is usually safest.
2. If outside in the open, you should move at right angles to the tornado's path.
3. If a communication system is available, use it to stay informed.
4. Keep calm.

Hurricanes. The hurricane is the most destructive type of storm. It causes damage through high winds, flood, and high tide. An extremely well-developed hurricane may be called a tropical cyclone or typhoon. It originates near the equator and is not technically a true hurricane until its wind velocity exceeds 74 miles an hour. Hurricanes generally move north away from the equator. Most of those that occur in the eastern part of the United States develop in the tropical latitudes of the Carribean, shift toward Florida, and finally start up the Atlantic Coast. Fortunately, most hurricanes usually weaken and dissipate

before moving far inland, but they can cause serious inland flooding.

Forecasting hurricanes is quite reliable today. The Hurricane Forecasting Service of the United States Weather Bureau has seven centers. Its research center is located in Miami, Florida. Once a hurricane is spotted, the information is sent to all U. S. Weather Bureau Stations. A hurricane watch is announced once the storm appears to be at least 30 to 36 hours away from the United States. When the winds of the storm are 74 miles per hour or more and the hurricane is expected to reach the mainland within 24 hours, a hurricane warning is issued. The following safety precautions are suggested:

1. Keep your radio on, and listen to the advisory warnings of the U. S. Weather Bureau.
2. If in the immediate area, stay off the road.
3. Attempt to protect your home by boarding up windows and doors.
4. Store as much safe drinking water as possible.
5. When warned to evacuate, don't hesitate.

Floods. Technology and research in flood control have reduced drastically the threat of floods even in the lowlands of the United States. Still, no region of this country is immune from floods, except the arid Southwest and the Great Basin. The financial losses because of floods average 350,000,000 dollars annually. This sum would be much higher were it not for the construction of dams, protective levees, storage reservoirs, and flood warnings. The Corps of Engineers of the United States Army has served as the major agency to develop flood control measures.

Except for flash floods, floods are a minor threat today to the safety of people because of reliable forecasting. The flood forecasting service of the U. S. Weather Bureau reduces flood damage by providing the opportunity to remove goods and evacuate people to safer places. Many more losses are further reduced by the efforts of the

American National Red Cross, the Coast Guard, and the Army Engineers in caring for persons driven from their homes. The flash flood may be diastrous, because water may rise several inches or feet in a short period of time. In a period of heavy rains, you should be aware of this possibility and be prepared to protect yourself against it.

VIOLENCE AND AGGRESSION

I Read the News Today Oh Boy—it told about a man avid to control everything he touches, carving his initials on the earth—and on his brothers. Hard, uptight man. For the national honor, you blew the guts out of a child this morning. I clubbed open the head of another for crying so loudly . . . . black, you know. Together, we can poison a whole species of animals, and it worries us a bit: DDT in mother's milk, now, that comes too close. The News: Man has at last collected enough power of various sorts to affect his own evolution, or to destroy himself. Either way, for the first time the choice is his. So far, we have not behaved as if we care to survive. We help each other a little, yes, but the real game is, be the boss. We gnaw at our bleeding flesh bit by bit, only dully curious about why it hurts so much.*

Accidents alone do not account for the many threats to our safe mode of living. The fear of violence is more real today than it has been in any other period of American history. Violence may occur at any time of the day or night or at any place. It may be committed by the sane and insane alike. It may occur within a family or between persons unknown to each other. Within this decade America has witnessed a phenomenal increase in crime and violence. Since 1963 three key leaders have been assassinated—John F. Kennedy, Martin Luther King, and Robert F. Kennedy. We have witnessed riots and violent student and labor revolts. Parents have been accused of rearing children in a violent manner. Courts are tabbed as being too lenient with criminal cases. Police forces are confronted with brutality charges. Television and other forms of mass media are indicted for programming violence.

Violence threatens to engulf most seg-

*Look **34:**21, January 13, 1970.

ments of American life. Violence is part of a struggle to resolve stressful and threatening incidents. America is also experiencing global problems with far-reaching overtones, which are progressing beyond our capability of understanding some of the relationships. The growth of inner-city ghettos, racism, labor and students in revolt, inflation, and crimes of all types relate to our safe mode of living. Social conflicts will continue to bring an increase in violence.

Television shows the way

The violence shown on television, both in news and in entertainment, breeds significant real-life violence, especially among the disorganized and the poor. This conclusion should not surprise you. The findings of the National Commission on the Causes and Prevention of Violence conclusively correlate television with violent behavior in our society, especially in children. Where meaningful social and moral values prevail, the young are not very likely to emulate the violence depicted on television. But among disorganized family units, where family, peer, and school-home relationships are poor, television was shown to be the most congruous replacement for real-life experience. The recommendations by the National Commission for reducing the problem cited were:

1. An overall reduction in programs that require or contain violence
2. Elimination of violence from children's cartoon programs—probably excluding the highly exaggerated violence of such films as "Popeye" and "Tom and Jerry"
3. Adoption of the British practice of scheduling crime stories, westerns, and adventure stories containing much violence only after children's bedtime
4. Permanent federal financing for the Public Broadcast Corporation to assist in offering high-quality alternatives to violent programs for children
5. Intensified research by networks into the impact of violence on television

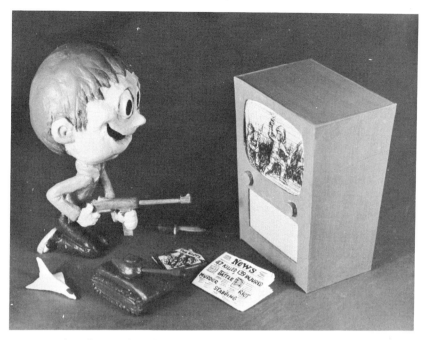

Fig. 5-1. Research indicates that the portrayal of excessive violence as entertainment may create excessive violence in real life. (Courtesy Martin Webster.)

Television does show the way to bigger and better things, to adventures into the unknown, to the moon and back, into the mysteries of current and future phenomena —and the many facets of violence, individually and collectively. Involved are not only people but also the makeup and influences of the environment in which they find themselves. Television takes you to the scene; it descriptively and candidly explores the violent behavior of real individuals and groups; and finally, it challenges you personally to respond. If you respond as a member of the "silent majority," the chances are that your response will be a passive, introspective one that will not result in overt action. But you represent the "vocal minority," your convictions will probably motivate you to take some appropriate action that will not only enhance your safe mode of living, but also that of your family, friends, and the entire human race.

Living your own life

The various relationships of the individual to himself, others, and his environment are described in Chapter 1. Rarely if ever is it possible to live one's own life without affecting other people or things. Any harmonious civilization, especially a democratic one, exists and is sustained by an intricate system of checks and balances that delimit an individual's basic freedoms. The great issue here is to increase the possibility that one may accomplish a task according to the standards that are tolerable both to the individual and to the environment and group in which one lives. Rather than withdrawing from our social context, it is important to be able to cope with those things and people that are responsible for the frustrations. This coping is generally interpreted as the successful struggle to realize our goals while maintaining our ability to adjust to the contest of our environment. Your attitude toward freedom may be to do as you please regardless of the manner in which it relates to others. We hope this is not the case.

In Chapter 2 you were asked the question "What do you fear?" Your response to this question has broad implications for your personal sense of survival in an allegedly hostile world. It is generally proposed that you don't fear too greatly the gun, knife, acid, or other instruments of aggression, as violence. Most of you fear other people and the other somewhat uncontrollable components of your world. People fear the unknown or the unpredictable. Who is suspect? Known criminals, drug addicts, hippies, Black Panthers, Ku Klux Klansmen, communists, and a host of other similar categorical types. What is suspect? Hurricanes, tornadoes, pollution of various forms, and other natural catastrophes.

The term "living your own life" has multiple meanings for your understanding of violence and aggression as related to a safe mode of living. This safe mode is most frequently threatened by the inability of individuals to cope with themselves or their relationship to other people, systems, or things in their environment.

The vast majority of violence is not executed by persons who are simply living their own lives. Predicting who will commit murder, for example, is a difficult task, for more than 90% of the murders committed are not premeditated, and about 80% of these involve an acquaintance or a member of the family. On the other side of the issue, it is known that some individuals who have witnessed sanctioned violence and aggression committed in the name of justice, law, order, duty, or moral obligation resort to violence themselves as an honorable means of coping with their problems. Herein is at least the partial basis for major threats to our safe mode of living. Violence to a rioter may be a means to accomplish objectives impossible to obtain through nonviolent means. Violence may breed counterviolence. The composite of these leads to supression. Suppression may lead to general rebellion or catastrophic revolution. Living whose life? All of this affects yours.

Reducing the conflicts

Reduction media—procedures or programs for reducing unsafe behavior and hazards—are quite difficult to identify, and once identified they often become impossible to administer. We have reviewed some of the more obvious means of reducing accidents in recreation activities and in the home. They are simple and clearly defined, and they are generally capable of good execution. One of the important problems in reducing violent acts is inability to deal with the nonadapting, noncoping people in our world.

If the major conflicts are to be reduced, the major instruments of violence and aggression need to be managed. There is a high relationship between the excessive use of alcohol and homicide. Similarly, there is a high relationship between guns and homicides and suicides. It is unlikely that human conflicts will be reduced significantly without preventive measures in the mental, emotional, and social domain. Violence and aggression seem to be deeply engrained in human behavior, and the major obstacle to reducing these conflicts is our slowness to change our violent mode of coping with our problems.

Do you really want to change? There might not be any news the next time you read.

SAFETY, LAW, AND ORDER

Safety in a dynamic environment is linked to law and order. The theme of this relationship encompasses much more than the use of law enforcement officers or courts to maintain civil order.

Laws may be interpreted as civil, criminal, natural, physical, mental, and emotional. Civil laws are those laws enacted by civil agencies, such as city councils, state legislatures, or the Congress of the United States. Criminal laws and contracts are derived in basically the same manner. These laws help people live together by establishing regulations and courts to settle disputes that may lead to disorder or have resulted in disorder.

These laws are designed to (1) maintain order and progress, (2) promote justice and the general welfare, (3) protect individual liberty and rights, and (4) protect society from harmful acts of individuals.

The implications of these purposes are far-reaching in health and safety. The evolving trauma of the ecologic imbalance that apparently exists may ultimately be traced either to poor laws, ordinances, codes, and regulations, or to the lack of will or inability to enforce them. The examples are many. Codes that were written in the early 1900's governing the free-enterprise interests of industrial complexes are often still on the books. Why haven't they been changed where the need dictates? The possible answer may be elusive. The body responsible for the change may not recognize that a change or revision is necessary, or it may assume that it is essentially satisfactory because of the monetary or political gains rendered by the industry or groups involved.

Consider the case of a large industrial complex employing ten thousand people in a city whose total population is 100,000. The city council passes an ordinance that requires an economically unbearable burden to be placed upon the industrial complex. The ordinance is designed to improve the environmental quality of the community. This decision was made in behalf of the citizens' health and safety. Rather than disobey the law, if it couldn't be changed, the industry decides to relocate. What may happen to the community? What is your response to law and order for health and safety in this case?

Your neighbor's property has several big oaks on it. Each autumn, when the leaves start falling, the neighbor rakes them into high piles and burns them. This is clearly in violation of your local city fire code. The burning of the leaves in your city is considered a safety hazard. Would you report him to the civil authorities and insist that he be restrained from threatening your safe environment?

These examples are cited to emphasize again the need for personal involvement in the solution of environmental safety problems. Far too many people often rely on others to cope with the problems that potentially relate directly to them. Safety in a dynamic environment is dependent upon the sincere efforts of individuals to maintain and protect the safe state.

Liability

You are generally liable for negligence when you fail to act as a reasonably prudent individual would under certain circumstances. In other words, negligence may be interpreted as the failure to conform to a standard of conduct required by law, for the protection of other persons against unreasonable risk of harm. However, the obligation to act reasonably is not the same for all types of persons, and the nature of the conduct obligated toward various individuals is not the same. Hence, against a trespasser or suspected burglar on your property, you have a duty to act without negligence. But the degree of negligence that is reasonable in this case is unequal to what it would be toward someone you invited to your home, and whose arrival you expected.

Some of your legal and personal obligations to maintain safety in a dynamic environment are:

1. Conduct your operations on your property so as not to injure any visitor.
2. Make known to visitors on your property the existence of hidden dangers.
3. "Attractive nuisances," such as swimming pools or swing sets, are to be safely secured.
4. Be sure you have reasonable liability insurance to cover your home, automobile, yourself, and other possible sources of negligent factors.
5. When lending your car to another person, remember that you may be held liable for his negligence.
6. Negligence is easier to establish in an act committed against a child than against an adult. When you drive, watch for children playing in the streets.

7. Parents are generally accountable for the acts of their children. The limits of accountability vary from state to state.
8. You may be accountable for the actions of your pets.
9. Remember the neighbor cited earlier. Any carelessness in handling a fire that causes personal or property damage is negligence in most states.

These are representative of the many things that should be known by the health- and safety-informed citizen. As a last factor, nuisances and how they might be dealt with should be considered. Nuisances may be public or private. A public nuisance is a minor criminal offense that causes inconvenience or damage to the exercise of certain public rights. A private nuisance is an interference with the ownership or possession of land or other property that causes substantial injury.

Suppose the family next door keeps a dog that barks or howls all night. The dog is tied up and is restricted from trespassing on your property but keeps you and your family awake every night. Keeping the dog is interfering with your right to the peaceful enjoyment of your property and may be abated by law. All kinds of health and safety annoyances that affect you may be

eliminated. So long as the interference is substantial and unreasonable, you may have it ended by a number of means. You may go to the person, group, or business responsible for the nuisance to get relief. If this fails, you may go to court and obtain damages for the nuisance or sue for a permanent injunction preventing the continuation of the act. But you should also remember that one who abates a nuisance personally may be liable for any damage caused in excess of what is required to abate it.

THE TASK

Our highly industrialized and complex country creates many threats to one's stable relationship with his dynamic environment. In spite of these hazards, present public attitudes toward a safe mode of living are not firm enough to reduce many of them. Public opinion does not fully demand functional regulations against those who threaten to destroy the safe environment, such as against the drunken driver. The causes and the possible solutions to those factors that threaten our safety may best be sought through three dimensions—the *skills* you employ, your *attitudes* toward maintenance of the safe state, and your *involvement* in promoting safety in a dynamic environment.

CHAPTER 6

Substances endangering health

Many substances found in the world to-day promise to endanger not only our health but our very existence. Some of these substances we cannot avoid. Some represent dangerous gifts bestowed by nature on man, and some were here long before man arrived to influence the ecologic balance. Some, such as combustion engine wastes, industrial pollutants, and nuclear residues, are concomitants of our chosen way of life. Some, such as the pesticides, promise to control the ravages of insects and so to produce more abundant harvests. And some are self-chosen, inflicted by man on himself, such as drugs, alcohol, and tobacco. In the case of each of these substances, benefits to man accrue, but each represents a serious danger to man as well.

DRUGS

I knew that for every hour of comparative ease and comfort its treacherous alliance might confer upon me *now,* I must endure days of bodily suffering; but I did not, could not, conceive the mental hell into whose fierce corroding fires I was about to plunge.

WILLIAM BLAIR, young English immigrant to the U. S., in July 1842 issue of *The Knickerbocker.*

Can't think. Can't think. Can't think. . . . . You really get messed up, boy, on that stuff. You might hear it sooner or later, Mom, but I'm sorry, Mom, Dad, and Bill. Sorry that your little boy has turned into an LSD addict.

I been getting pretty stoned lately, and you just don't know what's real and what isn't real. You really don't. All I can say is I had to find out myself—kind of poor excuse, you know—I really shouldn't have taken any dope at all—any acid, or I shouldn't have started off with any

grass, either. Course, grass isn't bad—it's the acid that got to me.

Words recorded by a 19-year-old male prior to committing suicide and read at his funeral February 1970.

A brief history

Drugs to relieve pain have been used in most civilizations extending back to the earliest recorded history of man. The juice of the poppy, opium, was used to relieve pain before the days of ancient Greece, perhaps first in Mesopotamia 5,000 years ago or by the Sumerians in 7,000 B.C. There is conjecture that its effect was known to Stone Age man. Arab traders are said to have introduced aspirin into the Orient, but its use became widespread there only after English and Portuguese merchants used it to aid in exploiting the Asians. Coincident with the beginning of the Christian era, it was used to treat hysteria.

But drugs, again particularly opium, have been used since the earliest of times for a second purpose, that of indulgence. The power of opium to reduce anxiety, gloom, and despair and to provide escape from boredom and loneliness was apparent at least by the ninth century, B.C., as reflected in Homer's *Odyssey.*

Around the world the use of opium spread, sometimes as a medicine, often as a drug of indulgence. In either case, its addictive qualities were not understood until early in the nineteenth century. By then a few physicians suspected the possibilities of addiction but ironically treated those so addicted with one of two newly discovered opium alkaloids, morphine (1805) or codeine (1832). Such treatment, of course, simply transferred the addiction from one drug to another.

Nearly a century later, in 1898 Dressen, a German chemist, extracted heroin from opium with the hope that it would relieve pain without addiction. This, too, was a vain hope.

In 1843 the spread of narcotic addiction was spurred by the invention of the hypodermic needle. It arrived in this country in time for the Civil War and, through the medium of morphine used as a pain deadener for thousands of wounded soldiers, gave rise to what became known as "soldier's illness," that is, narcotic addiction. Before the war ended, the drug addict had learned to take his drugs orally, rectally, or hypodermically, and in powder, liquid, or smoke form. Further refinements such as "dropping" (administered with an eye dropper directly into the eyes) have come on the scene since then.

Drug use, almost until the twentieth century, was viewed with but little criticism. Persons "enslaved by the habit" were pitied rather than condemned, and the drug was blamed, not its user. Gradually, the public, but more particularly the medical profession, began to recognize the true problem, and in 1901 the American Pharmaceutical Association appointed a special committee to learn the extent of the public's addiction. The committee reported the problem to be appalling. The evidence mounted. Personal histories of drug addiction, newspaper exposés, and the professional fears of physicians brought people to see addiction either as an illness or a vice. Since drugs were still available without controls, their relation to crime was not yet understood.

But controls were obviously necessary as the rolls of addicts grew. Finally in 1909, Congress passed a bill that prohibited the importation of opium, its preparations, and derivatives except for medical purposes. This law, although endorsed by all states but one, was poorly enforced, and the addiction problem increased. Seeking more effective control of drugs, Congress passed the Harrison Act in 1914. This legislation attempted to control the production, manufacture, and distribution of narcotic drugs, and made dispensing of drugs illegal except by written prescription. As a consequence, the addict was cut off from his previous easy access to drugs, and when even the few clinics that were opened across the country to dispense drugs to addicts as a part of treatment were closed in the face of public criticism, he was forced to turn to the black market, the underworld, and to crime in order to feed his need. Illegal drug traffic mushroomed, and the need for control by means other that legislation became obvious.

In 1929 Congress authorized construction of hospitals at Lexington, Kentucky and Fort Worth, Texas, where drug addicts could be treated in a controlled setting. These two institutions continue in operation today. By the mid-1940's, as a consequence of international treaties, vigorous law enforcement, enlightened treatment, and more effective drug-abuse education, the number of known drug addicts had been reduced to less than 60,000. However, rising addiction rates in the 1950's, especially among younger people, brought on new and more stringent legislation. The Narcotic Drug Control Act of 1956 set the mandatory minimum penalty for a first violation of the Harrison Act at 5 years with no possibility of probation or parole. If the threat of such a severe penalty had any effect, it was not apparent, as the problem ballooned to epidemic proportions during the 1960's.

Habituation, addiction, and dependence

The Expert Committee on Drugs Liable to Produce Addiction of the World Health Organization differentiates drug habituation from drug addiction by the following characteristics.

Drug habituation is characterized by:

1. A desire but not a compulsion to continue the drug because of a sense of well-being

2. No real tendency to tolerance or dosage increase
3. Psychologic (or mental) dependence on the drug but no physical withdrawal symptoms
4. Detrimental effects limited primarily to the individual

Drug addiction is characterized by:

1. An overpowering desire or compulsion to continue the drug and to use any means to obtain it
2. A tendency to increase the dosage
3. Both psychologic (mental and emotional) and physical dependence with withdrawal symptoms if the drug becomes unavailable
4. Detrimental effects both to the individual and to society

Of course, society is made up of individuals, so what is bad for the individual certainly ultimately affects society; thus the distinction between drug habituation and drug addiction is an arbitrary one of degree only. Every drug addict has gone through the stage of drug habituation; a fortunate few stop there.

The terms habituation and addiction have frequently been used interchangeably over the years. Because a real difference was originally perceived between the two, as seen above, the misunderstanding often led to semantic difficulties that clouded the issues. Consequently, the World Health Organization now is trying to substitute the term "dependence" for both habituation and addiction, although a distinction between the two terms continues to have value, as will be seen shortly in the case of tobacco habituation. Drug dependence is viewed as "a state arising from repeated administration of a drug on a periodic or continuous basis."

Most likely all three terms will continue to be used. Medical circles favor the term "dependence" because it is more inclusively descriptive. Legislative and law enforcement bodies favor "habituation" and "addiction," since the laws are couched in these terms.

All drugs fall into one of five categories: narcotics, sedatives, tranquilizers, stimulants, and hallucinogens.

Narcotics (opiates)

Opium is the primary source of most narcotics. Morphine and codeine are derived from opium. Heroin (scag, smack, the big H, horse, dope, junk, stuff) is a morphine derivative; meperidine and methadone are synthetic morphinelike drugs; and paregoric is a preparation containing opium.

Narcotics act as depressants to certain areas of the brain and other parts of the nervous system. They reduce hunger, thirst, the sex drive, and feelings of pain. Withdrawal sickness occurs when an addict ceases using the drug of choice; he may sweat, shake, get chills, diarrhea, nausea, and suffer sharp abdominal and leg cramps. Recent findings show that the body's physical dependence on any narcotic lasts much longer than previously thought. As the statistics make clear, pure or large doses can and do result in death.

Methadone maintenance for those addicted to heroin (the most abused of the narcotics) has been recommended as a way to wean people from the more potent drug. At the same time, it is far less expensive: a user may need $50 a day to meet his craving for heroin, whereas the equivalent quantity of methadone costs only 15¢. This method of treatment, pioneered in New York City in 1964 by Drs. Vincent Dole and Marie Nyswander is criticized in that it substitutes one addiction for another. Those who support it contend that the addict need not become a criminal to feed his addiction, and that use of methadone in this therapeutic manner eases heroin withdrawal and blocks heroin's euphoric effects. Longer evaluation is needed for this type of substitution before we will understand its true value.

The most accepted means of helping the drug addict is through a small, controlled, therapeutic community. Examples of these are California's famed Synanon, New York's city-run Phoenix and Horizon Houses,

Table 6-1. Summary of relevant drug information

Drug	Effect	Legal control	Medical use	Physical dependence/ psychologic dependence/ tolerance	Form of illegal administration	Effects of abuse
Morphine	C.N.S. depressant	Harrison Act	Pain relief	yes/yes/yes	Orally, injection	Drowsiness, stupor, pinpoint pupils
Heroin	Depressant	Harrison Act	Pain relief	yes/yes/yes	Injection, sniffed	Same as morphine
Codeine	Depressant	Harrison Act	Cough and pain relief	yes/yes/yes	Orally (cough syrup)	Same as morphine
Paregoric	Depressant	Harrison Act	Sedation, offset diarrhea	yes/yes/yes	Orally, injection	Same as morphine
Meperidine	Depressant	Harrison Act	Pain relief	yes/yes/yes	Orally, injection	Same as morphine, also excitation, tremors, and convulsions
Methadone	Depressant	1953 amendment to Harrison Act	Pain relief	yes/yes/yes	Orally, injection	Same as morphine
Cocaine	C.N.S. stimulant	Harrison Act	Local anesthetic	no/yes/yes	Injection, sniffed	Extreme excitation, tremors, hallucinations
Marihuana	Hallucinogen	1937 Marihuana Tax Act plus subsequent restrictive legislation	None	no/yes/no	Orally, smoked	Drowsiness or excitability, dilated pupils, laughter, talkitiveness, hallucinations
Barbiturates	Depressant	1965 Drug Abuse Control Amendments	Sedation, sleep, epilepsy, high blood pressure	yes/yes/yes	Orally, injection	Drowsiness, staggering, slurred speech
Amphetamines	Stimulant	1965 Drug Abuse Control Amendments	For mild depression, antiappetite, narcolepsy	no/yes/yes	Orally, injection	Excitation, dilated pupils, tremors, talkativeness, hallucinations
LSD	Hallucinogen	1966 Drug Abuse Control Amendments	(Medical research only)	no/yes/yes	Orally, injection	Excitation, hallucinations, rambling speech

Adapted from materials in Drug abuse: escape to nowhere, Philadelphia, 1967, Smith, Kline, and French Laboratories.

Table 6-1. Summary of relevant drug information—cont'd

Drug	Effect	Legal control	Medical use	Physical dependence/ psychologic dependence/ tolerance	Form of illegal administration	Effects of abuse
Glue, paint thinners, lighter fluid	Depressant	No Federal controls; some states control sale of glue	None	?/yes/yes	Inhaled	Staggering, drowsiness, slurred speech, stupor

Marathon House in Providence, R. I., and, of course, the two federal narcotics hospitals at Lexington, Kentucky, and Fort Worth, Texas. These federal hospitals are far more conservative than the others. The program of treatment in all of these centers is to detoxify the effects of the drugs, then to rehabilitate the drug user by restructuring his ego and life pattern. Full treatment takes 18 to 36 months, but unfortunately the individual may return to addiction. We don't yet know how to break the dependence of any more than a minority of those afflicted.

Sedatives

The sedatives are a family of drugs that relax the nervous system and induce sleep. Best known are the barbiturates, first produced in 1846, from barbituric acid. They range from the short-acting, fast-starting pentobarbital (Nembutal) and secobarbital (Seconal) to the long-acting, slow-starting phenobarbital (Luminal), amobarbital (Amytal), and butabarbital (Butisol). The slow-acting barbiturates, called downers, goofballs, and barbs, are most commonly abused.

Barbiturates in overdose will kill; more people die from an overdose of a barbiturate than from any other drug. Death usually comes from paralysis of the respiratory center of the medulla. The reticular formation of the brain stem, or medulla, is the portion most concerned with awareness. Our reaction to stimuli helps keep us awake and aware of what is going on. In sleep the reticular formation reduces its activity. Under the influence of a barbiturate the reticular formation reduces its activity still further. The action of the nerves, skeletal muscles, and heart is depressed. The rate of breathing is reduced, and blood pressure drops. An overdose will paralyze the reticular formation, and death will follow unless first aid is quickly administered.

Barbiturates have valuable medicinal applications. They are used for epilepsy, high blood pressure, insomnia, and to treat a variety of mental disorders.

Symptoms of barbiturate overdose include slurred speech, staggering or unsteady gait, sluggish reactions, erratic emotions reflected in alternating tears and laughter, irritability, belligerence, and euphoria. Chronic users develop a tolerance to the drug. Abrupt withdrawal is dangerous and should always be supervised by a physician. In barbiturate withdrawal, unlike narcotic withdrawal, convulsions are possible and can be fatal. Delirium and hallucinations, similar to the delirium tremens of the alcoholic, may also be present.

Other nonbarbiturate depressants are used medically, although their use may occasionally be abused. These include glutethimide (Doriden), ethchlorvynol (Placidyl), ethinamate (Valmid), and methyprylon (Noludar). These are controlled legally under the Drug Abuse Control Amendments of 1965.

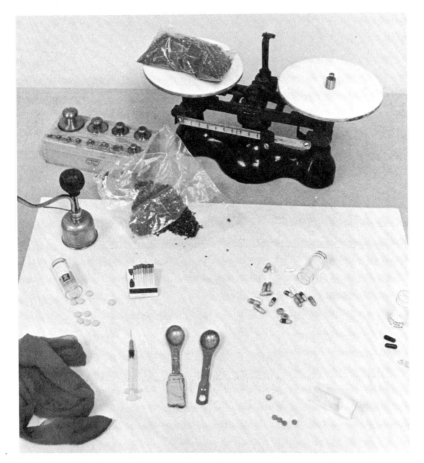

Fig. 6-1. Confiscated drugs. Clockwise, from top, scales for measuring marihuana; drugs available only by prescription; amphetamines; pills containing LSD; heroin paraphernalia including spoon, hypodermic syringe, and a stocking to be used as a tourniquet; Class A narcotics and marihuana pipe.

Tranquilizers

As long as 3,000 years ago inhabitants of India learned that when emotions ran wild and became destructive, the root of snake hemp, or rauwolfia, would quiet agitation without producing sleep. In recent times and particularly since the 1950's tranquilizers have completely changed the care and treatment of the agitated patient. Today, straightjackets, water baths, and isolation rooms are rarely required, because of the quieting effects of the tranquilizers. Through their use the daily friction of life can be eased and functioning made almost normal.

Generally, there are two groups of tranquilizers. The so-called major tranquilizers are those used in antipsychotic therapy.

Phenothiazine (Mellaril) and reserpine (Chrysoserpine) are of this type. They are not likely to produce dependence, and abuse is rare.

The second group, the minor tranquilizers, are seldom used to treat psychosis but are used widely in cases of emotional disorder. Drugs of this group, especially meprobamate (Equanil, Miltown) and chlordiazepoxide (Librium), are often abused. Dependence on these does develop. In addiction they can also produce jaundice, rashes, extrapyramidal symptoms, such as severe tremors, and may cause severe depressions with suicidal tendencies. Driving can be extremely hazardous while one is under their influence. The use of tranquilizers combined with alcohol and a sedative have been the cause of death in more than a few cases; this combination is certainly a potent, lethal one.

Stimulants

Drugs in this category directly excite the central nervous system. A widely used stimulant is caffeine, found in coffee, tea, cola, and other common drinks. The effects of caffeine are mild, and except for chronic heavy coffee drinkers, its use is seldom abused. More powerful by far than caffeine and certainly abused extensively are the amphetamines and cocaine.

The amphetamines, first produced in the 1920's, are known best for their ability to offset fatigue and sleepiness and to curb appetite in medically supervised weight reduction programs. They also are used, under a physician's direction, to relieve the mild depression that sometimes accompanies menopause, convalescence, grief, and senility. The immediate physical effects of amphetamines on the body include increasing heart rate, rising blood pressure, palpitations, and dilating pupils. They also cause dry mouth, sweating, headache, diarrhea, and paleness. Persons on large doses of amphetamines appear withdrawn, with dulled emotions. They seem unable to organize their thinking.

The most commonly used stimulants are amphetamine (Benzedrine), dextroamphetamine (Dexedrine), and methamphetamine (Methedrine). They are more commonly referred to as pep pills, bennies, and speed.

Physical dependence on stimulants does not develop, but a psychologic dependence most definitely does. Persons so affected find mental and emotional relief in stimulation and so turn to the amphetamines for their effect. Tolerance to these drugs does develop so that larger and larger doses are required to feel the effects.

Under the influence of these drugs, a person is pushed to do things beyond his physical endurance. Once the effects wear off, he is left exhausted and depressed. Heavy doses may cause a temporary mental derangement accompanied by auditory and visual hallucinations. To heighten the effects, a practice known as "speeding" the injection of liquid Methedrine directly into a vein is followed by some amphetamine abusers. Critical serum hepatitis and death have been the all too often tragic consequences of this practice. Long-term heavy users of amphetamines are usually irritable and unstable and, as with other drug users, reflect varying degrees of social, intellectual, and emotional breakdown.

Enough amphetamine is produced each year to provide each American with more than 25 doses. Since many persons seldom use a stimulant in capsule form, many others are consuming sizeable quantities. More than 20% of all medical prescriptions for mood-affecting drugs are for stimulants; but beyond these legal outlets, more than half the total supply enters nonprescribed, illegal channels. Businessmen, housewives, students, athletes, truck drivers, and many others use them seemingly without discrimination or concern for the total physical and mental consequences.

Cocaine comes from the leaves of the coca bush found in South America and is not to be confused with the cacao tree from which cocoa and chocolate are derived. In years past cocaine was used as a local anesthetic, but more recently, less toxic drugs have replaced it for this purpose.

Cocaine acts as a stimulant to produce excitability, talkativeness, and to reduce fatigue. It dilates the pupils and increases the heartbeat and blood pressure. As with the amphetamines, stimulation is followed by depression, and in overdosage death can result. It does not produce physical dependence nor does tolerance develop. Psychologic dependence is strong, and the desire to reexperience the intense hallucinatory effects of cocaine leads to its chronic misuse.

Hallucinogens

Dream images, distorted perceptions, and hallucinations are the effects of the several drugs classified as hallucinogens (also sometimes referred to as psychotomimetics, dysleptics, or psychedelics). These include mescaline, lysergic acid diethylamide (LSD), psilocybin, dimethyltryptamine (DMT), peyote, and STP (named by users after the motor fuel additive, but actually is DOM, an experimental compound developed by the Dow Chemical Company). As a group these drugs have no medical value except in research. The extent to which they have been abused in recent years is awesome.

Marihuana is a hallucinogen with a confused background. Although chemically different from all other hallucinogens, it produces similar effects. Although it is *not* a narcotic, its control under the Marihuana Tax Act of 1937 is similar to the controls imposed on the narcotics. Similarly, the marihuana laws are enforced by the Federal Bureau of Narcotics. This connection explains why marihuana users, and especially pushers, have received such severe legal punishment since the narcotics laws were first established.

Marihuana is found worldwide and is subject to greater abuse than any other dangerous drug. It grows in the flowering tops and leaves of the Indian hemp plant, *Cannabis sativa*. In India it is known as bhang or ganja, in the Middle East as hashish, in South Africa as dagga, and in South America as maconha or djamba. In this country its equivalent slang includes pot, tea, grass, weed, mary jane, hash, and kif. When abused, marihuana may be smoked, sniffed, or ingested; the most rapid effects take place when it is smoked. The leaves and flowers of the plant are dried and crushed or chopped into small pieces and smoked in short cigarettes (reefers, joints, sticks) or pipes.

The more obvious physical reactions to marihuana include rapid heartbeat, lowering of body temperature, and reddening of the eyes. It also changes blood glucose levels, stimulates the appetite, and dehydrates the body. Other effects of marihuana are less clearly understood. By irritating the frontal lobes of the brain, it frequently produces hilarity, lowers inhibitions, and produces lack of motivation, carelessness, distortion of emotional responses and sensations, and impairment of judgment and memory. One or two reefers may produce intoxication. Usually, the effect is felt quickly and can last from 2 to 4 hours. Some users, however, experience no change in mood at all. The social setting appears to be as influential as the drug itself in the changes that take place in those who use it. Repeated use appears to lower the sensory threshold for both optical and auditory stimuli; light is painful, and noises become acute. Sleep disturbances are common with hallucinations and delusions that predispose to antisocial behavior; anxiety and aggression is the result of intellectual and sensory derangements.

There is increasing evidence that marihuana may have severe effects beyond those described above. It may be much more than a "benign euphoriant" that occasionally triggers obnoxious behavior. Psychosis has been precipitated by the continued use of marihuana, but just what brain lesions are responsible for bizarre disturbances are not known any more than we know the brain lesions involved in the major psychoses. These conditions are not fatal, so few brain specimens have been available for examination. Those that do occur are frequently so subtle that they may escape postmortem examination just as have the lesions of the major psychoses. When our physiologic methods of studying the live and working brain have improved, we will find major chemical changes in the cells of the brain of hallucinogenic users as well as psychotics, but as yet our methods of study are too gross.

One group of eleven psychiatric patients were studied before and after they became marihuana users. All were diagnosed as schizophrenic after becoming chronic users. Severe social disability, including failure to complete school, delinquency, and participation in a drug subculture, occurred in the ten who continued to use the drug. Fortunately, one patient used it only once in the history of the study.*

*Milman, D. H.: The role of marihuana in patterns of drug abuse by adolescents, J. Pediat. **94**:283, February 1969.

In another study* adverse acute and schizophrenic reactions were reported in fifteen college students who used a combination of marihuana, LSD, and amphetamine.

Although much more reliable research on marihuana needs to be done, the legal and medical professions are becoming more convinced with time that its deleterious effects far outweigh its euphoric benefits. In remarks before the Commonwealth of Massachusetts Drug Dependency Conference on March 12, 1969, Chief Justice Tauro of the Massachusetts Supreme Court noted that in his experience there was no substantial controversy among reputable and informed authorities on the following points concerning marihuana.

1. Marihuana is universally recognized as a mind-altering drug that produces euphoria.
2. To produce euphoria is the primary cause of marihuana use in the U. S.
3. The euphoric state causes a lessening of psychomotor coordination and produces a distortion in perceiving time, distance, and space.
4. The habitual use of marihuana is prevalent in people with inadequate personalities, in neurotics, and in psychotics. These people will go to great lengths, including crime, to ensure a supply of the drug.
5. Marihuana tends to exaggerate or aggravate a preexisting neurotic or psychotic state.
6. There is no acceptable worthwhile medical use for marihuana, nor is it a part of any recognized Western religion.
7. Marihuana has had a growing attraction for the young thrill-seeker.

Similarly, the Council on Mental Health of the American Medical Association recently recommended a five-point policy on marihuana:

1. Cannabis is a dangerous drug and as such is a public health concern.
2. The sale and possession of marihuana should not be legalized.

3. The handling of offenders should be individualized.
4. Additional research on marihuana should be encouraged.
5. The AMA should continue its educational programs to all segments of the population with respect to the use of marihuana.*

Lysergic acid diethylamide (LSD) was synthesized in 1938 from lysergic acid present in ergot, a fungus that grows on rye. It is the most potent of the hallucinogens; a single ounce will provide 300,000 usual doses. In popular slang it is referred to as acid. A quantity amounting to a speck has effects that last for hours. It is taken in sugar cubes, on food, or by licking an object into which a quantity of LSD has been injected.

The physical alterations caused by LSD are clearly understood. It increases the pulse and heart rate, causes a rise in blood pressure and temperature, and dilates the pupils. Other effects include shaking of the hands and feet, cold sweaty palms, alternate flushing and paleness of the face, shivering and chills, irregular breathing, nausea, and loss of appetite. Tolerance to the behavioral effects of LSD may develop after extended use, but physical dependence does not occur. Psychic dependence does not seem to be severe; users will partake when LSD is present but do not experience a serious craving when it is not available.

Why is LSD popular as a drug of abuse? Without question, users enjoy the severe alterations that take place in their physical senses. Under the influence of LSD, one sees walls move and become three dimensional, unusual patterns are seen, and colors become extremely acute. Synesthesia, one sensory experience translated into another, may occur. Thus, the color red may develop a beat, and music may seem as the rainbow. Past events in one's life may be conjured, and some users have claimed transcendence. Simultaneous opposite emotions are not uncommon; happy-sad, elated-depressed, and tense-relaxed may be all rolled together in a collage of sensations. The normal feeling of

*Kuler, M. H.: Adverse reactions to marihuana, Amer. J. Psychiat. **124:**674, 1967.

*Delegates declare marihuana dangerous, Amer. Med. News, December 15, 1969.

boundaries between body and space may be lost. Death has occurred when a user, under the effects of LSD, believed he could fly.

Users experience both "good trips" and "bad trips," and there is no way to predict which will take place. Consequently, even controlled research with the drug is unpredictably dangerous. Evidence of "bad trips" is accumulating rapidly. One survey of 21 reports up to June 1967 contains the details of adverse reactions to LSD.* These include 142 cases of prolonged psychotic reactions, 63 nonpsychotic reactions, 11 spontaneous recurrences, 19 attempted suicides, 4 attempted homicides, 11 successful suicides, and 1 successful homicide. Another study, a survey of 2,700 medical and related professionals in the Los Angeles area, reported 2,300 adverse reactions between July 1, 1966, and January 1, 1968.† The exact number of LSD users having adverse reactions is not known, but the serious circumstances of those that do has made this hallucinogen less popular than it was 10 years ago.

Sidney Cohen, an authority on hallucinogens, classifies the adverse reactions of LSD as follows:

I. Psychotic disorders
  A. Accidental LSD intoxication, children as well as adults.
  B. Chronic LSD intoxication—slurred speech, ataxia or inability to walk properly, impaired coordination, and euphoria.
  C. Schizophrenic reactions—incoherence, agitation, bizarre behavior, and persistent hallucinations; symptoms persist for days or months.
  D. Paranoia—prolonged megalomaniacal state.
  E. Acute paranoid states—these are transient, but while one believes in his omnipotence, injuries or death to either self or associates can occur.
  F. Prolonged or intermittent LSD-like psychoses, such as hallucinosis.
  G. Psychotic depressions—the drug may activate aggressive impulses and weaken the ability to control these. Agitation and feeling of anxiety and guilt become overwhelming.
II. Nonpsychotic disorders
  A. Chronic anxiety reactions—time distortion, visual alterations, body image change, depression, difficulty in functioning may accompany a feeling of anxiety.
  B. Acute panic states—"hellish" LSD experiences occur not infrequently. In addition to overwhelming panic, there is a loss of control. At such times, people may run away or commit acts which injure themselves or others.
  C. Dyssocial behavior—loss of values and aspirations, loss of interest in reality or life.
  D. Antisocial behavior—defiance of social rules and regulations.
III. Neurologic reactions
  A. Convulsions.
  B. Permanent brain damage.*

Scientific evidence that LSD causes serious genetic and developmental abnormalities is conflicting. A number of studies have shown that there is decided chromosomal damage in the offspring of mothers who had used LSD during pregnancy.† Other studies have shown no significant increases in the chromosomal aberration rate before

---

*Smart, R. G., and Bateman, K.: Unfavorable reactions to LSD, Canad. Med. Ass. J. **97:**1214, November 11, 1967.

†Ungerleider, J. J., and others: A statistical survey of adverse reactions to LSD in Los Angeles County, Amer. J. Psychiat. **125:**352-356, September 1968.

*Cohen, S.: A classification of LSD complications, Psychosomatics **7:**182-187, May–June 1966.

†Cohen, M. M., Hirschhorn, K., and Frosch, W. A.: In vivo and in vitro chromosomal damage induced by LSD-25, New Eng. J. Med. **277:**1043-1049, November 16, 1967; Irwin, S., and Egozcue, J.: Chromosomal abnormalities in leukocytes from LSD-25 users, Science **157:**313-314, July 21, 1967; Nielsen, J., and others: Lysergide and chromosome abnormalities, Brit. Med. J. **2:**801-803, June 29, 1968.

and after use of LSD.* Its conflicting nature notwithstanding, the data provide sufficient evidence to justify the expectation that further studies may confirm the significant alteration of chromosomal material caused by use of LSD. The same may be said for the abnormal fetal development (teratogenesis) effect of LSD.

But if chromosomal damage and possible psychosis were the only concerns, many would argue that the risks are no greater than many other things we do regularly anyway and that the enjoyment is far more. How else can the psychologic processes be released in so wonderful a manner? How else can the miraculous nature of perception be viewed for the wonder it is? The color red, the sound of the word red, the concept of redness, and a red object all mingle under the influence of LSD in a manner that philosophers claim to suspect we have always used. If this were the only effect, we might be up there riding the high wind with everyone else, at least occasionally. The dangers are extreme, however, and cannot be denied or controlled.

First, the sad thing about LSD and other strong hallucinogens, as opposed to marihuana, is that psychologic effects outlast by weeks, and sometimes months, the disappearance of the drug from the system.

I have known some scholars who, after taking a single dose of morning glory seed concoction and having a wild trip lasting for a day or two, were literally unable to get back to serious work for about three months, although they functioned pretty well socially within the week. Their complaint was that, with respect to critical arguments, it was as if they had been clubbed with a dull mallet. Students at MIT who have taken only one dose of LSD have reported return trips to me, and, on reviewing their school performance, I could see a significant change for quite a while after. I except those who went psychotic after one dose and speak only of those who did not show any "bad" effects afterward.

The blunt fact is this: if someone came to a neurologist complaining of a disordered perception

of the sort had under LSD, the most probable diagnosis would be an affection of the temporal lobe of the brain, or the temporoparietal region. Further, if the man said it was episodic (return trips), occurring for no obvious reason, the neurologist would suspect a focal lesion in that part of the brain. Here, where we are assured that the drug has been excreted, but effects similar to those of focal lesions persist, what is a neurologist to think? I shall not pursue this matter further, but instead only remark that disorders in judgment and perception last for a long time after a dose of psychedelic drugs. Furthermore, this disorder may be such that the man cannot judge he is disordered (like the drunk who insists that he is sober enough to drive home).*

The second danger, and by far the more important, is the fact that LSD influences behavior adversely long after its chemical residual has left the human body.

What recommends alcohol or pot as an intoxicant is that within a day after the binge you can make a judgment comparing how you were the day before yesterday with how you felt yesterday. On this basis you can either decide to have it again or not, but the choice is made with your full faculties. In the case of LSD or DMT or some of the more protracted and frightening new compounds, you do not have your judgments returned so rapidly that you can compare validly the imperfect with the pluperfect view.

Thus it is that students, already somewhat pressed, already subject to the far less than idealistic tenor of our schools and the nature of our society, on taking such compounds can become easily recruited to the hippies, and turning on, drop out.

It is this feature that makes the hippie movements (as contrasted with mere eccentricity) dangerous. Hippies, in one form or another, have always been with us; they are, in a way, appealing, for they reflect the beachcomber, the people of Tortilla Flats, and all the other romantic pastoral types we all dream of being for a while. But they have never before had so strong a recruitment of the young as now when they have the judgment-dissolving drugs, the psychedelics, coupled with the extraordinary rearward force of a diseased society. I admit that it is a moral judgment on my part to say that it is a better thing to confront the world, terrible as it is, than to retreat from it to limbo. It is a matter of free choice that a

---

*Jjio, J. G., Pahnke, W. N., and Kurland, A. A.: LSD and chromosomes, J.A.M.A. **210:**849, November 3, 1969.

*Lettvin, J.: You can't even step in the same river once, Natural History **76:**6, October 1967.

Table 6-2. Comparative strengths of the hallucinogens

Hallucinogen	Comparative strength*	
Marihuana (leaves and tops of Cannabis sativa, swallowed)	30,000	mg.
Peyote buttons (Lophophora williamsii)	30,000	mg.
Nutmeg (Myristica fragrans)	20,000	mg.
Hashish (resin of Cannabis sativa)	4,000	mg.
Mescaline (3,4,5-trimethoxyphenelethylamine)	400	mg.
Psilocybin (4-phosphoryltryptamine)	12	mg.
STP (2,5-dimethoxy-4-methyl-amphetamine)	5	mg.
LSD (D-lysergic acid diethylamide tartrate)	0.1	mg.

Adapted from Cohen, S.: Pot, acid, and speed, Med. Sci. **19**:31, February 1968.

*Each of the dosages indicated has an equivalent effect.

Table 6-3. Amounts of LSD (seven samples) and STP (two samples) in samples analyzed

Sample	Alleged chemistry	Actual chemistry	Amount	
1	LSD	LSD	50	μg
2	LSD	LSD	80	μg
3	LSD	LSD	80	μg
4	LSD	LSD	100	μg
5	LSD	LSD	110	μg
6	LSD	LSD	200	μg
7	Mescaline	LSD	283	μg
8	Mescaline	STP	3.7	mg
9	Mescaline	STP	4.8	mg

From, Cheek, F. E., Newell, S., and Joffe, M.: Deceptions in the illicit drug market, Science **167**:1276, February 27, 1970. Copyright 1970 by the American Association for the Advancement of Science.

man should decide between lethe and hell. But the choice should be made on the basis of fully informed comparison, and I claim the drugs to be vicious because their effects last so long as to bias that choice. It is equivalent to asking a lobotomized man, or a patient after prolonged psychotherapy, aren't you happier now? I hold stacking the cards to be unfair and immoral.*

Table 6-2 indicates that marihuana is the weakest and LSD the strongest among the several hallucinogens. Serious side effects, including death, have been attributed to each of the drugs shown in this table.

Persons who buy hallucinogens illegally (many are sold legally in the form of cough syrups, cold tablets, and sleep inducers, although their indiscriminate use is a serious medical concern) seldom purchase the quantity claimed. Usually the buyer gets far less than he pays for, but too often he gets far more. Also, the substance purchased often is not what it is claimed to be. Table 6-3 summarizes seven samples of LSD and two samples of STP that were believed by the users to contain about 250 mg of LSD or a comparable quantity of mescaline.

ALCOHOL

Candy
Is dandy
But liquor
Is quicker

These words by Ogden Nash succinctly describe the lure that alcohol has for millions of people. Although it is classified as a drug and its action on the human body is to depress all of the life processes, alcohol is an accepted part of our culture, legally purchased, and used by those of age. Despite its dangers, control of alcohol is primarily an individual matter. You alone will decide whether you will master or be mastered by alcohol. You may choose to abstain, to use alcohol socially and with discretion, or to use it beyond acceptable social and discretionary boundaries. Certainly, alcohol is a substance that can erode individual life and threaten our whole culture. As such, it is, along with all other drugs, a serious threat to our ecologic balance.

Every man's poison

Alcohol, from the old Arabic term *al-kohl,* has two meanings as currently used. First,

*Ibid., pp. 11-12.

Table 6-4. Source, manufacturing process, percent alcohol, and caloric content of selected alcohol-based drinks

Beverage	Made from	Malting	Distillation	Percent alcohol by volume	Calories per fl. oz.
Beer	Cereals	yes	no	4- 6	10-18
Ale	Cereals	yes	no	6- 8	16-21
Hard cider	Apple juice	no	no	8-12	10-20
Wine	Grape juice	no	no	10-22	18-50
Whiskey	Cereals	yes	yes	40-55	60-90
Brandy	Wine	no	yes	40-55	60-90
Rum	Molasses	no	yes	40-55	60-90
Gin	Neutral spirits, plus juniper berries, orange peel, etc.	no	usually	40-55	60-90
Vodka	Neutral spirits	no	no	40-55	60-90

it is used generically to describe a large group of organic compounds that contain a hydroxyl (-OH) group attached to a carbon atom. Examples are methyl alcohol (wood alcohol) and isopropyl alcohol (used in rubbing alcohol), both highly toxic to humans. Second, alcohol means a specific compound, C_2H_5OH, known as ethyl alcohol, grain alcohol, or ethanol. Ethyl alcohol is the alcohol used in all "spirited" beverages and is the form of alcohol we are talking about in the remaining discussion of this topic.

Ethyl alcohol is a clear, thin liquid with a pleasant, mild odor. It mixes with water in all proportions, is many times more soluble in water than fat, and is virtually insoluble in dry proteins or minerals. Its small molecular size explains its rapid diffusion throughout the body, once ingested.

Alcohol is produced whenever yeast acts upon the sugars contained in and produced by nature. The conversion of sugars to alcohol by yeast is called fermentation and is expressed in a simple chemical formula:

$$C_6H_{12}O_6 \xrightarrow{\text{Yeast}} \underset{\text{Ethyl alcohol}}{2C_2H_5OH} + \underset{\text{Carbon dioxide}}{2CO_2}$$

Cereals, berries, and fruits are among the sources of natural sugar used to produce beer and wine. Hard liquors require a subsequent artificial distillation process. Grains such as rye, wheat, barley, and corn provide the raw materials for most of the alcoholic drinks consumed in this country.

Table 6-4 summarizes the source, process, percent alcohol, and caloric content of several alcoholic substances.

Entering the body. Alcohol is absorbed very quickly from the stomach and intestine because of its low molecular weight and high solubility in water. Approximately one-third of the alcohol entering the stomach will be absorbed directly into the body within one-half hour. If it remains in the stomach for an hour (unlikely under normal digestive action but possible experimentally) about two-thirds will be absorbed within an hour. Other liquids and food in the stomach will retard the rate of absorption. Absorption from the small intestine is even more rapid than from the stomach.

Alcohol can enter the body through portals other than the digestive tract, but seldom and usually only in small amounts. Alcohol in contact with a break in the skin, as would be possible in the case of dermatitis, for example, can be absorbed. Virtually no absorption is possible through the unbroken skin. Human beings can tolerate air containing about 2% alcohol vapor and will absorb approximately 60% of this via the lungs. Fifteen percent alcohol in an enema solution is absorbed rapidly from the bowel. Alcohol injected into the urinary bladder is absorbed very slowly because of the poor circulation of blood through the bladder wall. Absorption of alcohol by vein is possible up to a 20% solution. Glucose and alcohol are sometimes given in combination intravenously to meet certain emergency nutritional needs.

Physiologic effects. In the body alcohol is oxidized to acetaldehyde, a highly toxic substance, but present in this form only briefly; to acetic acid, a mild, harmless substance; and finally to carbon dioxide and water. This occurs at a nearly uniform rate. A 150-pound person will oxidize ½ to 1 fluid ounce of 100-proof whiskey per hour (the indicated proof is twice the percentage of alcohol by volume). A heavier person would oxidize proportionately more alcohol per hour, a lighter person proportionately less. There is some relation between oxidation rate and basal metabolism. People with hyperthyroidism often are able to oxidize alcohol at a higher than average rate. However, there seems to be no change in the rate of oxidation when thyroid extract is administered to persons having normal thyroid activity. Exercise, exposure to cold, and various types of shock have no known effect on the rate of oxidation. Some research suggests that the ingestion of sugar in the form of fructose, but also increased protein intake, may step up the rate of alcohol combustion. On the other hand, experimental evidence of the effect of glucose and insulin, administered either singly or in combination, on the oxidation rate of alcohol is conflicting.

Alcohol often is used as an appetizer because of its capacity to stimulate the flow of gastric juices and initiate muscular action of the stomach. In limited amounts it appears to aid digestion; in excessive amounts it slows and even blocks digestion. If gastric or duodenal ulcers are present, alcohol will aggravate these conditions.

Alcohol is almost exclusively an energy food; one gram contains 7 calories, or 200 calories per ounce. Since food intake is seldom reduced, except in the case of the extreme alcoholic, the calories in readily oxidized alcohol provide the necessary energy, and those in the food are stored as fat. Thus, a normal diet supplemented by alcohol will be fattening.

The most serious effect of alcohol is on the central nervous system. Although it is popularly termed a stimulant, alcohol is mainly a depressant. It acts first on the cortical functions of the brain and then gradually affects the medulla. Thus, judgment, memory, learning, and awareness of environment are the first functions to be altered. The presumed stimulatory effect of alcohol occurs when control of the lower brain by the cortex is depressed, and our usual social restraints are cast aside. As more alcohol is ingested and the level of concentration in the blood increases, progressively more primitive parts of the brain are affected until, with very high concentrations, death results when the respiratory and circulatory centers are paralyzed.

Other parts of the body come under alcohol's influence. In moderate amounts alcohol causes the vessels of the skin to dilate, resulting in the characteristic flushed appearance. In excessive amounts when stupor occurs, the skin becomes pale and cold because of impaired circulation. Two to three ounces of hard liquor will cause a 5% increase in pulse rate, blood pressure, and total blood flow. Heavy drinkers develop cirrhosis of the liver (a hardening, granulation, and contraction of the tissues) more often than moderate and nondrinkers, caused as much by their overall faulty diet as by the alcohol itself. Alcohol causes a marked increase in the volume of urine caused, for the most part, by its action on the pituitary gland (its antidiuretic action is depressed) and by the reverse osmotic effect that alcohol in the bloodstream has on all the body's cells. Loss of fine muscle coordination occurs with small amounts of alcohol; larger amounts cause staggering gait, thick speech, and finally complete paralysis of voluntary muscles and coma. As muscular efficiency is lowered, reaction time is increased, and the person so affected becomes a menace to our dynamic environment (see Chapter 5). In large dosage alcohol reduces the ascorbic acid and the cholesterol content of the adrenal glands, thus impairing the "fight or flight" protective function that these glands serve.

The therapeutic effects of alcohol have been appreciated for many years. In part these are physiologic in nature: as a sedative to relieve aches and pains, to relax tensions and reduce irritability, and to whet a poor appetite and provide supplementary calories. At the same time its effect is also euphoric. Its capacity to tranquilize, to make almost anyone actually feel better no matter what the problem, introduces us to the psychologic effects of alcohol.

Psychologic effects. Why do people drink? Is it to relax their tense and apprehensive feelings? Is it to make them better able to cope with personal problems? Is it to reduce their feelings of loneliness, or perhaps to reduce the burden of guilt they may carry, or to celebrate a happy occasion for pure pleasure and out of good spirits? All of these and more emphasize the complexity of the phenomenon of why people drink.

The behavioral psychologist explains that people drink basically to reduce their fears and tensions and that the reduction becomes the reinforcement that encourages them to drink again in subsequent similar circumstances.

Actually, we know very little in a precise, scientific way about the psychologic effects of alcohol. How alcohol will cause a person to behave is a function of the individual, the task, and the amount of alcohol consumed. Since the combination of these three is subject to great variation, it is not surprising that the available data tends to be conflicting. It seems, depending on the study you read, that alcohol may facilitate, may depress, or may have no effect on behavior. But there is no denial that it can and does change people. It pervades our culture and holds several million unwilling and other-directed persons in its liquid grasp.

Alcohol in our culture

The acceptance of alcohol in our culture is such that few persons remain complete abstainers throughout life. Where do you place yourself in the progression of statements that follow?

1. As far as I know I have never tasted alcohol in an identified form, nor do I intend to.
2. I tried it once or twice, but didn't like it.
3. I've had an occasional drink with friends.
4. Whenever alcoholic drinks are offered, I accept.
5. I have bought and used liquor on many occasions.
6. I don't really pay attention to how much I drink at any one time.
7. I love it any time, any place.
8. I'm dependent on alcohol.

The social drinker. The eight statements above are on an obvious continuum from complete abstention to complete subjugation. At no time in your life should you find yourself below category 5. Many persons, probably half the adult population, belong in category 1 or 2. They do not use alcohol themselves and should be appreciated for this characteristic. Ridicule of their position is certainly not appropriate nor mature.

Those persons in categories 3, 4, and 5 are among the more than 80 million social drinkers in our country today. For most of these, drinking reduces the tensions that are a concomitant part of our busy life. It relieves self-consciousness, loosens the tongue, and transforms strangers into friends. The pleasant glow that a small concentration of alcohol in the body creates is the feeling that all social drinkers desire. That it should or does go beyond this is not the case for most people.

One study of 2,766 persons indicated that 1,744 (65%) used alcohol on occasion.* Of these, 38% did so for reasons of sociability. Others said they drank to keep other people company, because they had been brought up with it, to celebrate important occasions, and for business reasons. Still others drank for personal rather than social reasons: "makes me feel good," "quenches

---

*Riley, J. W., Marden, C. F., and Lifschitz, M.: The motivational pattern of drinking, Quarterly Journal of Studies on Alcohol, September 1948, pp. 353-362.

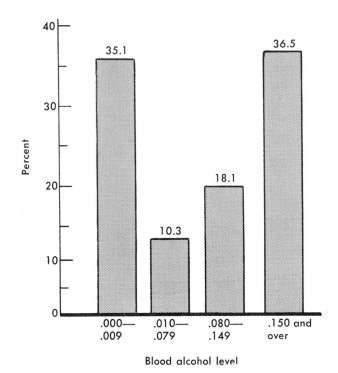

Fig. 6-2. Percent distribution of 507 driver fatalities in Wisconsin, by blood alcohol level, February 1, 1968, through May 30, 1969. Drivers with more than .08% blood alcohol level are definitely under the influence; thus, 54.6% of fatal accidents in Wisconsin during the period indicated were caused in part or whole by alcohol. (From Laessig, R. H., and Waterworth, K. J.: Involvement of alcohol in fatalities of Wisconsin drivers, Public Health Rep. **85**:537, June 1970.)

thirst," "health reasons," "I like it," "stimulates appetite."

Numerous studies of high school students reveal that from 33% to 86% have some experience with alcoholic beverages.* These same studies, however, report that most of this confessed experience is sporadic, especially for girls.

But an unfortunate number of persons slip beyond the point of drinking for sociable or controlled personal reasons only.

The social drunkard. The effects of alcohol become obvious when consumption is

*Chappel, N. N., and others: The use of alcoholic beverages among high school students, New York, 1953, Mrs. John S. Sheppard Foundation, Inc.; University of Kansas: Attitudes of high school students toward alcoholic beverages, New York, 1967, Mrs. John S. Sheppard Foundation, Inc.; University of Wisconsin: Attitudes of high school students toward alcoholic beverages, New York, 1956, Mrs. John S. Sheppard Foundation, Inc.

more rapid than metabolism. When this occurs the person very quickly becomes intoxicated, a fact soon obvious to everyone. Our culture tolerates intoxication to a ridiculous degree. At a party the intoxicated person is tolerated, even accepted, as long as he (or she) does not become physically or otherwise obnoxious. We wish that the intoxicated person would not drink so much, and we even tell him to take it easy; but we usually don't do anything about it until we carry him, unconscious, to the nearest bedroom or waiting car.

Most social drunkards are persons who can control their drinking but don't. They are irresponsible persons and a very real menace to society as well as to themselves. For example, our toleration and the consequent danger is most evident in the statistics of automobile accidents where drinking is a factor (Fig. 6-2). Our courts are far too lenient with those who drive while under the influence of alcohol. But the courts respond to the pressures of society, and society ("There but for the grace of God go I") remains blithely tolerant.

Social disorganization. The heavy drinker first loses the respect of his friends, working associates, and family. At social gatherings those who know and love him come to fear the behavior they are certain he will manifest. At his place of business the competence he once demonstrated gives way to blundering failure, and his very livelihood is threatened. At home there is a tenseness broken at more and more often intervals by nagging, argument, apology, recrimination, shouting, and occasional physical abuse. Love finds it difficult to survive under such circumstances.

In recent years recreational patterns have changed to keep pace with other changing patterns in society. Leisure hours have increased while the personal and emotional rewards from work have decreased for many. For many, work has become impersonal, commercial, and passive. In order to enjoy leisure a person must be creative, but many find this impossible. For them, drinking becomes a passive way of relieving their tension and of enjoying their leisure without having to be creative.

But it is important that alcohol be seen in its proper relation to social problems. One writer has summarized this relationship as follows:

1. Social problems arise out of the ongoing social processes of a society. Alcohol does not create them.
2. All behavior is learned in a social context and, depending on the characteristics of that context, deviant or nondeviant behavior will be the outcome. Deviant behavior is not caused by alcohol.
3. All personalities emerge as a result of relationships with other members of the society and, depending on the nature of their relationships, these personalities can or cannot adapt to changes in the social system. Depending on the place of the person in the social system, his flexibility or inflexibility will permit or mitigate against his continuing comfortable functioning. Pathological personality disturbances are not caused by alcohol.

4. Alcohol is used in our society because its use is integrated with other social patterns and because it performs a function both for the individual and for society as a whole. Restricted to such a context, its use does not constitute a problem.
5. Society's definition of the use of alcohol as a problem arises not from alcohol per se or from the behavior which accompanies its use, but (a) from the culture's value system; (b) from the incompatibility between the excessive use of alcohol and the individual's effective participation in social institutions; and (c) from the inefficiency of social controls.
6. Society's reaction toward the excessive use of alcohol may contribute to pathologic personality problems and to socially disapproved behavior, depending on the individual's adaptation to this societal reaction.*

The above points make clear that alcohol in itself is not the problem. We once thought it was, but Prohibition proved us wrong. The problem lies in people and how they react to their problems, to society, and to alcohol, whether they be abstainers, moderate drinkers, or excessive drinkers.

Effects on the family. The above points on social disorganization tell us to be cautious in our indictment of alcohol per se. Nonetheless, heavy drinking is not likely to ensure a happy family. In fact, available data on drinking and the family indicates that those who develop drinking problems at some time during their lives are less likely to have been married and, if they do marry, are likely to have been involved in one or more marital failures. If drinking problems arise during marriage, the marriage is more likely to be terminated.

Family conflict, always present in varying degrees within and between families, is intensified and blurred when drinking is involved. The following events inevitably occur.

1. When the response to interpersonal difficulties is excessive drinking, the

---

*Jackson, J. K.: Assumptions regarding social disorganization and alcohol, in McCarthy, R. S., editor: Alcohol education for classroom and community, New York, 1964, McGraw-Hill Book Co., p. 154. Copyright 1964 McGraw-Hill Book Co. Used with permission of McGraw-Hill Book Co.

conflict is not as amenable to resolution.

2. The drinking interferes with the performance of family roles during each drinking episode, causing anxiety. The anxiety causes further disruption, leading to more problems and still more drinking. Thus the spiral tightens.
3. Since the excessive drinking is socially undesirable, the family's shame and guilt is intensified.
4. The conflict heightens; the drinking becomes more often and more excessive; and the extra-family roles become impaired. These may include problems with the police and illness; job performance may suffer; and the children may withdraw from friends and do poorly in school.
5. All family problems, whatever their nature or origin, become focused in the struggle to control the drinking.
6. The community may be drawn into the family's problem and add to its complexity.*

Excessive drinking does not a happy family make. Where the two coexist, one need only wait a while before asking, "What family?"

Alcohol and crime. Police spend nearly three-fourths of their time handling people who have been drinking excessively. Drunkenness is usually the charge, and many persons arrested have been arrested for being drunk on previous occasions. The heavy drinker commits misdemeanors more often than felonies and is more likely to commit unlawful acts against other persons than against property. As many as 25% of those in prison for felonies were inebriated when they were apprehended. Eighty to ninety percent of all inmates blame their imprisonment on alcohol.

But if alcohol is the cause of crime, it is perhaps no more so than it is the cause of

*Adapted from Bacon, S. D.: Excessive drinking and the institution of the family, in Alcohol, Science, and Society, Quarterly Journal of Studies in Alcohol, New Brunswick, N. J., 1954, pp. 223-248.

family disintegration and social disorganization. Alcohol certainly makes bad problems worse, but there is inconclusive evidence that it is the direct cause for the serious problems of our culture.

Alcoholism

We doubt that you saw yourself below category 5 on the eight-point continuum previously presented (p. 145). If you did, you're in trouble. But even if you didn't, you should understand the phenomenon of alcoholism. It's a sickness that any one of us might develop.

Both the American Medical Association and the World Health Organization hold alcoholism to be a specific disease entity. The courts now recognize it legally as a disease and thereby have shifted responsibility for the care of many alcoholics from law enforcement agencies to the medical profession.

Any heavy drinker may soon be an alcoholic if he is not already. Alcoholism is a type of drug dependence; it is pathologic; and it seriously affects the patient's health and impairs his relationship to his environment.

Causes. Would that alcohol had a single cause. We know, however, that it is the consequence of physiologic, psychologic, and social factors in combination that gives rise to the disease.

A number of theories have been advanced to explain alcoholism in a physiologic context.

1. It is the result of abnormal sugar metabolism.
2. It is caused by metabolic disturbances that trigger a craving for alcohol.
3. The malfunctioning of the endocrine glands causes its onset.
4. Dietary defects result in a metabolic deficiency that gives rise to alcoholism.

At the present time these are only theories; and if there is a basic physiologic cause, it is yet to be discovered. Nonetheless, it is certain that one or more physiologic deficiencies contribute significantly to alcoholism.

The psychologic dimension is no less complicated. A wide variety of emotional and mental illnesses are found among alcoholics. Many alcoholics display a decided dependency reaction—almost complete dependence masked by seeming independence. Also, most alcoholics resent responsibility and maneuver away from it with great skill. Alcoholics' aspirations exceed their capabilities by a wide margin, and alcohol is viewed as an attractive escape. Self-destructive impulses are more prevalent among alcoholics, and certainly many of them literally and knowingly drink themselves to death.

Alcoholism has sociologic foundations that are also influential. In countries where drinking to excess is generally discouraged, alcoholism is a relatively minor problem. In the United States where society tends to approve drinking and the inebriate is kindly tolerated, we have a serious alcoholic problem. Society's reaction to the alcoholic conveys the idea to him that "life is tough; if you must escape, alcohol is as good a way as any to do it."

Young adults want to belong, but such membership should not include a regular diet of alcohol. For many it does, and a dependency often develops before the victim is aware of what is taking place within himself.

Extent. There may be as many as six million alcoholics in this country, maybe more. Those so affected seem to be increasing; certainly total alcohol consumption is increasing year by year. Alcoholism is more prevalent in large cities, but this may be more a function of alcoholics' gravitating to the cities for anonymity rather than any negative influence the city may have over the country in this regard. Of the eight states with the highest rates of alcoholism, seven are located in the industrial Northeast (New Hampshire, Massachusetts, Connecticut, Rhode Island, New Jersey, New York, and Delaware). The eighth state, California, also highly industrialized—and densely populated—has the highest rate of alcoholism.

More men than women are known alcoholics, the presumed ratio being about 4 : 1. In recent times the women's liberation movement seems also to have included alcoholism; prevalence of alcoholism among women appears to be greater today than it was 10 to 20 years ago. Whether this observed increase is a function of greater visibility recently achieved by women, where once the extent of their sickness may have been protected by the home, or whether it is a real increase is not yet clear.

Industrial studies have estimated that alcoholics lose an average of 22 more working days a year than the nonalcoholic, are victims in twice as many accidents, and have a life expectancy that is 12 years less.

Treatment. The treatment of alcoholism is exceedingly complex. Common illnesses always demand attention, and one or more specific disease entities may also influence the course of treatment.

Of general and just concern is the need to isolate the patient from alcohol. This can be done on a voluntary or forced basis. Many patients voluntarily commit themselves into alcohol deintoxication units of state or general hospitals. Here they are restrained and given various tranquilizers, such as hydroxyzine (Vistaril) and prochlorperazine (Compazine), to relieve nausea, motor excitement, vomiting, and anxiety, and an anticonvulsant, such as diphenylhydantoin (Dilantin), to control their withdrawal symptoms (alcoholic tremulousness, alcoholic hallucinosis, alcoholic convulsive seizures, and delerium tremens) while they are "drying out." Acute intoxication is a severe condition. The importance of expert medical supervision during the deintoxication phase cannot be overemphasized.

Coincident with the "drying out" process is the need to initiate a balanced nutritional program. Alcoholics usually have poor nutrition, tending instead to drink their food. Consequently, their diet is high in calories but lacking in all other important nutrients. They are dehydrated and emaciated and may even have to be fed intravenously for a period if food will not stay in their stomachs.

Once past the primary rehabilitation stage, the patient still needs careful supervision. He naturally begins to feel good and can be released to the custody of family, friends, or a halfway house. The latter represents a pattern originated in the 1950's. It is a semicustodial institution that bridges the gap between hospital care and the demands of everyday life. Therapy is continued in the halfway house, but the patient can be in the community in nearly all normal respects for much of the time. As the patient's well-being improves, his confidence to handle alcohol in a self-directed manner returns, and he will take a drink to prove himself, unless counseled otherwise. He must not be permitted to drink. When he does, he has taken the first step backward and is on the road to his next binge. Alcoholics, once rehabilitated, may never again touch a single drop of alcohol. If they should, the odds are overwhelming that the disease will recur.

A number of deterrent drugs have been used in recent years to good effect. Disulfiram (Antabuse) is one of these. When the drug is taken regularly, alcohol in the body causes a highly unpleasant reaction characterized by transient hypertension, flushing, nausea, vomiting, and occasional collapse. The effect of the drug is to arrest the metabolism of alcohol at the acetaldehyde stage. This highly toxic substance produces the unpleasant reactions just described. If the drug has this effect, the patient will remain abstinent and continue his recovery therapy.

Another method similar to the use of disulfiram is known as the aversion, or conditioned response, method. With this method the patient is allowed the alcohol he desires, but it is altered so as to make him severely ill. He associates his illness with drinking and will even become ill when he simply thinks about alcohol. Psychodrama and hypnosis are other therapy techniques that are used, depending on the patient being treated.

At least three voluntary organizations have been developed to offer assistance to alcoholics and their families. Alcoholics Anonymous (A.A.), founded in 1934, is made up of former alcoholics. Its strength is in the moral and spiritual support that older members give to the newer ones who are beginning their rehabilitation. Al-Anon offers help to the families of alcoholics so they may better understand the problem and the various methods of support that the patient must receive from those close to him if he is to recover. Al-A-Teen, similar to Al-Anon in program thrust, is made up of the children of compulsive drinkers.

A number of specific disease entities may be brought on by long-term alcoholism and will require specific treatment as part of the overall therapeutic procedure. Included among these diseases are:

1. *Alcoholic polyneuropathy.* This condition is vague in its manifestation. However, it includes weakness, numbness, pain, and paresthesia (abnormal sensation without objective cause). More specific symptomatology includes wasting of the leg muscles, calf tenderness, and motor and sensory impairment, especially of the lower extremities. Treatment is long term with diet therapy, pain sedation, and gentle muscle massage indicated.

2. *Wernicke's encephalopathy.* Wernicke's disease is an acute condition with ataxia, ocular abnormalities, and mental confusion with ataxia, ocular abnormalities, and mental confusion the paramount characteristics. Mortality is about 15% mostly because of such complicating conditions as heart failure, hepatic coma, and infections. Vitamin B, especially thiamine, is the indicated treatment.

3. *Korsakoff's psychosis.* Here the patient suffers serious memory and learning impairment; he is inert, apathetic, and disinterested in his surroundings, and is not aware of his memory defect. Although Korsakoff's psychosis might occasionally develop in the malnourished alcoholic patient independent of prior conditions, it usually follows the onset of Wernicke's disease. Recovery is seldom complete, and there is no affirmed therapy.

4. *Alcohol amblyopia.* Visual failure,

typically a painless blurring of vision that continues indefinitely, occurs in some alcoholics. Vitamin therapy will usually eliminate the condition.

From Noah to now—and beyond

Noah was the first tiller of the soil.
He planted a vineyard; and he drank
of the wine, and became drunk, and
lay uncovered in his tent.

GENESIS 9:20, 21

The time span from Noah to now covers many years, and for at least that long alcohol has influenced man's behavior. Without question, it will be with us an equal number of years—and more—into the future. Certainly for the present, it is and will remain an integral part of our culture. Our challenge is to harness the medicinal and social benefits of alcohol. But that is the challenge of all substances in the modern environment that endanger health.

TOBACCO

Tobacco is a dirty weed,
I like it.
It satisfies no normal need,
I like it.
It makes you thin,
It makes you lean.
It takes the hair right off your bean,
It's the worst darned stuff
I've ever seen,
I like it.

G. L. HEMMINGER

In the contradiction of these lines is found the devil's fork. On one hand, there is the statistically significant evidence that smoking, especially cigarettes, contributes to the onset of many diseases and shortens the life span, at least for the heavy smoker, by as much as 8 years. On the other hand, there is the bald fact that millions continue to smoke for reasons of presumed pleasure or real habituation or both, and over a million people, mostly teenagers, join the smoker's ranks each year.

Smoking and disease

Until this century the cigarette was virtually unknown. Tobacco was burned in

cigar form and in pipes, chewed, and taken through the nostrils as snuff. Between 1900 and 1909 only 4.2 billion cigarettes were produced annually in the United States. By 1968 this production figure had climbed to 580 billion cigarettes.

As cigarette consumption rose, the voices of concern, at first faint, grew in number and volume. In 1936 two New Orleans surgeons, Alton Ochsner and Michael E. De-Bakey, observed that nearly all their lung cancer patients were cigarette smokers. In 1938 Raymond Pearl, the noted John Hopkins medical statistician, reported that smokers had a shorter life expectancy than those who did not smoke. Dr. Pearl published a table based on the life histories of 6,813 men (2,094 non–tobacco users, 2,814 moderate smokers, and 1,905 heavy smokers). The results of his study, as seen in Table 6-5, led Dr. Pearl to conclude that smoking is definitely associated with a reduction in the length of life and that the degree of reduction is proportional to the amount of tobacco used. Note also that in the middle years, 30 to 50, the chances of a man's dying are 15% greater for a moder-

Table 6-5. Tobacco smoking and length of life*

Age	Nonusers	Moderate	Heavy
30	100,000	100,000	100,000
35	95,883	95,804	90,943
40	91,546	90,883	81,191
45	86,730	85,129	71,665
50	81,160	78,436	62,699
55	74,538	70,712	54,277
60	66,564	61,911	46,266
65	57,018	52,082	38,328
70	45,919	41,431	30,393
75	33,767	30,455	22,338
80	21,737	19,945	14,498
85	11,597	10,987	7,865
90	4,573	4,686	3,392
95	1,320	1,366	938

From Pearl, Raymond: The search for longevity, Scientific Monthly **46**:462-483, May 1938.

*The number of survivors at 5-year intervals, starting at the age of 30, of (1) 100,000 white males who were nonusers of tobacco, (2) 100,000 who were moderate smokers but did not chew tobacco or take snuff, and (3) 100,000 who were heavy smokers but did not chew tobacco or take snuff.

ate smoker and 98% greater for a heavy smoker than for a nonsmoker.

Experimental evidence to support Pearl's position came in 1939 when A. H. Roffo of Argentina reported that he had produced cancer by painting tarlike tobacco extracts on the backs of rabbits. In the 1950's and 1960's several thousand historical, prospective, and experimental studies were conducted on the subject of smoking and health, caused partly by trends in tobacco consumption and partly by trends in death rates. Widespread concern for the decided increase in deaths that appeared to be linked to smoking prompted the Surgeon General to establish a special committee to review all the studies and to report the indicated interrelationships of smoking and health. This report, *Smoking and Health,* was released in January 1964. It was followed in 1967 by a second report, *The Health Consequences of Smoking,* which reviewed more than 2,000 research studies published between 1964 and 1967. Subsequent reports in 1968 and 1969 added to this information.

In summary, these studies have concluded the following:

1. Days of work lost increase in direct relation to the amount smoked. Those who smoke half a pack of cigarettes a day lose one more day per year than nonsmokers; those who smoke two packs a day lose three days per year more than nonsmokers.

2. Days of bed rest required similarly increase: 5.1 for nonsmokers, 6.8 for those who smoke 1 to 10 cigarettes a day, 5.6 for those who smoke 11 to 20 cigarettes, 7.0 for those who smoke 21 to 40 cigarettes, and 8.8 for those who smoke more than 41 cigarettes per day.

3. Among females there is a similar work loss and increase in bed rest required in relation to the amount smoked.

4. Death rates for all causes are nearly 70% higher for cigarette smokers than for nonsmokers. Those who smoke more than 2 packs a day have a 120% higher death rate than nonsmokers.

5. Cigarette-smoking males have a higher coronary disease death rate than nonsmoking males. This death rate may be 70% to 200% greater, depending upon the presence of other known risk factors for coronary disease. Females have a similar increase in their death rate profile if they smoke.

6. Cigarette smoking is the most important of the causes of chronic nonneoplastic bronchopulmonary diseases (chronic bronchitis, emphysema) in the United States.

7. Lung cancer death rates continue to rise sharply. Those who smoke less than one pack a day have mortality rates as high as 10% greater than nonsmokers, and smokers of more than one pack a day have mortality rates as high as 30% greater than nonsmokers. Similarly, the death rates from cancers of the oral cavity, larynx, esophagus, kidney, urinary bladder, and pancreas are all considerably higher for smokers than nonsmokers.

8. The oral cavity suffers additional trauma beyond cancer because of excessive smoke. Gum inflammation, bony-tissue destruction, and loss of teeth are all more common among smokers than nonsmokers. Solomon has reported that women smokers, ages 20 to 39, have twice the chance of losing all their teeth than women who do not smoke; the same holds for men ages 30 to 59.*

9. Babies born to smoking mothers average half a pound less than those born to nonsmoking mothers. Spontaneous abortions, stillbirths, and premature deliveries are higher among pregnant women who smoke.

Triggering lung cancer

Normally, the lining of the bronchial tubes of the lungs includes two layers of cells. The first layer consists of columnar cells (they look like columns) with a few goblet cells (they look like wine goblets) interspersed. The goblet cells secrete a sticky fluid to the surface. The columnar

*Solomon, H. A., and others: Cigarette smoking and periodontal disease, Medical Bulletin on Tobacco **6:**4, December 1968.

Trachea

Innominate artery

Left common carotid artery

Right lung upper lobe

Subclavian artery

Arch of aorta

Left lung upper lobe

Pulmonary artery

Right lung middle lobe

Heart

Right lung lower lobe

Left lung lower lobe

Diaphragm

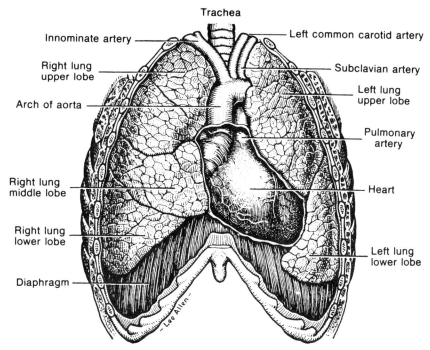

Fig. 6-3. Illustration of organs of thoracic cavity. Part of pericardium has been removed to expose heart. The heart and lungs are both affected by inhaled smoke. Tars in smoke deposit on the epithelium of the bronchioles and clog the alveoli. The cilia are paralyzed, and mucus accumulates. Coughing ruptures the alveoli and small encapsulating capillaries, forcing the heart to pump blood through a smaller number of capillaries, against increased pressure, on a reduced oxygen supply. (From Tuttle, W. W., and Schottelius, B. A.: Textbook of physiology, ed. 16, St. Louis, 1969, The C. V. Mosby Co.)

cells contain short hairlike cilia that protrude to the surface and with a whiplike motion move the sticky fluid (mucus) toward the throat, where it is either swallowed or expectorated. The second layer is composed of small, round cells with relatively small nuclei, called basal cells. Beneath these two layers of cells is a thin webbing of tiny fibers, called the basement membrane.

The action of the cilia is extremely important. In moving mucus up the tubules to the throat, foreign particles that reach the lungs via the air inhaled are eliminated. Tobacco smoke, however, inhibits the whiplike movement of the cilia, and if excessive, may even paralyze this movement completely. Thus, the tars in tobacco smoke are allowed to accumulate on the lining of the bronchial tubes.

As the tars build up, three changes have been observed to occur in the bronchial epithelium: hyperplasia (an increase in the number of layers of cells, as with a callus on the hand), reduction in the number of ciliated columnar cells, and changes in the nuclei of the cells. When the nucleus of a cell is altered and through division this alteration is replicated, a cancerous condition exists. The nuclei of cancer cells are usually large, irregular in shape, and have an abnormal number of chromosomes. When atypical cell formation first begins, these cells are found only in the epithelium layer. As they proliferate, however, they penetrate the basement layer and invade the underlying tissue. A carcinoma, or tumor, composed of cells with atypical nuclei, develops. This grows to considerable size and spreads to other parts of the body.

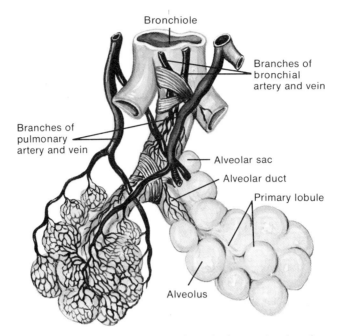

Fig. 6-4. Illustration showing termination of bronchiole in alveolar duct and sacs and relationship of blood supply to these structures. Bronchioles clogged by tars are subject to the proliferation of epithelial cells with atypical nuclei. The tiny air sacs formed by terminal expansion of the bronchioles are called alveoli. Oxygen enters the bloodstream, and carbon dioxide is given up by the alveoli. When the bronchioles constrict and the alveolar tissue is destroyed, the rate at which the lungs can exchange oxygen and carbon dioxide is reduced. Emphysema and other abnormal conditions develop. (From Tuttle, W. W., and Schottelius, B. A.: Textbook of physiology, ed. 16, St. Louis, 1969, The C. V. Mosby Co.)

It appears that exposure to tobacco smoke produces a change in the local environment of bronchial epithelium, which favors the survival and replication of cells with atypical nuclei. Thus, the development of cancer results from natural selection under conditions of greatly altered environment. Normal cells are best adapted to an environment free of tobacco smoke, whereas cells with atypical nuclei are best adapted to an environment that includes smoke.

Cancer is but one of several conditions that tobacco smoke appears to trigger. Lung infections, emphysema, and coronary artery disease also occur at significantly higher rates among smokers than among nonsmokers.

Tobacco habituation

If smoking, particularly cigarettes, is so directly tied to disease, why do people develop and continue the habit? This question and its answer constitute the second point on the devil's two-tined fork.

Earlier we discussed the distinction between addiction and habituation. Tobacco use is an habituation in that once established, there is little tendency to increase the dose; psychic but not physical dependence is developed; the detrimental effects are primarily on the individual rather than society; and no characteristic abstinence syndrome is developed upon withdrawal.

But why does the habit develop in the first place? In the case of children and adolescents, mimicry of adult behavior definitely is a factor. That smoking contributes to peer group membership is no less important. Nicotine is also a stimulant of the nervous system, which is the attraction for many. Beyond these reasons a number of psychologic factors appear to enter the picture; manipulating the cigarette and sucking on it is similar to the early breast or bottle experience; it gives people something to do, gracefully, in social situations; the optical perception of the smoke is pleasantly and mildly hypnotic; and some claim is made for the capacity of smoking to build self-confidence.

It is important to make clear that neither nicotine nor tobacco comply with any of the requirements considered necessary to demonstrate drug addiction. In fact, heavy smokers may cease abruptly and, while retaining the desire to smoke, experience no significant symptoms of withdrawal. What is observable to others as they watch a friend who struggles to break the habit is any one or several of a gamut of mild symptoms: in some, insomnia, anxiety, tremor, palpitation, and restlessness occur; in others, there is diminished excitability manifested as drowsiness, amnesia, impaired concentration and judgment, and diminished pulse. Although these withdrawal symptoms are reported to continue for days, weeks, or even months, they never constitute a threat to life.

Smoker's Anonymous doesn't exist, but it might sometime in the future. One wag has described its function as follows: "When you feel like smoking, you call two friends and they come over and drink with you." Beyond the humor of this joke is the point that consumable substances that are one person's weakness may be another person's strength. Such is the nature of most substances that endanger health.

CAFFEINE AND OTHER XANTHINES

The xanthines, caffeine, theophylline, and theobromine are mild drugs that can cause habituation. Caffeine is the familiar drug found in coffee; theophylline and caffeine are the drug constituents in tea; theobromine is in cocoa. Caffeine is the strongest of the three, theobromine the weakest.

Caffeine is a strong alkaloid that dilates the blood vessels, stimulates intestinal peristalsis, and increases both respiration and heat production. Also, it elevates the mood slightly and relieves fatigue.

Moderate use of coffee, tea, cocoa, cola (which also contains caffeine), or other xanthine-containing drinks is not harmful to most people. In excessive amounts they may cause nervousness and insomnia. If cardiovascular problems are present, the consumption of coffee and tea may be controlled or discontinued. What effect the xanthines have on life span, if any, is insignificant and impossible to measure.

ACCIDENTAL POISONING

In contrast to "nature's dangerous gifts" of drugs, alcohol, and tobacco, which are intentionally used for their physical and mental effects, many poisons usually found in the home are occasionally accidently ingested. The list grows longer almost by the day: deodorants, depilatories, detergents, pesticides, petroleum products, stimulants, sedatives, and many others. Unfortunately, the younger age group is the one most usually affected.

Prevention, of course, is the primary concern. Necessary precautions include the following:

1. Keep all drugs, poisonous substances, and household chemicals away from the very young, the very old, and the emotionally disturbed.
2. Do not store poisonous substances on the same shelves with food or in food-identified containers.
3. Do not leave discarded or outdated medicines in regularly accessible areas.
4. Never give medicine to children under the guise of candy.
5. Read *all* labels before using.
6. Never take or give any ingestant in the dark.

When you know that someone has accidentally taken a poisonous substance, the unabsorbed poison should be removed from the stomach as soon as possible. To induce vomiting is commonly believed appropriate, and it is if the situation does not contraindicate. Vomiting should *not* be induced if the victim is unconscious, is in convulsions, has severe pain, or is known to have swallowed acid, strychnine, or a petroleum product. When vomiting is appropriate, this can be done by giving a glass of milk first and then inducing gagging by inserting a finger down the throat. Three or four tea-spoonfuls of syrup of ipecac (not usually in the home but should be) will usually produce prompt vomiting. Ingested acids may be neutralized by any of the following substances: 8 to 20 teaspoonfuls of milk of magnesia, a diluted sodium bicarbonate solution, 4 tablespoonfuls of aluminum hydroxide gel. To neutralize an ingested alkali, 1 or 2 glassfuls of lemon or orange juice may be administered.

The poison should be identified as soon as possible, and the container saved. It should be taken with the patient to the nearest emergency hospital service, or a physician should be called if this is the more rapid way to get expert assistance. Over 200 poison control centers in the country offer another avenue of assistance. Since 1953, when the first center was established in Chicago, these centers maintain an up-to-date list of the poisons in most substances and will give you valuable emergency instructions by telephone, together with a specific antidote if there is one. Such a center is most likely available to you.

PESTICIDES

To set the tone for her book *Silent Spring,* Rachel Carson used the following two passages.

> The sedge is wither'd from the lake,
> And no birds sing.
> KEATS

> I am pessimistic about the human race because it is too ingenious for its own good. Our approach to nature is to beat it into submission. We would stand a better chance of survival if we accommodated ourselves to this planet and viewed it appreciatively instead of skeptically and dictatorially.
> E. B. WHITE

Keats, writing a century and a half ago, saw beauty being raped. The sober words by White, less poetic but equally chilling, voice the present concerns felt by increasing numbers. For Miss Carson and for us, pesticides provide an awesome example of our present predicament and potential doom.

A pesticide is an agent to kill pests. Under this broad category fall such terms as insecticides, rodenticides, fungicides, miticides, and herbicides, which are agents used specifically to kill insects, rodents, fungi, mites, and plants.

Although there had been sporadic concern for the increasing reservoir of pesticide pollution before the publication of *Silent Spring* in 1962, Rachel Carson's book brought all arguments into the open. Where once pesticides were touted as a means to "control the environment" in man's behalf, they were seen, overnight, as a worldwide menace.

Registered death

There are over 45,000 pesticides registered with the Department of Agriculture; approximately 1,000 of these are actually in use. Before World War II, most pesticides were inorganic compounds, with arsenic as the prime example. Arsenic is a highly toxic mineral occurring widely in association with the ores of various metals. It was the first recognized carcinogen (producer of cancer) and has caused many epidemics of arsenic poisoning. Much sickness and some deaths have been caused by arsenic-contaminated wells in various sections of the country, even to the present day.

Most modern pesticides fall into one of two large groups of organic chemicals. One is known as the chlorinated hydrocarbons, with DDT the prime example. The other group has organic phosphorus as its base and is illustrated by the familiar malathion and parathion.

Biologic magnification

Although DDT (dichlorodiphenyltrichloroethane) was synthesized by a German chemist in 1874, its properties as an insecticide were not discovered until 1939. Since then it has been used worldwide to control various pests, and through the 1950's was viewed as harmless by most of those who promoted or used it.

Evidence began to mount, however, that suggested a problem with continued indiscriminate use of DDT. Although DDT provided quick extermination of pests, nature's balance appeared to be upset. To understand the long-term effects of DDT, Clear Lake near San Francisco was carefully studied. This was a large weedy lake populated by gnats, called midges, that irritated fishermen and local residents. A chemical closely related to DDT was applied to the lake in amounts of 0.02 of one part per million parts of water in order to control the midges. This was equal to a few drops in a railway tank car of water. Thirteen months later analysis of the insecticide residues showed that there were.

1. 10 parts per million of insecticide in the lake's plankton
2. 903 parts per million of insecticide in the fat of plankton-eating fish
3. 2,690 parts per million of insecticide in the fat of fish-eating fish
4. 2,134 parts per million of insecticide in the fat of fish-eating birds (Most of the fish-eating birds had died.)

This process has become known as biologic magnification. Small life forms collect tiny bits of DDT, which is very soluble in fat but not in water. When the small forms are eaten by larger forms, the DDT, with a half-life of 10 years, goes along in the fat and is concentrated in the larger form's fat. DDT is attracted to fat like filings to a magnet. Throughout the food chain, from gnat to frog to bass to birds, the DDT endures and is passed along for over 10 years.

The intricacies of ecologic balance

Commercial and sport fishing on the Great Lakes, once extensive, very nearly became extinct after the St. Lawrence Seaway was opened in 1959. The lakes were invaded by alewives, a St. Lawrence River fish of low nutritional value, and by the parasitic lamprey. By the mid-1960's fishing was at a low ebb.

Fishery ecologists shifted the balance when they stocked Lake Michigan with Coho salmon, indigenous to the Northwest but a mortal enemy of the lamprey. The

lampreys quickly disappeared, and the other revived species of fish took care of the alewives. Commercial and sport fishing improved.

In March 1969 the FDA tested Coho salmon caught in the Great Lakes. It found 13 to 19 parts per million of DDT with traces of the more potent dieldrin in all Coho salmon tested. Seventeen tons of the salmon were ordered seized, and a new problem confronted the fishing industry. The FDA had set DDT limits for fish sold commercially, containing 3.5 parts of insecticide per million; this was raised to 5 parts per million in late 1969, but the Coho salmon were still dangerously contaminated.

How much is too much?

If a man eats one-fourth pound of salmon with 21 parts per million of DDT, he gets 2.52 milligrams of DDT. To study the effect of various levels of DDT in man, a Public Health Service test was conducted on volunteers in a Federal prison. No immediate effect could be detected with 35 milligrams of insecticide consumed daily for 21 months. When the dosage was increased to 154 milligrams daily, burning and itching of the face, tongue, and lips developed. These amounts would appear to lull the unsuspecting. Yet man stores DDT just as animals do. Individuals with no known exposure have been shown to store 5 to 8 parts per million, agricultural workers 17.1 parts per million, and workers in insecticide plants as high as 648 parts per million. Even the lower figures are above the level at which damage to the liver and other organs or tissues may begin. In animal experiments, 3 parts per million inhibits an essential enzyme in heart muscle; 5 parts per million brings about necrosis, or disintegration of liver cells.

As many as 200 deaths per year are attributed to pesticide poisoning, mostly of young children, mostly by accident. Nonlethal pesticide poisoning may run as high as 50,000 cases a year and may be higher. But questions of the long-term effects of pesticides remain unanswered. Data compiled by the World Health Organization suggest that liver damage and protein and sugar metabolism disturbances are initiated by excessive pesticide intake. The spectre of cancer also looms as a consequence. A number of chemical pesticides are known to produce cancers in mice. Although the medical community is reluctant to make the direct transposition to human beings, Dr. Malcolm M. Hargraves of the Mayo Clinic commented on the research of the National Cancer Institute to *Medical World News* in 1969:

Since the advent of pesticides in 1947, I've seen and taken inquisitive personal histories of 1200 cases of blood dyscrasias and lymphoid diseases. Every patient at some time or another had great exposure to a pesticide, an herbicide, a paint thinner, a cleaning agent, or the like. . . . I've had several cases demonstrating their involvement in blood marrow depression, sudden prothrombin changes, liver insufficiency, and thrombocytopenia purpura.

Geneticists at the Oak Ridge National Laboratory in Tennessee and the Jackson Laboratory in Maine are conducting intensive research on the relationship between pesticides and cancer; they have called this "our number one health problem." Cancer in an existing population is bad enough, but it may prove minor beside the possibility of genetic change, which pesticides portend to cause.

Breakthrough

Much of our difficulty resides in the fact that the chlorinated hydrocarbons and organic phosphorus compounds are so stable. As stated earlier, the half-life of DDT is 10 years. The potential for immense reserves to build up in any living system are therefore great. If a means could be found to trigger earlier natural breakdown of these complex poisonous molecules once they escape to the free environment, part of our present problem could be solved.

In a speech before the Wisconsin chapter of the American Public Works Association in 1970, Carl L. Klein, Assistant Secretary of the Interior for water and quality re-

search, said: "We think we can get to the pocket of the problem. We may have found a way to turn off pesticides when we need to." Under a government-financed project the Aerojet General Corporation has experimented with a method that involves removing three chlorine atoms from each particle of one particular pesticide and combining chlorine atoms of other pesticides. Thus, the effective characteristics are retained, but the pesticide is short lived in nature and undergoes disintegration. Work on this breakthrough continues. We hope it will prove successful.

AIR POLLUTION

Are we fighting a losing battle with man-made air pollution? If you fly occasionally, notice the murky haze that hangs over most cities nearly every day: New York, Chicago, Los Angeles, Kansas City, even Knoxville, and Portland (Maine and Oregon), as well as many, many others. The fallout over these cities increases each year: an average winter day in New York City produces an estimated 335 tons of particulate matter; in Kansas City dustfall in the winter measures more than 67 tons a square mile a month. Where does it come from?

The processes of pollution

Civilization maintains three air-contaminating activities: attrition, vaporization, and combustion.

Attrition is simple friction. It is the wearing down of shoe bottoms, automobile tires, knives as they are sharpened, and many others, all caused by friction-producing activities. The industrial processes of sanding, grinding, demolishing, drilling, and spraying are prime examples of pollution via attrition.

Vaporization occurs when a substance such as gasoline changes from a liquid to a gas. This may happen as a consequence of heat or pressure or through natural evaporation of volatile materials. (A volatile material is one that readily evaporates at normal temperatures.) Most odors, offensive or otherwise, are caused by vaporization.

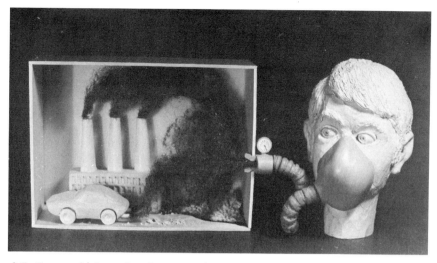

Fig. 6-5. Our world is a closed system. The poisons we release to it are significant and constitute a real threat to personal health. (Courtesy Martin Webster.)

Combustion is the major contributor to our air pollution problem. Combustion is the process of burning, that is, the chemical combination of certain substances with oxygen, and the product is energy plus waste materials. We covet the energy and are plagued by the waste materials. Furnaces, internal combustion engines, the diesel engine, jet-propelled engines, and incinerators expel combusted pollutants to the atmosphere with relatively little control to date.

Nature, with the help of man, creates still another form of air pollution, and one that is not yet completely understood: photochemical smog. Originally the term referred to a combination of smoke and fog, as was common in London. In Los Angeles the term was used before what occasioned there was completely understood. Now we know that the Los Angeles smog is caused by the action of sunlight on automobile emissions. The sun's energy is absorbed by nitrogen dioxide in the presence of some hydrocarbons. The compound then breaks into nitric oxide and atomic oxygen. The atomic oxygen reacts with the oxygen molecules of the atmosphere to form ozone and with other constituents of automobile exhausts to form a variety of products. Hundreds of chemical transformations occur,

and many undesirable chemicals result, including peroxyacyl nitrate (PAN) and formaldehyde.

The sources and types of pollutants

There are five primary sources of air pollution: transportation (your car plus the ninety million other vehicles, plus trains, airplanes, motorcycles, etc.), industry (the pulp and paper mills, iron and steel mills, petroleum refineries, smelters, chemical manufacturers, and others), power plants, space heating, and refuse disposal. Table 6-6 is an estimate of the type and amount of major pollutants from each of these sources per year.

Although these figures tend to be impressive, the figures have limited use. They are worthwhile when standards for control are being set, when the effectiveness of methods of control are being examined, or when the existing danger at any given time is being evaluated. But it is more important to know the concentration of pollutants in the air at a specific time and place. The level of pollution might rise to the immediately dangerous level and necessitate quick action. If that level is approached anywhere, authorities need to be aware of it. The Federal Air Quality Act of 1967 gives the Secretary of Health, Education,

Table 6-6. National sources of major air pollutants (millions of tons per year)

Source	Carbon monoxide	Sulfur oxides	Hydrocar-bons	Nitrogen oxides	Particulate matter	Miscellane-ous other	Total
Transportation	66	1	12	6	1	*	86
Industry	2	9	4	2	6	2	25
Power plants	1	12	*	3	3	*	20
Space heating	2	3	1	1	1	*	8
Refuse disposal	1	*	1	*	1	*	4
Total	72	25	18	12	12	4	143

From Air pollution primer, New York, 1969, National Tuberculosis and Respiratory Disease Association, p. 34.
*Less than 1.

and Welfare the right to close down polluting sources at any spot in the nation where and when an emergency prevails.

The following list is of the major categories of pollutants and their related compounds that are sampled regularly in our atmosphere. (Consult your chemistry text for a complete analysis of each.)

Sulfur and its compounds are a major reason for many pollution problems. These include: sulfur dioxide (SO_2), sulfurous acid (H_2SO_3), sulfuric acid (H_2SO_4), sulfur trioxide (SO_3), and hydrogen sulfide gas (H_2S).

Carbon is a main constituent in organic fuels. Its contribution to pollution is tremendous: soot or simply finely divided carbon particles, carbon monoxide (CO), and carbon dioxide (CO_2).

The hydrocarbons contain both carbon and oxygen in various combinations. Two groups of hydrocarbons are of the greatest importance: (1) the olefin or ethylene series, and (2) the aromatic, benzenoid, or benzene series. The olefins appear not to have any direct effect on animal life; the aromatics appear to be carcinogenic. Most dangerous in the latter group is benzpyrene.

Nitrogen oxides are still another ingredient in the pollution picture. There are several, but only two are considered pollutants: nitric oxide (NO), and nitrogen dioxide (NO_2), a dangerous gas. The latter combines with water vapor or raindrops to form nitric acid (HNO_3).

Fluoride compounds also pollute when the discharge is excessive at an industrial source.

Finally, the products of photochemistry (action of sunlight on all the above pollutants) are a major cause of eye irritation, breathing difficulty, vegetation damage, deterioration of materials, and decreased visibility. Some of these have been discussed briefly earlier: oxidant, ozone, PAN, and the aldehydes.

Effects of pollution

Several episodes provide us with examples of extreme pollution. In December 1930 in Belgium's industrial Muse Valley 62 persons died during a 3-day smog. In January 1931, 592 persons died in Manchester, England, because of smog. In 1948 in Donora, Pennsylvania, half the town's population of 14,000 became ill during a 4-day smog, with 22 deaths. A great smog blanketed London in 1952 and left dead 4,000 more than would have normally been expected. A recurrence in 1956 caused another 1,000 deaths. In New York City in November 1953 there were 220 deaths caused by heavy air pollution; in 1963 an episode caused 350 deaths; and in 1966, again in New York City, 168 deaths were registered during a Thanksgiving weekend episode of heavy air pollution. Periods of stifling smog that completely envelope a city are on the increase. More deaths than we would normally expect are on the increase. These gross statistics are irrefutable.

Can we be sure at the person level that the smog, or polluted air in general, is a long-range deterrent to health? Epidemiologic surveys, clinical studies, industrial research, laboratory experiments, and even

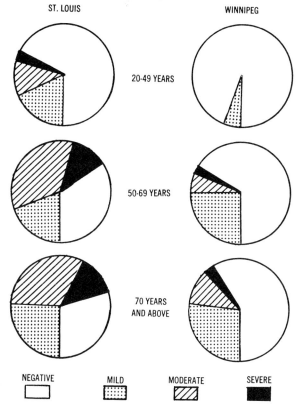

ST. LOUIS   WINNIPEG

20-49 YEARS

50-69 YEARS

70 YEARS
AND ABOVE

NEGATIVE   MILD   MODERATE   SEVERE

Fig. 6-6. Prevalence of emphysema, as found in a 1960-66 postmortem examination of the lungs of 300 residents of heavily industrialized St. Louis, Missouri, and an equal number from relatively unpolluted Winnipeg, Canada. The subjects were well matched by sex, occupation, socioeconomic status, length of residence, smoking habits, and age at death. The findings clearly suggest a link between air pollution and pulmonary emphysema. (From National Tuberculosis and Respiratory Disease Association: Air pollution primer, New York, 1969, The Association.)

information derived from accidents are providing increasing evidence of a statistical relationship. Proof positive of a direct cause-and-effect relationship is still over the horizon.

Scientists now believe that air pollution may actually alter the body's responses to infectious diseases. Specifically, the following changes occur.

1. Certain irritants can slow down and even stop the action of the cilia and thus leave the epithelial cells without protection (recall now the tobacco discussion).

2. The irritants can cause the production of increased or thickened mucus, cause a constriction of the airways, induce swelling or excessive growth of the cells that form the lining of the airways, and cause a loss of cilia or even of several layers of cells.

3. As a consequence, breathing may become more difficult, and foreign matter, including bacteria and other microorganisms may not be effectively removed, thus resulting in respiratory infection.

Pollution has been linked to respiratory disease, both acute and chronic. Epidemiologic studies in Nashville, Tennessee (1960), Los Angeles (1961), Cumberland, Maryland (1950), as well as studies in Great Britain, Japan, and the U. S. S. R. have shown a close correlation between air pollution and allergic disorders, acute upper respiratory infections, influenza, bronchitis, and heart and vascular diseases. The common cold is more prevalent among those subjected to excessive pollution.

The more severe chronic respiratory diseases—bronchial asthma, chronic bronchitis, pulmonary emphysema, and lung cancer—also are higher among smog-bound dwellers. Fig. 6-6 compares the prevalence of emphysema in polluted St. Louis with relatively unpolluted Winnipeg, Canada.

Air pollution control on an area-wide basis of many hundreds or thousands of miles must be planned even beyond national boundaries. Sulfur dioxide freed in Germany floats over Sweden and is precipitated as sulfuric acid in rain. In Poza Rica, Mexico, an accident at a sulfur-producing factory spilled hydrogen sulfide into the atmosphere during a fog-patched inversion. Within half an hour enough hydrogen sulfide escaped and remained in the air to kill 22 people and cause 320 to be hospitalized.

Before you take that next breath, will it be a safe one? Probably. But what about tomorrow, next winter, next year? Are you concerned? You should be. We all should be.

WATER POLLUTION

How strange that we should conclude our chapter on substances endangering health with a brief discussion of water. We take for granted the fact that drinking water is a faucet-turn away, and yet it may not be. Too long we have used our rivers and lakes as open sewers, and now we must scramble to restore a healthful balance. Pollution in our municipal water supplies serving two-thirds of the population, and tragically, also in many deep-well water supplies, may be one or more of the following types.

1. Oxygen-demanding wastes are the traditional organic wastes contributed by home sewage and industrial wastes of plant and animal origin. Also included are wastes from food processing, paper mill production, and tanning. These wastes are usually destroyed by bacteria if there is sufficient oxygen present in the water. But when the wastes are excessive, the oxygen is depleted and fish die.

2. Disease-causing agents include infectious organisms that are carried into surface and ground water by sewage from cities and institutions. Usually chlorine gas is fed into the water during primary treatment of sewage to kill disease-causing bacteria.

3. Plant nutrients are the substances in the food chain of aquatic life, such as algae and water weeds, which support and stimulate the growth of aquatic life. Nitrogen and phosphorus are the two chief nutrients present in small amounts in natural water, but much more is contributed by sewage, certain industrial wastes, and drainage from fertilized lands. Biologic waste treatment processes do not remove the nutrients; in fact, they convert the organic forms of these substances into mineral form, making them more usable by plant life. As a consequence, the algae and water weeds reproduce to the point of choking off all other life.

4. Synthetic organic chemicals are the detergents, the synthetic organic pesticides discussed earlier, and synthetic industrial chemicals. Most of these are toxic to fish, cause taste and odor problems, and resist conventional waste treatment.

5. Inorganic chemicals and mineral substances include mineral salts, acids, solid matter, and many other chemical compounds. The sources of pollution include mining and manufacturing processes, oil field operations, agricultural practices, and natural sources. The largest single source of acid in our water comes from mining operations and mines that have been abandoned. (Our plunder of the land comes back to haunt us, with serious health consequences.)

6. Sediments are the particles of soils, sands, and minerals that wash from the land into our streams and lakes. Sediments are a problem because of their sheer magnitude in our waterways. They fill stream channels and reservoirs, erode power turbines and pumping equipment, blanket fish nests and food supplies, and reduce the amount of sunlight penetrating the water. Sunlight is required by green aquatic plants, which produce the oxygen necessary to normal stream balance.

7. Radioactive substances result from the mining and processing of radioactive ores; from the use of refined radioactive materials in power reactors and for industrial, medical, and research purposes; and from fallout following nuclear weapons testing. This last source has ceased to be important since international agreements to limit testing went into effect.

Although the Atomic Energy Commission has a superb record (26 years of operation without a reactor accident in the country), the chances for accidental radioactive release increase steadily. Today nuclear energy accounts for about 1% of all energy produced in this country; it is expected to represent close to 30% by 1980. We now have 85 nuclear-powered ocean vessels and will build another 46 in the next few years. Trucks travel over our highways carrying radioactive materials, and people are increasingly working with or using nuclear fuels and radioisotopes.

8. Heated water loses its capacity to absorb oxygen. Power plants and industry use large quantities of water for cooling and then return the water, at a raised temperature, to streams and rivers, thus raising their temperatures. With less oxygen, the water is not as efficient in assimilating oxygen-consuming wastes and in supporting aquatic life.

Seldom is a body of water polluted by only one of these eight wastes. Generally, pollution is the consequence of several different wastes in combination, thus making the task of treatment quite difficult.

How extensive is water pollution? In June 1970 the Illinois State Health Department announced that not one lake or river in the state was safe enough for swimming. Lake Erie, once a beautiful body of water, has been declared "dead"; that is, it will no longer support life. The Hudson River is an open sewer and cannot be used as a source for drinking water with present treatment capabilities despite its flow of 30,000 gallons per second. Similarly, the Connecticut, Merrimac (Massachusetts), Willamette (Oregon), Ohio, and Mississippi Rivers, plus many, many more have been despoiled

perhaps to the point of no return, unless we change our ways.

The Water Quality Act of 1965, which established water quality standards for all interstate streams, coastal waters, and lakes, and the Clean Water Restoration Act of 1966, which increased Federal financial aid to cities to help build the necessary treatment plants, provide us with the appropriate legislation. With the cooperation of local municipalities and state water control agencies, it is hoped that a conventional secondary treatment level (reducing the biochemical oxygen demand in wastes by 85%) will be achieved in nearly all parts of the country by 1973. In order for this to happen the interest of many people, at the local level, must be peaked enough to support bond issues proposed for modernization and increase in water treatment facilities. You soon will have the option to vote for or against such an issue. It matters little where you locate; there will undoubtedly be a water problem. How will you respond?

A MATTER OF CHOICE

We've touched on a few problems that are primarily of a personal nature and some that are of a community-wide nature. Each problem constitutes a danger to personal health. Against some we can take direct action in order to *control* their *influence* on our person—if we wish to. Others require that (1) we work through community organizations and (2) we exercise our privilege to vote whenever necessary if we are to *influence* their *effect* to our person. All dangerous substances remain within our capacity, as individuals and as responsible members of a community, to control. Drug addiction, alcoholism, use of tobacco, ravaged lands, and polluted waters will remain or disappear as we decide at the personal level.

ON MAINTAINING YOUR BALANCE

The substances that endanger our health are numerous. They permeate our environment and remind us constantly of their presence. Often it is difficult for us to maintain our balance, and we may lose it to a clearly observable degree (as with the alcoholic or the drug addict). There is good evidence that all of us, especially if we live in metropolitan areas, are being affected deleteriously, by way of the air we breathe, the food we eat, and the water we drink, even when we strive with diligence to continue wise and beneficial personal health habits.

Is it worth the effort to fight these problems? Why not? Certainly there is much to lose if you abdicate personal effort, and there is much to gain if you don't.

CHAPTER 7
The impingement of disease on man

The delicate balance between man and his environment is tenuous at best. Man is in competition with many agents—biologic, chemical, physical, and mechanical—that seek to disrupt his equilibrium. When disequilibrium occurs, the consequence, unless checked, will be progressive disintegration beginning with the loss of homeostasis and leading through disease and disability to death.

Our discussion of disease to this point has been secondary to the positive health principles we have presented. But disease is, either directly or indirectly, very much a part of our lives. We need to understand its nature and extent if we are to reject, remove, reduce, or retard its ravaging effects.

NATURE OF DISEASE

Disease, taken literally, means the lack or absence of ease. It is any malfunctioning of the body and includes, among others, those conditions caused by the lack of some nutrient (Chapter 4), those that manifest in some form of mental ailment (Chapter 2), those that are communicable, and those that are caused by some loss or degenerative impairment of the cells. This chapter will focus on the communicable and degenerative diseases.

Disease in retrospect

Recorded history tells us that man has long viewed disease as one of the mysteries of life. Primitive people accepted disease as an evil and engaged in forms of voodoo, quarantine or banishment, tribal dancing, and the use of noise and smoke to drive these evil spirits away. As recently as 100 years ago night airs were described as the cause of epidemics, and "knowing" people resorted to the burning of pitch and the firing of cannon as combative measures.

Without a real, scientific base earlier civilizations often took effective measures to restrict the spread of disease. The Minoans (5000 B.C.) and the Cretans (3000–1800 B.C.) constructed drainage systems, water closets, and water-flushing systems. The Egyptians of 1000 B.C. had a fetish for personal cleanliness, and the Jews developed the Mosaic law, the first formal hygienic code.

The early Greek civilization exalted the human body. Attention was given to personal cleanliness, exercise, and diet; and the concerns of environmental sanitation were deemphasized to some extent. Ill and diseased persons were ignored, banished, or even deliberately destroyed. To be sick was a sign of weakness, and weakness was not compatible with nor did it contribute to the goals of Greek society.

The Christian church gained power in the early centuries following Christ's death, and a philosophy that elevated the soul, even to the rejection of the body, became prominent. At this time sickness, pain, and disease were viewed as obstacles; the greater the obstacle, the more sure was man of a happy existence after death. As a consequence, personal and community health were almost ignored, thus adding fuel to the potential for the wildfire spread of disease. And spread it did. Cholera, leprosy, bubonic plague, tuberculosis, and smallpox caused the premature death of millions of people throughout Europe and Asia. Quarantine and the 40-day detention of ships in certain Mediterranean ports to prevent the spread of the Black Death (bubonic plague) were established without knowledge as to how the disease was really spread. Consequently, rats continued to transmit the disease from man to man between ports. In the 40 years from 1320 to 1360 alone, bubonic plague accounted for 13 million deaths in China; India was decimated; and 10 to 15 thousand died daily in Cairo when the disease was at its peak.

Man has been chained to his environment until almost modern times. The ravages of communicable diseases over many centuries made him the victim of much suffering and a short life span. Mental disorders and degenerative diseases were also his fare, but their significance is lost because of the awesomeness of the more acute communicable diseases.

The Renaissance (1500-1700 A.D.) offered a glimmer of hope. Through the brilliant efforts of such men as Andreas Vesalius (1514-1564), founder of the science of anatomy; Ambroise Paré (1510-1590), distinguished surgeon; William Harvey (1578-1657), discoverer of the circulatory system; and Antonj van Leeuwenhoek (1632-1723), inventor of the microscope, knowledge slowly accumulated that later contributed to even more significant discoveries.

The eighteenth and nineteenth centuries included events that contributed directly to the dramatic increase in life expectancy that has taken place in the twentieth century. Notable contributions were made by Giovanni Morgagni (1682-1771), the first great pathologist; Simon Tissot (1728-1797), medical author and physician; Edward Jenner (1749-1823), discoverer of the first effective smallpox vaccine; and the triumvirate of Louis Pasteur (1822-1895), Robert Koch (1843-1910), and Emil von Behring (1854-1917), founders of the science of bacteriology and world escorts into the modern era of preventive medicine. Scientific advances during this time included the stethoscope, the clinical thermometer, the x-ray, anesthesia, and the antiseptic method. Germ theory was established; the theory of evolution shook the academic world; and genetic theory hovered in the wings.

The natural history of disease

In the early years of the twentieth century increasing knowledge about pathogenic organisms allowed health officials to exercise control procedures directed at the three variables of the disease process: characteristics of man (host), characteristics of the pathogen (agent), and the characteristics of the surroundings (environment) that contribute to the interaction between host and agent. This concept of interaction, the biologic explanation of communicable disease, was used by public health workers in the early 1900's to bring the serious diseases under control. Since then, and particularly in the past 20 years, the concept has been extended to other diseases affecting man, such as obesity, mental disorders, and even accidents. Today disease (and the qualifier "all," though not yet appropriate, may soon be) is viewed ecologically and is based on the three premises of the biologic laws:

1. Disease is the consequence of an imbalance between agent and host.
2. The degree of imbalance depends on the nature and characteristics of the agent and host.
3. The nature and characteristics of the agent and host are affected by the nature of the physical, social, economic, and biologic environment.

Two living organisms interact in communicable diseases; one living organism and a nonliving disease agent interact in noncommunicable diseases. This process of interaction may be divided into two parts, prepathogenesis and pathogenesis.

Prepathogenesis. Long before a person is involved with a specific disease, precipitating events must take place. For example, the condition of obesity is of sufficient seriousness in affluent societies to warrant its identification as a disease. Before the necessary disease agent—a food supply that greatly exceeds individual needs—can affect

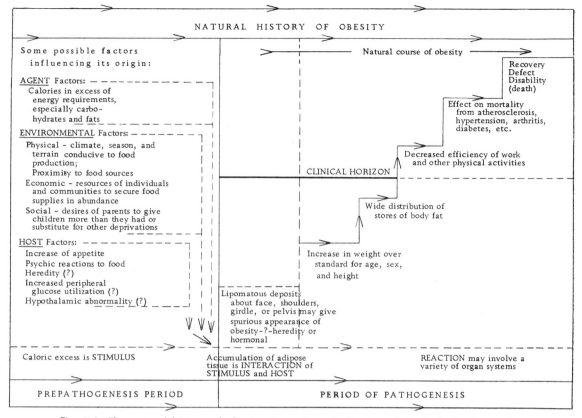

Fig. 7-1. The natural history of obesity. (From Leavell, H. R., and Clark, E. G.: Preventive medicine for the doctor in his community, ed. 3, New York, 1965, McGraw-Hill Book Co. Copyright 1965 McGraw-Hill Book Co. Used with permission of McGraw-Hill Book Co.)

one individual, there must be technologic control of the environment so that production of all necessary nutrients exceeds the society's needs for sustained periods of time. Status symbols attached to food by the society must also contribute to its characteristics as an agent, as must individual insecurity, fear, frustration, and the lack of accomplishment, which are satisfied psychologically through increased food intake. Given the presence of these factors, the second aspect of the disease process will occur.

Pathogenesis. The natural course of a disorder, or period of pathogenesis, refers to those events that occur from the time of the individual's first interaction with a disease-inducing stimulus through resultant changes in form or function to the time of recovery, disability, or death. In obesity,

food supply (agent) in excess of need, accompanied by pressures (environment) that create psychologic and/or physiologic needs in the individual (host), results in excessive food intake and an insidious gain in weight. Obesity itself precedes and is related to other serious conditions, such as heart disease, circulatory disorders, endocrine disease, and joint disease. These latter consequences are discussed later in this chapter.

The two processes of prepathogenesis and pathogenesis together comprise the natural history of a disease. In Fig. 7-1 some of the elements in the natural history of obesity are illustrated.

Current state of knowledge about disease

The modern status of knowledge about disease is a dramatic contrast to that of earlier times. Much of the mystery and confusion about disease that once prevailed has been eliminated. When only a century ago we knew very little, today over 100 communicable diseases that affect man, ranging from actinomycosis to yaws, are understood; and various control measures have been described. Vaccines have been developed against no fewer than 12 important viral infections, including smallpox, rabies, yellow fever, three forms of encephalomyelitis (Western, Eastern, and Venezuelan), both Japanese and Russian encephalitis, certain respiratory viruses including influenza A and B and adenovirus, poliomyelitis, rubeola (measles), rubella (German measles), and mumps. Most of these vaccines have been developed since Enders introduced practicable cell culture technology in the late 1940's. Others will be developed in the immediate years ahead as the science of immunology expands.

In the future, however, vaccines may not prove to be the most effective means of controlling the viruses that plague man. A process known as the interference phenomenon (the presence of one virus that limits or excludes infection by a second, unrelated virus) has received considerable attention since 1957 when Isaacs and Lindenmann showed that such activity was mediated by a protein called interferon. They demonstrated that interferon was produced by virus-infected cells. This discovery is important, because the conventional antibody immune mechanisms may have little to do with the early stages of recovery from viral infections. Thus, interferon appears to be a line of defense that warrants further investigation. The great hope is that the interferon mechanism, with its broad spectrum of antiviral activity (as opposed to the specificity of vaccines), will provide control of those viral infections in which the number of serotypes is so great that successful control by vaccines is impossible. The common cold is the most obvious example.

INFECTIOUS DISEASES

Man is host to a wide variety of organisms. Most of these are harmless or even beneficial; others could be harmful given the right conditions, but remain neutral to man most of the time. A small percentage of all the organisms that man comes in contact with are seriously harmful unless measures are taken to reduce or offset their effect.

Classification of disease-producing organisms

The agents that cause disease in man may be classified into four groups: (1) organisms with plantlike characteristics, (2) organisms of animal origin, (3) the rickettsiae, and (4) the viruses.

Plantlike organisms. The yeasts, molds, and bacteria are the major categories of plantlike organisms that affect man. Examples of infections caused by yeasts or molds are thrush in infants and ringworm (which occurs on the scalp, foot, in the nails, and other parts of the body) in children and adults. Bacteria are by far the most numerous of the unicellular plants that cause disease. Several types have been described: (1) round organisms called cocci (streptococci, staphylococci, pneumococci, meningococci, and gonococci), (2) rodlike organisms called bacilli (which cause typhoid, paratyphoid, whooping cough, diphtheria, tuberculosis, leprosy, undulant fever, tularemia, tetanus, dysentery, and plague), and (3) spirallike organisms called spirilla (which cause syphilis, yaws, and Weil's disease).

Infections by animals. Primitive one-celled animals classified as protozoa give rise to infections in man. The principal ones cause amebic dysentery and malaria. Multiple-celled animals infest rather than infect, but nonetheless are especially harmful. The most important of these is a large intestinal roundworm that causes ascariasis. Trichinosis is a second example.

Rickettsiae. The rickettsiae occupy a position intermediate between bacteria and viruses. They differ from bacteria in that they require living cells for growth and differ from viruses in that with one exception they are retained by the Berkfeld filter.

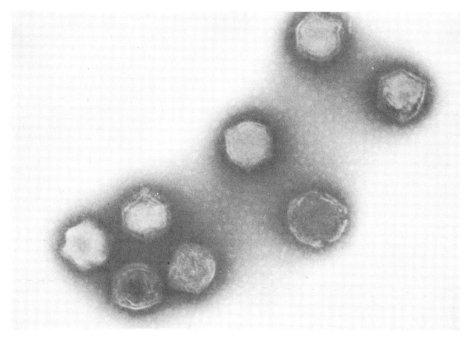

Fig. 7-2. An electron photomicrograph of a virus. (X100,000.) (From Brown, W. V., and Bertke, E. M.: Textbook of cytology, St. Louis, 1969, The C. V. Mosby Co.)

Over 40 rickettsiae have been identified, but only a few of these are pathogenic to man. Principal among these are: (1) the spotted fever group (Rocky Mountain spotted fever, African tick fever, rickettsial pox), (2) the typhus group (endemic typhus, Brill's disease, scrub fever), (3) Q fever, and (4) trench fever.

Viruses. As the techniques of microbiology have improved, particularly with the advent of the electron microscope, our knowledge about viral disease has correspondingly increased. Nearly 200 viruses have been identified, and there is scientific confidence that many more yet remain unknown. Tremendously small in size (more than 6,000 polio virus particles could form a single line on the head of a pin), most viruses have been elusive to study; for this reason microbiology is truly one of the frontier sciences today. Common diseases caused by viruses are measles, rubella, smallpox, chickenpox, mumps, poliomyelitis, hepatitis, herpes zoster, rabies, and mononucleosis.

Factors in control

The control of infectious disease is difficult even with our present knowledge, but the task is made easier as we understand the intricate relationship between the agent, the host, and the environment.

Agent. As indicated in the previous section, the number of plants and animals of microscopic size that threaten man's equilibrium is large. Any agent that adversely alters our health status is said to be pathogenic (recall that the second stage in the natural history of a disease is called pathogenesis).

Three factors enable pathogenic organisms to debilitate and even bring death to man. The first is their rapid rate of multiplication from one to many billions within a few hours and the tremendous material burden this places on the host as a consequence. The second is their ability to interfere with the normal function of certain organs by destroying tissue. More serious than either of these, however, is the third—the production of poisonous substances known as toxins. These vary in effect. Some interfere with the central nervous system, others with normal red cell production, and so on, rather than with the body as a whole. As a consequence, there are specific symptoms that alert the physician as to the primary cause of infection, depending upon the manner and site affected.

Most pathogenic organisms multiply rapidly and invade tissue; some produce toxins. Their capacity to do these, however, varies. The botulinus organism is very toxic but less invasive. Slightly less toxic but more invasive are tetanus (0.0005 ml. of tetanus will kill a guinea pig), diphtheria (0.002 ml. has a similar effect), streptococci, and staphylococci organisms. At the other end of the continuum, the tubercle bacillus is not very toxic but invades and destroys tissue extensively.

Host. Fortunately, man is not completely passive to the affront of pathogenic organisms. The first line of defense is comprised of the skin, mucous membranes, and digestive tract lining. Few agents can penetrate the skin to the deeper structures unless through a break. Some invasion is possible along sweat gland ducts or hair follicles, but this is usually not serious. Usually the skin acts to destroy bacteria unless encumbered by dirt or other media. The mucous secretions of the digestive tract, nose, and lungs trap bacteria. The cilia of the respiratory tract beat foreign particles up to the throat where they are swallowed to be destroyed in the stomach by gastric juices. A few organisms survive these barriers and multiply in the intestine. Normally these are present in the feces.

The second line of defense is performed by cells known as macrophages. Each part of the body has its own specialized macrophages (also called phagocytes, or reticuloendothelial cells). These wander about over surfaces and through tissues, gobbling any particles that are large enough and have a surface charge enough opposite to be held fast and engulfed. In most cases digestion and destruction of the ingested agent follows. Should the "leftovers" be detectable to the host as foreign matter, or should something interfere with macrophage function (such as alcohol, other toxins, and other duties making simultaneous demands),

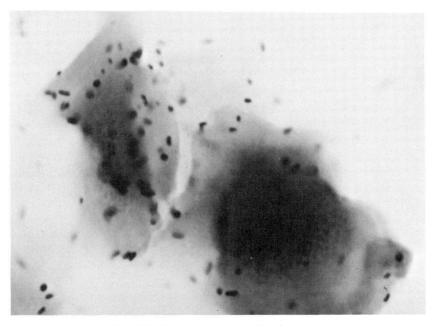

Fig. 7-3. Macrophages engulfing bacteria.

there will be opportunity for the third line of defense to come into play.

The immune reaction, our third line of defense, warrants a discussion of some detail.

The immune reaction. Early in the eighteenth century many people, believing that smallpox was inevitable, deliberately exposed themselves to the organism. It was both fashionable and dangerous then to be inoculated, since the agent was the genuine smallpox (variola) virus. The serum from a pustule of a person only mildly affected was used; and if the inoculated person lived, he was protected for life.

In 1796 Edward Jenner published the results of an experiment that was to make inoculation against smallpox much safer. He observed that milkmaids seldom contracted smallpox and inferred a relationship between cowpox and smallpox from this fact. To test his observation he scratched some serum from the pustules of a cow's udder into the arm of a boy. A mild infection resulted, with a lesion of smallpox at the site of the scratch. Subsequent attempts to infect the boy with smallpox failed. Without knowing exactly how it occurred, Jenner had observed immune reaction; the boy had developed an acquired immunity that was specific for smallpox.

An acquired immunity develops in the presence of a foreign protein called an antigen. In reaction to the antigen the body produces specific proteins called antibodies, which destroy or neutralize the antigen. Thus, the toxins of bacteria are destroyed by antitoxins, which the body produces in reaction to the toxins.

The antibody reaction is not immediate. There is first a latent period of nearly a week before many antibodies appear. Then the volume of antibodies gradually increases (primary response) to a level usually not adequate for guaranteed protection. Following the primary response, another injection of the antigen triggers a tremendous increase in antibody production (secondary response). Depending upon the antibody level considered desirable, subsequent in-

jections will induce additional secondary responses. The volume of antibodies is reduced over time, and periodic boosters are needed to maintain protection.

Exactly why an antigen produces an antibody is not known. One theory holds that the information for synthesis of a specific antibody is always present in the genetic makeup of each person but remains latent until stimulated by the antigen. Present knowledge of protein synthesis and the transfer of information during cell division seems to support this theory, but much remains to be discovered before the total process is understood.

A vaccine, of course, is a commercially prepared mixture of antigens that is strong enough to produce antibodies but weak enough so that most harmful effects of the disease do not develop. Depending upon the vaccine, toxicity is reduced in the following ways:

1. Only a small amount of the toxin is present.
2. Both toxin and antitoxin are given in order to protect the person while the antibody reaction is taking place.
3. Heat and chemicals destroy the harmful properties without destroying the antigen's ability to trigger antibody production. (This vaccine is called a toxoid.)
4. The live agent is attenuated (toxicity is reduced) by long periods of growth in test tubes or in an alien host. (Rabies and Sabin poliomyelitis vaccines are examples.)

We have been talking to this point of active acquired immunity. Passive acquired immunity, although much less satisfactory, is also possible. Once a person is known to have contracted some diseases, the time it would take to develop antibodies may be too long to provide the necessary protection. In this case the antibodies produced by another animal or human are injected into the exposed person in a form called serum. Although protection is immediate, it is also temporary, usually diminishing and disappearing within a few weeks. The blood serum of previous polio victims was used extensively to protect vulnerable groups in the early 1950's prior to the advent of the Salk and Sabin vaccines.

Brief mention needs to be made of natural immunity: the inherited resistance to a specific disease. Measles once was virulent; today it is relatively mild. Tuberculosis, diphtheria, and influenza are further examples of diseases to which one may be naturally immune. Over many generations, the less hardy succumb to certain diseases, while the more hardy pass their "ability to survive" on to their offspring. The consequence is a race more resistant to specific diseases.

The immune reaction, whether active or passive, is quite specific. Protection developed against diphtheria, for example, does not protect against any other disease. We must carry the antibodies to combat or neutralize the antigens of all diseases for which we wish protection. So it becomes a challenge to medicine to provide the many vaccines necessary and a task for the individual to maintain the necessary level of protection against each.

If we fail in the first instance, it is because we lack the scientific breakthrough, as was the case for a long time with rubella (German measles). Prior to 1969 we had no vaccine, and many congenital (present at birth) defects resulted in babies whose mothers had contracted the disease while pregnant. By fall 1969 a vaccine had been developed and was being used widely.

If we fail in the second instance, where vaccines are available, it is because of lethargy and inattention to personal health needs. The outbreak of diphtheria in Florida in late 1969 makes clear the fact that epidemics of diseases believed under control will occur if we ignore responsibility. In widely separated counties (Dade, Duval, Jefferson), Florida suffered an outbreak of epidemic proportions that claimed several lives. School surveys as a consequence revealed that as many as 40% of the students had never been immunized against diphtheria or any other disease.

Specificity of protection obviously has its drawbacks. If protection of a more general nature could be developed, we might then have a fourth line of defense. This may be a possibility. Earlier we mentioned the substance known as interferon. It deserves recall again now.

Disease-producing organisms often are unable to multiply as they would like. The reason seems to be because of the presence of interferon in the host cells, which perhaps reduces the supply of adenosine triphosphate (ATP), which is necessary for the cell to conduct the important processes of phosphorylation and oxidation. Without ATP the most virulent disease agents cannot reproduce and so become benign. Interferon has been isolated and identified as a protein. Its production in the host is triggered by the initial infection and is at peak concentration as soon as 3 days later. In contrast, antibodies cannot peak until at least 8 days after infection.

Experimental study to date indicates that there is only one kind of interferon and that this is effective against many viruses. Thus, specificity is not a problem with interferon as it is with the immune reaction. Many known but uncontrolled diseases are virus caused. Research suggests that many others, not yet described, may also be virus caused. When interferon is completely understood, this fourth line of defense against disease may prove to be our best. Routine use of safe, reliable inducers of interferon is not too far away; eventually different kinds of interferon may be synthesized. Much experience is yet to be gained as to optimal doses and timing of administration of interferon-inducing chemicals into the human body.

Environment. Man is but a small part, albeit a powerful one, in a large ecologic system. The environment, of course, is a most significant part of this system, especially in the context of disease. Quarantines, inspection of food supplies, elimination of insect pests, testing of dairy herds, supervision of milk pasteurization, filtration and chemical treatment of water supplies, and sanitary disposal of sewage are all measures to control disease that we take for granted. Each influences a small part of the environment. Each has been controversial at earlier times but gradually has won approval as our understanding of the disease process increased.

Perhaps the most important factor in disease control has been the increasing tendency toward cleanliness. At the community level we demonstrate this through procedures such as restaurant inspections, better aseptic techniques in hospitals, and constant monitoring of commercially prepared foods. At the personal level, bathing, hand washing, and careful clothes maintenance are obviously important. Unfortunately, many persons choose to ignore these important relationships in the agent-host-environment triangle, to the detriment of themselves and others.

Extent of problem

Some infectious diseases are classified as being acute. These are characterized by rapid onset, severe symptoms, and relatively short duration. Included for statistical purposes under this general heading are some of the parasitic diseases, a variety of respiratory conditions, and digestive disorders. Acute diseases accounted for 41% of all deaths in 1901, but in 1966 this proportion fell to 8%. Pneumonia and influenza, which together constituted 12% of all deaths and was the leading cause in the early years of the century, now ranks fifth, causing less

than 3% of all deaths. Diarrhea, enteritis, and the communicable diseases of childhood (measles, scarlet fever, whooping cough, and diphtheria), which once took an enormous toll of children's lives, are rarely listed today as causes of death. Death from typhoid fever and poliomyelitis has also been reduced to a vanishing point. Currently, the chances of eventually dying of an acute disease are 6 in 100 for both males and females at birth. After adolescence this likelihood drops to about 4 in 100 through the middle years and then rises slightly at the advanced ages. Table 7-1 shows the number and rate for acute conditions by general types and age groups for 1968.

Although the changing picture of acute conditions specifically and infectious conditions generally has been favorable, we will probably always be confronted with possible recurrences. The hard fact is that all diseases ever present with us in the past are still with us today, most only sporadically; but many remain endemic, epidemic, or even pandemic (that is, worldwide, as in the case of Asian flu in 1957 and again in 1968-69). Table 7-2 summaries the incidence of selected infectious conditions at 5-year intervals over the past 25 years.

As pointed out earlier, there are over 100 infectious conditions that have been described. Each has had a significant effect on man's health history. Those shown in Table 7-2, a cross section of the total group, have been selected for their significance in the past and even today to man's ecologic

Table 7-1. Acute conditions—number and rate by type and by age group for 1968 in the United States

Age group	Number of conditions				Rate per 100 population			
	Infective and parasitic	Respiratory		Digestive	Infective and parasitic	Respiratory		Digestive
		Upper	Other			Upper	Other	
Under 6	9,935	29,171	15,033	3,248	43.8	128.5	66.2	14.3
6-16	15,944	36,959	28,312	4,776	36.0	83.4	63.9	10.8
17-44	10,958	36,067	46,876	7,066	15.7	51.6	67.1	10.1
45 +	4,755	20,974	25,082	4,301	8.1	35.9	42.9	7.4
Total	41,592	123,171	115,304	19,390	21.3	63.0	59.0	9.9

Adapted from Statistical abstract of the United States: 1970, ed. 91, Washington, D. C., 1970, U. S. Bureau of the Census.

Table 7-2. Incidence at five-year intervals, 1945-1965 and 1968, of selected infectious conditions in the United States

Condition	1945	1950	1955	1960	1965	1968
Botulism	not known	20	16	12	19	7
Diphtheria	18,675	5,796	1,984	918	164	260
Hepatitis	not known	2,820	31,961	41,666	33,856	45,893
Influenza*						
Malaria	62,763	2,184	522	72	147	2,317
Measles (rubella)	146,013	319,124	555,156	441,703	261,904	22,231
Poliomyelitis (acute)	13,624	33,300	28,985	3,190	72	53
Salmonellosis	649	1,233	5,447	6,949	17,161	16,514
Tuberculosis (new cases)	not known	not known	76,245	55,494	49,016	42,758
Typhoid fever	4,211	2,484	1,704	816	454	395
Venereal diseases						
Gonorrhea	313,363	286,746	236,197	258,953	324,925	464,543
Syphilis	351,767	217,558	122,392	122,003	112,842	96,271
Other	10,261	8,187	3,913	2,811	2,015	1,486

Adapted from Statistical abstracts of the United States: 1970, ed. 91, Washington, D. C., 1970, U. S. Bureau of the Census.
*Reported cases of influenza vary widely depending on the agency reporting or the sample taken. Unquestionably, several hundred thousand cases occur each year in the U. S.

relationships. Each is discussed separately below.

Botulism

The term food poisoning applies to certain illnesses acquired through consumption of food. It includes food intoxication caused by chemical contaminants (heavy metals, fluorides, and others), by toxins produced by organisms carried by food (staphylococcal toxins, botulinus toxins), and by a number of organic substances occurring in natural foods which in themselves are harmful to man (certain mushrooms, mussels, eels, and other sea foods).

Of all types of bacteria food poisoning the most deadly is botulism, an intoxication caused by the saprophyte *Clostridium botulinum*. Symptoms of the disease include weakness, dizziness, headache, and constipation, soon followed by dropping eyelids and visual disturbances. Difficulty in swallowing and loss of voice occur. In nearly two-thirds of all cases death results from respiratory failure or pneumonia within 3 to 7 days after onset. Absolute rest and use of serum containing polyvalent botulinus antitoxin, types A and B, constitute the best understood treatment.

The bacillus responsible for the disease is capable of producing heat-labile neurotoxin. It grows in the absence of oxygen in decaying animal or vegetable matter or in improperly sterilized foodstuffs, such as navy beans, meats, olives, asparagus, and string beans. The host food must contain protein.

Although we know little about its incidence prior to 1900, the prevalence of home canning methods then undoubtedly resulted in many more cases than occur today. Modern commercial canning techniques practically eliminate the danger of botulism, although occasional incidents demonstrate the need for constant surveillance. In 1969 a can of Spanish anchovies sold in Virginia was found to contain botulism toxin that could cause fatal food poisoning. In that same year, 9 outbreaks of botulism involving 15 cases with 5 deaths were reported to the National Communicable Disease Center. Both commercially and privately prepared foods were involved. Indicted foods included fish cured in seal oil and buried underground 6 months by some Eskimos, home-canned chicken soup causing type B botulism, vegetables, fruit preserves, improperly cooked hamburger, and commercially prepared chicken livers causing type A botulism.

Diphtheria

Diphtheria is caused by the Klebs-Löffler bacillus, a rod-shaped organism that varies considerably in size. It is prevalent throughout the world but occurs primarily in the temperate zones. In the United States the incidence is greatest in the late fall and early winter, usually peaking in December.

The throat is the primary site of infection. Toxin given off by the bacillus there is transmitted by the bloodstream to other parts of the body, with the nervous system and heart muscle primarily affected. The toxin is neutralized by substances produced by the victim's own defense system or by an antitoxin injected for treatment. Commercial antitoxin is prepared from the serum of a horse previously injected with diphtheria toxin. Prior to the development of antitoxin 1 in every 3 persons contracting diphtheria died; today none need die if given antitoxin in time. Unfortunately, a number of cases are not diagnosed in time, and a case fatality of nearly 10% has changed little in the past 50 years.

Prevention is dependent upon active immunization of children by the injection of a modified diphtheria toxin called diphtheria toxoid. The immunity so produced is an active immunity and is sustained for 5 to 10 years. It is recommended that children 3 to 6 months of age receive diphtheria toxoid as part of a combined immunization that also includes whooping cough, or pertusis, vaccine; tetanus toxoid (the familiar DPT combination); and poliomyelitis vaccine.

The incidence of diphtheria today is not what it once was. In the 1930's more than 30,000 cases and 3,000 deaths were recorded in a single year. In 1965, 164 cases were identified in the United States. Nonetheless, statistics suggest that adults, particularly young parents, are ignoring their responsibilities to themselves and their offspring in not obtaining the proper primary and booster immunizations. Between November 1968 and November 1969 there were 27 cases of diphtheria with 4 deaths in Phoenix, Arizona. In the same period there were 90 to 100 cases, with 4 deaths in Travis County, Texas. During late 1969 three large areas in Florida reported several cases and 4 deaths among unimmunized children. Florida officials estimated that only 88% of its population had been vaccinated and that many children were among the unprotected. In 1969 across the country there were 213 cases reported, almost exactly equal to the previous 5-year median of 214 cases. These figures seem small, yet diphtheria would completely disappear if everyone were properly immunized.

Hepatitis

Infectious hepatitis is a term that has several synonyms: catarrhal jaundice, epidemic hepatitis, "yellow jaundice," infectious jaundice, and a few others of a more technical nature. All refer to a condition of acute hepatitis (inflammation of the liver) caused by one or more filtrable agents, believed to be viruslike in their characteristics but otherwise not yet identified. Symptoms of the disease include fever, anorexia (loss of appetite), nausea, malaise, and abdominal discomfort, followed by jaundice (yellowing of the skin) approximately 5 days after onset.

Person-to-person contact is the mode of transmission of infectious hepatitis, with respiratory spread possible. It may also be contracted during transfusion of whole blood, injection of blood serum or plasma from infected persons, and by accidental contamination of syringes or needles with traces of blood. Contaminated water, milk, and food, including oysters and clams, have been the source of innumerable epidemics.

No specific treatment for infectious hepatitis is recommended except restriction of physical activity and a diet high in protein and carbohydrates and moderate (no more than 125 grams daily) in fat. Happily, over 90% recover in about 3 months if they follow sound medical advice. Some patients suffer extended illness for as long as a year and still enjoy complete recovery. A few subsequently develop one or more of several varieties of chronic hepatic disease, but this is usually a consequence of other complicating conditions, such as alcoholism or amebiasis. Less than 1% of all cases are fatal.

There is clear evidence that infectious hepatitis is on a gradual increase. In 1969 there were 48,085 reported cases as compared with 45,578 in 1968. The 5-year median, 1964-68, was 37,652. What these figures portend for the future is not known. But, they do emphasize the need, for this reason among many, to maintain safe water, milk, and food.

A second form of hepatitis, known as serum hepatitis, is of some concern. Also called homologous serum jaundice, serum hepatitis is caused by a different virus (virus B) than infectious hepatitis (virus A). Although its symptoms are essentially the same as infectious hepatitis, it has a longer incubation period (approximately 80 to 100 days as compared with 25) and a higher fatality rate (12% compared with less than 1%).

In years past, serum hepatitis was a more serious problem than it is today. Since its medium for transmission is blood, improved and more sterile techniques for taking, processing, and donating blood have markedly reduced total incidence. Nonethless, 5,359 cases were reported in 1969, including many that were fatal. Many of these were the consequence of using contaminated needles or syringes in drug experimentation or addiction.

Influenza

In the days of Elizabeth I, people of fashion referred to influenza as the "Gallant's Disease" or the "Jolly Rant." During the disastrous pandemic of 1918-19, it was known as the "Spanish flu" or "the grippe." Many refer to it today as the "Hong Kong flu."

The influenza virus has been under scientific observation since 1933 when type A was first isolated in England. Type B was identified in the United States in 1940, and vaccines were introduced soon afterwards. In 1947 a new virus strain, type A-1, made its appearance. Although no major outbreaks resulted, it was found that existing influenza vaccines were almost completely ineffective against this strain. Modifications made the vaccine protective again, a procedure that had to be repeated in 1955 when the type B virus changed its characteristics.

By contrast, the A-2 virus was seriously pandemic in 1967. Better known as "Asian flu," the A-2 virus caused more than 60,000 deaths in the United States beyond those expected. Many of these were in the very young and very old age categories, and the primary cause often was other than influenza itself (for example, pneumonia); but the indirect cause for most of these was influenza. Although vaccines were changed again to add A-2 components (and further modified to include the Japanese strain discovered in 1962 and the Taiwanese strain discovered in 1964), it has been obvious that since the A-2 strain has developed, many more people are getting influenza.

Today we associate influenza with the city of Hong Kong, where the current variation of the disease burst forth in July 1968. When it struck Hong Kong, brought there from central China, its dangerous nature was quickly apparent. One in every five persons living in Hong Kong came down with it (that is, nearly 800,000). There were 32 deaths directly attributed to influenza, and at least 100 more died from related complications. During August it spread to Singapore, the Philippines, Taiwan, and Indonesia, and finally came to this country on September 2 via a serviceman who had been stationed in Hong Kong.

Health officials believe that the principal strain of influenza that will affect us in the first few years of the 1970's will be the Hong Kong variety. But there is also clear expectation that new strains will develop in the future. As these appear, scientists will need to produce new vaccines quickly enough to head off epidemics.

There is only one thing certain about the influenza virus—it is an exceptionally unstable organism. Outwardly, the effects of influenza continue to be much the same. You suddenly have chills, fever, head-

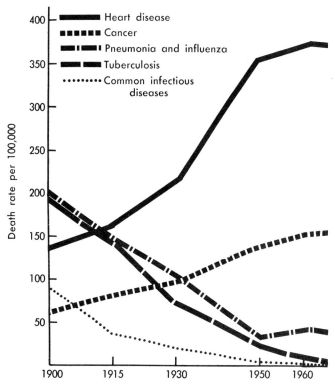

Fig. 7-4. Trends in selected causes of death, United States, 1900-1966. (From U. S. Public Health Service.)

ache, sore throat, muscular pains, and often a lingering cough. But the virus that gives you these symptoms is in a continuous state of change. Unfortunately, with each change we have to develop a new vaccine or else suffer sickness of epidemic nature. As a consequence, it has been difficult to produce effective vaccines against the disease. Even after receiving the vaccine, a person could still come down with the flu; the vaccine provides about 60% protection.

It takes about 2 weeks for immunity to be built up in the body following a flu shot. But if you are vulnerable to the virus and are exposed to it (communicated during the first 3 days after a person is clinically ill with the disease), you could come down with it yourself within 24 to 72 hours.

The ease and speed with which the virus spreads are factors that make influenza one of the most difficult problems faced today in the field of communicable disease preven-

tion. Fortunately, we have developed a few lifesaving aids over the years. These include the antibiotics, such as penicillin, which, although not effective against the flu virus, can be used to treat pneumonia and other serious complications. We also have an "early warning system." Constant surveillance is maintained by the National Communicable Disease Center of the U. S. Public Health Service, the World Health Organization, and other cooperating agencies. As to passive immunity, of course, after an epidemic begins, human sera are available from those who are in the convalescent stage.

Nonetheless, there is one sure prediction about influenza—it is going to continue to plague us unpredictably for many years into the future.

Malaria

The incidence of malaria in the United States over the past 25 years is a clear example of the global nature of communicable disease. In the mid-1940's the World Health Organization estimated that there were over 300 million people with malaria in the world. The United States reported 62,763 of these in 1945, a figure made greater than normal by infected World War II soldiers returning from the Pacific theater of operations. In the face of these alarming statistics a concerted effort to reduce the worldwide incidence was initiated by the World Health Organization. Consequently, within a few years there was a significant reduction, as reflected, for example, in the fact that as recently as 1965 there were only 106 cases in the U. S. with all of them but two originating outside the country. The curative drug, primaquine, has been very effective in treating and reducing existing cases.

But in the late 1960's the influence of Vietnam had brought about an upswing in U. S. malaria cases. Again, returning servicemen infected overseas caused the total incidence to rise sharply. In 1969 there were 3,216 reported cases as compared with 2,370 in 1968 and a 1964-68 5-year median of 559. These figures are not alarming, but they do underscore the need for continued surveillance. Although a real outbreak of malaria is unlikely in this country, a reservoir of infected humans is one of the necessary prerequisites.

The causative agent of malaria is a pathogenic protozoan transmitted by a mosquito. An infected female Anopheles mosquito is the definitive host linking infected and uninfected human beings. Four varieties of the infective agent cause the disease in man: *Plasmodium vivax; P. malariae; P. falciparum;* and *P. ovale.*

The disease is characterized by episodes of indefinite malaise followed by chills and rising temperature, usually accompanied by headache and nausea and ending with excessive sweating. After a period of seeming relief lasting from 1 to 3 days, depending on the type of malaria present, the cycle of chills, fever, and sweating is repeated. Untreated, primary malaria attacks will last from 1 week to a month; relapses may occur regularly for several years after infection.

The environment must be satisfactory for the Anopheles mosquito to thrive. Warm, damp, dark spaces, and swampy terrain are especially conducive to its reproduction. Such sites have been the focus for worldwide preventive measures. Where efforts to spray with DDT and to dry swamplands have been concentrated for 3 or 4 years, the incidence of malaria has been reduced to nearly zero.

But the very use of DDT (Chapter 6), almost indiscriminantly in the first years after evidence of its dramatic effect on organisms harmful to man, now causes us to reevaluate the problem. As it has been widely used for many health reasons, including the destruction of the Anopheles mosquito, many ecologists warn us that the level of DDT in the world, in soil and water, is dangerously close to, if not above, nature's threshold of tolerance. If this is so, the effect on future generations, although not yet clear, can only be harmful. We hope we are not too late with current efforts to reduce or ban the use of DDT.

Measles

Another viral disease, this one primarily affecting children, is measles, or rubeola (also called regular measles or red measles). Measles is a severe disease among malnourished children in underdeveloped countries, with a case fatality rate of 5% to 10%; but in the United States it is relatively mild and rarely is a direct cause of death. Resulting complications, however, such as pneumonia (causing over 90% of related deaths), encephalitis, and middle-ear infections cause several hundred deaths each year. Probably 80% to 90% of those who reach age 20 have had measles. A first attack usually assures a lifetime of immunity.

Vaccines are available in three forms. A single injection of a live, attenuated virus induces active immunity in 95% of susceptible children for at least 5 years. A second form of vaccine is inactivated virus; three doses of this at monthly intervals are required. A third form is the inactivated and live viruses in combination; one or two doses of inactivated vaccine are followed in 1 to 3 months by one dose of live, attenuated vaccine.

All infants should be immunized at 9 to 12 months of age. Also, children who are institutionalized and those with cystic fibrosis, tuberculosis, heart disease, and asthma and other chronic pulmonary diseases should be especially protected. Adults rarely need to be immunized. It is not advised to use the live, attenuated vaccine in cases of pregnancy, leukemia, generalized neoplasms, immunosuppressive therapy, and in the presence of severe illnesses. Measles-immune globulin is recommended for susceptible infants and exposed children under 3 years of age.

The dramatic effect of measles vaccine is made clear in the following statistics. In the early 1960's nearly 5 million children a year were stricken with measles, and more than 30,000 were hospitalized for 300,000 hospital days. More than 5,000 of these children developed encephalitis, and 1,600 were left with permanent mental retardation. In addition, measles caused nearly 500 deaths a year. In 1968, however, because of the widespread use of measles vaccine, there were only 220,000 actual cases of measles, with a corresponding decline in its tragic complications.

Sometimes confused in the public's mind with rubeola, but actually quite different from it, is the less severe disease known as rubella or "German measles." This fact of confusion warrants a brief discussion of rubella here.

Rubella is virus caused, is relatively mild, but highly communicable. Two or three weeks after exposure the disease manifests in a rash and may be accompanied by low-grade fever and malaise. Usually the rash begins on the face and neck as small, irregular, pink eruptions that tend to coalesce. As the rash spreads to the trunk it frequently begins to clear on the face.

Although rubella is endemic, with a seasonal peak in the late winter and early spring, its greatest impact has been felt during explosive epidemics that have occurred at irregular intervals (Fig. 7-5). The disease occurs primarily in young children and teen-agers but has a high attack rate among young adults. This has been the basis of the rubella problem: maternal infection during pregnancy. During the last severe epidemic of 1964-65, more than 30,000 children were

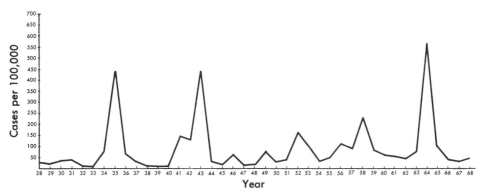

Fig. 7-5. Rubella incidence for 9 selected areas (Illinois, Maine, Maryland, Massachusetts, New York City, Ohio, Rhode Island, Washington, Wisconsin) in the United States, 1928-1968. These data suggest that major epidemics occurred throughout the country in 1935, 1943, and 1964. Periods of high incidence were also observed in 1952 and 1958. These periods of increased rubella activity have occurred at 6- to 9-year intervals, a moderately long and somewhat irregular cyclicity that contrasts strikingly with the regular 2-year periodicity observed in rubeola in the United States prior to the large-scale use of measles vaccine.

born blind, deaf, with heart defects, or with mental retardation because their mothers contracted rubella during the first 3 months of pregnancy. Studies cited at the 1969 International Conference on Rubella Immunization indicated that the cost to the U. S. economy from that one epidemic will eventually exceed $3 billion.

Only one strain of pathogenic organisms has been identified. This was accomplished in 1962 by two teams of scientists working independently. The isolation of the rubella virus in tissue culture made possible the characterization of the natural history of postnatal and congenital rubella and the development of rubella vaccines.

In 1966 Parkman, Meyer, and co-workers described completion of a small rubella vaccine trial in which they used a strain of rubella virus attenuated by 77 tissue culture passages in African green monkey kidney tissue culture. This strain, known as HPV-77, was evaluated in extensive programs involving children living in isolation units in institutions, families living in the community, and school boys exposed to a rubella epidemic. It proved highly effective and after further study was licensed by the U. S. Food and Drug Administration on June 10, 1969. Since then millions of children and young married women have been vaccinated, and the incidence of the disease today is on a decided downward trend. Since rubella per se is a trivial disease, however, the real proof of vaccine efficacy will be reduction of rubella-associated congenital birth defects. For this development the world waits anxiously.

Poliomyelitis

It is hoped that both types of measles will go the way of poliomyelitis, once a serious three-strain (types, 1, 2, and 3), virus-caused disease. Prior to 1954 polio was a scourge feared by everyone. Although never as serious in absolute numbers as many other diseases, its power to permanently maim and cripple often caused widespread panic whenever an epidemic was considered imminent. In the first half of the

twentieth century in the U. S. alone it struck down more than half a million children and young adults, killing 57,000 and crippling 300,000. Included among these was Franklin D. Roosevelt, who sponsored the March of Dimes in 1938. Research financed by the March of Dimes led to the eventual discovery of a vaccine in 1954, some ten years after Roosevelt's death. Polio cases averaged 38,727 a year between 1950 and 1954; in 1955, the year the Salk vaccine was licensed, there were 72 cases; and in 1969 there were only 17.

The development of a killed virus vaccine by Salk in 1954 and the later development of the first live virus vaccine by Sabin in 1961 has virtually eliminated the disease today. As long as children are immunized as recommended, in the first 6 months of life and with a booster whenever necessary, the disease should remain almost extinct.

Salmonellosis

Salmonellosis is a disease of bacterial origin that manifests primarily as acute gastroenteritis but occasionally as an enteric fever or a septicemia. Symptoms include sudden onset of abdominal pain, diarrhea, frequent vomiting, and fever. Recovery usually occurs 1 to 3 days after onset. Death occurs in about 0.8% of all cases.

Although there may be as many as 800 serotypes of salmonella involved in food poisoning, *S. typhimurium* is the most common; it and about six others cause most of the outbreaks in the United States.

Most outbreaks of salmonellosis occur in the warm months when poor or absent refrigeration allows the organisms to multiply rapidly. Many raw foods are consumed during these months, and cooked foods are often not brought to a temperature (160° F) sufficient to destroy the bacteria.

We acquire the organism from contaminated foods of animal origin, but particularly ground meat often including sausage, from turkeys and other fowl, and from related egg products. Commercial feed made from meat products often harbors the salmonella organism in large quantities. When these feeds are consumed by fowl, their meat and eggs become contaminated. The organism in turn is consumed by man.

The increase of salmonellosis in recent years (see Table 7-2) prompted the passage of a strong poultry inspection by Congress in 1969. Known as the Wholesome Poultry Products Act, it requires:

1. That the states establish inspection standards at least equal to Federal standards. Any state failing to do this will be subject to Federal inspection of all poultry plants within the state.

2. That, where requested, the Federal government give financial and technical assistance. Once a cooperative inspection agreement has been reached, the Federal government will pay 50% of the cost of the state's inspection program.

3. That if a plant is a threat to human health and the state does not take appropriate corrective action, the Secretary of Agriculture is authorized to provide Federal inspection immediately, even if the company sells only to customers within that state.

4. That the Secretary of Agriculture have authority over allied industries that could divert unfit poultry into the human food supply. This permits the USDA to review the records of transporters, brokers, cold-storage warehouse operators, and animal-food manufacturers.

5. That poultry storage and handling facilities be regulated to prevent adulteration or misbranding of poultry products.

6. That the Secretary of Agriculture be able to withdraw or refuse inspection services to a plant and detain and seize unfit poultry.

7. That the investigative authority of the USDA be increased.

These controls should help to reduce what seems now to be a rising reservoir of salmonella organisms in many of the foods we enjoy regularly.

Tuberculosis

Tuberculosis germs are relatives of the common oral streptomycetes and skin corynebacteria, one of which *(Corynebacterium diphtheriae)* is the agent responsible for diphtheria. Tuberculosis germs, however, are able to grow inside cells, and are protected from harm by a tough waxy coating. Thus, when the body's second line of defense (phagocytic cells) takes up invading tuberculosis bacteria, the germs can multiply and can even be carried from place to place inside host cells, via circulation of lymph and blood.

Tuberculosis bacteria gain entry chiefly via the respiratory passages, though they may also be ingested, and invade by way of the intestine. Thus, primary tuberculosis is apt to be pulmonary. (In the old days, when raw milk and uninspected dairy cattle were the rule, intestinal primary tuberculosis was not uncommon, especially in infants.) When the body arrests the invading germs, the disease does not progress; but since a walled-off focus of smoldering infection remains, it stands to break down in the future should a patient neglect proper hygiene. The result of breakdown is called disease reactivation. Reinfection tuberculosis can also occur.

Interestingly, the tuberculosis germs (mycobacteria) produce no known toxins. Most of their damage is caused by the usual allergic processes that occur in all normal human beings. When phagocytic cells do not completely digest the germs they take up, macromolecules of mycobacterial debris are left. Some of these provoke an allergic response in the host so that future exposures to these macromolecular antigens from mycobacteria produce allergic tissue responses, or allergic inflammation. In tuberculosis, most of the allergy is of the cellular type, as will be explained later in this chapter. Caseating granuloma is a typical sort of inflammation in tuberculosis by which pathologists may recognize, or suspect, either tuberculosis or a similar type of infecting organism from microscopic examination of tissues.

Mycobacterium tuberculosis is the species accounting for most tuberculosis throughout the world. Bovine and avian mycobacteria, named according to their major animal reservoirs, are also able to cause human disease.

Other species are atypical (unclassified, anonymous) mycobacteria.

Since allergy develops routinely in the presence of infection with mycobacteria, and since it persists for many years, it is possible to use skin tests to screen human populations in detecting which members have been or are presently infected. By this means, it can be shown that in urban areas 50% to 80% of the older population has had active tuberculosis. In other areas, and in younger age groups, the incidence of positive skin test reactions is less than 10%. In the United States young adults and older males seem to acquire the active disease at a higher rate than the rest of the population.

Prevention of tuberculosis lies in prompt identification and treatment of active cases. In close communities, as on shipboard and in institutions, viable tuberculosis germs can live in dust and be carried by air currents to all the neighbors. The more crowded the community, the more frequent should be its periodic health survey, with chest x-rays and skin tests administered for tuberculosis. When an active case occurs in a family, the whole family must be monitored more closely.

Treatment is now quite satisfactory for tuberculosis. Instead of a few years in a sanitarium, one now expects only a few months. Medicines are available that are taken by mouth as well as by injection; after disease germs are no longer being shed, one can return to his community and finish his course of oral medicines. Since public health funds and facilities are available for the management of tuberculosis in the United States, it need not be an expensive illness.

Because of the scarring and disturbed functioning left in lung areas infected by tuberculosis, and because not all cases are found early, it sometimes is necessary to have a damaged lung removed surgically. When too extensive for surgery, the fibrosis and emphysema are apt to be crippling. If spread to other organs—joints, growing

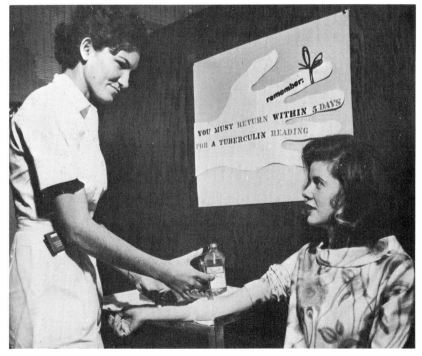

Fig. 7-6. The tuberculin, a simple test for tuberculosis, is a service of most public health programs. Have you had one lately? (Courtesy Health Department, Knox County, Tenn.)

ends of bones, kidneys, lymph nodes, bone marrow, and brain covering (meninges)— has occurred, they, too, may be permanently impaired. As with all diseases, the treatment is far more difficult than the prevention, when the cause of the disease is known.

Typhoid fever

Typhoid is a disease occurring almost exclusively in man. Intelligent human beings can prevent its occurrence, since it is only infectious by the oral-intestinal route; good sanitation regarding food and drink (especially milk and water) is essential for prevention of typhoid. Chronic carriers do exist, however, who shed in their stools the infectious organisms, *Salmonella typhosa*. If these persons were not food handlers, and should their excrement pass only to a private septic tank, no blame could be placed upon them for continuing the natural cycle of typhoid. Unfortunately, all adults are food handlers at one time or another, preparing food for others and sometimes failing to use soap and water after using the toilet. Furthermore, in many areas of the world, raw sewage is poured either onto the land (as fertilizer) or directly into the stream or river. It was our sad experience to learn that in our own community of Knoxville, which is a typical one, there still exist areas where "privies" empty onto stream banks; and at the opposite end of the social scale, a country club can be cited that for years has discharged raw sewage into our nearest recreational lake.

Though vaccination has been favored for years as the best approach to individual prevention of typhoid, it must be confessed that the rationale for this opinion is rather shaky and that many instances exist where vaccinated personnel have succumbed to the disease when swallowing sufficient numbers of typhoid germs in drinking water. We are grateful that chlorination of drinking water has been practiced in so many communities of the United States that it has become familiar and accepted, for chlorination does help considerably in preventing epidemic typhoid. The individual remains at the mercy of an infected food handler, however, who may or may not recall ever having had an illness compatible with typhoid. Periodic stool culture for Salmonella organisms should be required of all food handlers.

The disease, typhoid fever, has a variable asymptomatic period after germs are swallowed, depending on how many *Salmonella typhosa* organisms are in the intestines and able to begin to multiply; the average incubation period is 10 days. Gradual onset of symptoms occurs in the next 2 or 3 days, with headache, weakness, chills, fever, and abdominal pain developing slowly. Nausea, vomiting, constipation, diarrhea, and nosebleed may occur. Bronchitis is common. (Sounds like any "GI flu," but without a stool culture or blood culture for the typhoid germs, who would know the difference?) The usual case goes on to continued fever for the next 2 or 3 weeks. If not properly diagnosed and treated, however, complications, including gastrointestinal bleeding, intestinal perforation, pneumonia, osteomyelitis, and meningitis, may develop.

Treatment involves high doses of a very few special antibiotics, replacement of fluids and lost blood, and is best carried out in a hospital. Relapses are common. Public health follow-up is important to be sure that infectious organisms are not being shed by a patient otherwise perfectly well. There is good evidence that such chronic carriers of typhoid are only cleared after careful antibiotic treatment combined with removal of the gallbladder (where salmonellae can hide for years, unharmed and able to cause continued shedding of germs in the stool, as well as relapse in the patient).

Venereal disease

Gonorrhea. Gonorrhea is caused by a small, gram-negative (referring to the chemistry of its cell wall) diplococcus, *Neisseria gonorrhoeae*. It multiplies as an intracellular invader, destroys tissue, and can exist as a chronic infection with or without any preceding acute symptoms. As a chronic infection, it can pass during sexual intercourse to either member of the pair involved.

Tissues affected include any portion of the genital tract and lower urinary tracts of both sexes. There may or may not be a discharge of pus to the outside, though this is common. Equally common is pain, burning on urination, and urge to urinate more often (especially in males). Having gained a route upstream, the organisms can spread into the reproductive tracts, the urinary tracts, and the blood and lymph streams. In the male, the seminal vesicles, prostate gland, and testicles may be infected secondarily as the disease spreads; in the female, the uterus and fallopian tubes may be infected. Pelvic peritonitis can even occur in females, since the fallopian tubes open into the peritoneal cavity or can be perforated into the cavity as their walls are destroyed by gonorrheal infection.

An infected female birth canal can permit the germs to reach the nose, mouth, and eyes of a newborn infant. This had been a common occurrence for so many years that in 1884 the German obstetrician Credé, after much thought, began the practice of instilling 1% solutions of silver nitrate into the eyes of all newborn infants. This, or penicillin used similarly, has been effective in preventing blindness caused by gonorrhea acquired during birth. In recent years, however, with so much worldwide use of penicillin as treatment of gonorrhea, some strains have developed resistance of penicillin. Thus, we shall have to go back to silver nitrate, or some similar general protoplasmic poison against which bacteria cannot develop resistance.

This is all very well for the newborn, but what about the adult? First, of course it is far better simply to prevent infection (no sexual intercourse except with one partner, who likewise has no other sexual experiences.) Should one become infected, damage will have begun even before he seeks medical attention. Germs on the surface are easy to kill; germs that have already invaded the body are not. The individual may be allergic to the best available drug (peni-

cillin), or the gonorrheal strain might be resistant to penicillin. Physicians know other effective management; one should be sought and his advice followed.

Neglected gonorrhea in the adult can and does lead to sterility, urethral scarring and obstruction of urine flow, and a variety of complications in other organs: arthritis, peritonitis, endocarditis (infection of the inside of the heart)—serious results of a "little case of the clap," or "strain." Strict discipline for sex urges is far better than risking permanent joint, heart, or urinary tract disease, with crippling of function in these organs, or even death from endocarditis.

Syphilis. Less common than gonorrhea, but still present in every community, is syphilis. Public health measures, such as mandatory blood tests for syphilis (for marriage license or employment), have helped identify only the secondary, latent, and tertiary victims of the disease, not those who are most apt to spread it. A newly infected individual, feeling healthy and quite unaware of his or her chancre (or "hair cut" on or near the genitalia, mouth, or hand, which is the primary lesion of syphilis) may not have a positive reaction to blood tests even if by chance they are taken.

Syphilis, even more than gonorrhea, is a chronic infectious disease able to produce tissue damage in essentially every organ of the body. In certain areas (eye, brain, and spinal cord) it is extremely hard to cure with drugs. The organism responsible is a spirochete, *Treponema pallidum.* It is spread in exactly the same way as gonorrhea. Like gonorrhea, it can easily perpetuate itself; it is spread by sexual intercourse; and it doesn't kill its victims too fast. Each infected person can be counted on to infect others unless he refrains from sexual intercourse.

In around 10 days or more (sometimes up to 3 months) after sexual exposure, a small, insignificant-appearing sore may appear where sex partners' flesh met flesh during sex play or intercourse: this is often the genital area, but may be on the hand, mouth, breast, or any other part of the body. It may not be on the area visible to the infected person; especially in females the chancre may go unnoticed. A special dark-field microscope examination at this stage—primary syphilis—can prove the diagnosis, and treatment will follow; cure can be expected. A large dose of penicillin for 10 days is apt to be prescribed unless someone is allergic to penicillin.

Six weeks or so later, variable skin rash and other symptoms may occur; the rash may also occur in the mouth and throat, on the genitalia, or near the anus. Like the chancre earlier, the rash is contagious. But at this stage the affected person is apt to feel sick and to seek medical attention. He or she may have cough, fever, joint pains, and swollen lymph nodes (glands).

This stage, the secondary stage of syphilis, can look like measles, hives, or any other skin condition (except the blistery ones, like chickenpox and poison ivy). Reaction to the blood test is always positive in normal persons at this stage. If the infected person is not reinfected, he or she will not be able to transmit the disease after some 4 years—a nonsense statement, perhaps, since promiscuous persons are not apt to abstain from intercourse for 4 years, not even in prison.

Late syphilis is the form that produces the greatest tissue destruction. Medieval paintings of crowd scenes often included one or more hideously disfigured persons in the wake of syphilis. More important, since potentially fatal, are tissue losses in critical areas: heart, brain, spinal cord, stomach, liver, and throat, destruction that few painters have seen. Late syphilis may develop between the ages of 35 and 50 years, or later. There is no satisfactory treatment of late syphilis.

Between secondary and late syphilis is a stage, variable in duration, in which there are no symptoms of disease, but only a positive reaction to serologic tests: this is latent syphilis, the last stage at which treatment can cure the disease. This is the stage most often responsible for transmittal to the developing fetus as congenital syphilis. Such infants may succumb to the overwhelming infection or may survive, crippled and re-tarded, with progressive deafness or blindness; response to treatment is not good in these infants.

Other venereal diseases. The three remaining venereal diseases are less common and will not be fully discussed here. Chancroid, granuloma inguinale, and lymphogranuloma venereum are all infections that occur throughout the world. Chancroid's causal agent is related to the pinkeye and whooping cough germs. All are in the *Hemophilus* genus, requiring special culture media for growth in the bacteriology laboratory. Another, more distantly related bacillus, is the agent of granuloma inguinale. Lymphogranuloma venereum is caused by a virus-like agent akin to that of "parrot fever" (psittacosis) and trachoma. It is apt to produce large groin swellings, node rupture, and scarring. If caught early by the patient and promptly diagnosed and treated by his physician, the complications are not apt to occur. The early stage of each of these three types is indicated by a sore on the genitalia. All can be prevented by abstaining from sexual intercourse.

Summary

Venereal diseases require no vector other than the human animal. In this respect, the diseases resemble typhoid and tuberculosis. In contrast to the other infectious diseases, however, they require intimate body contact for transmission to other humans. No vaccines against VD exist. With all the infectious diseases, host allergy is responsible for the tissue damage and host immunity is responsible for protection from disease. Active immunization with a mild form of the disease, introduced via the natural portal of entry (such as live, attenuated polio virus administered orally), offers best protection, both individually and for the community at large, against those diseases for which vaccination is safe, simple, and cheap.

DISEASES OF MIXED CAUSES

In the previous section we have been talking about diseases of known cause: each is easily preventable if we use our wits and plan ahead. We are indebted to many astute physicians and related scientists for the useful knowledge handed down to us after having applied scientific methodology to the study of each disease. New infectious diseases are described yearly; doubtless some diseases of uncertain cause today will be shown to be caused by specific infectious agents in the future.

We now turn to diseases of mixed causes, where it is clear that hereditary and environmental factors are contributory, but less apparent as to how. Some of these diseases are of early onset and rapid progression, either in childhood or young adulthood; others, similar qualitatively, have delayed onset and may not present problems until middle age or later, such as diabetes mellitus or cataracts. The list is quite long of these illnesses. In general, the question is not so much "will I contract one of them" as it is "which one, how soon, and how severely?"

One might classify these disease of mixed causes according to the primary organs affected or by incidence and prevalence by age group, occupation, race, or class. For acute diseases, incidence is more important; for chronic disease, prevalence. (Incidence has to do with number of new cases, prevalence with numbers affected at any given time.) Most of the diseases of mixed causes are chronic, progressive, or intermittent in activity. Since it is the individual patient's personal complaint that prompts him to seek medical attention, in practice it is common for these disease to be grouped according to the particular medical or surgical specialty (or subspecialty) of those who have most regularly observed and managed patients presenting with these problems. Much confusion has resulted from this random manner of classification.

Seeking a qualified practitioner

Amid the confusion and lack of real knowledge so often found with these conditions, and in spite of the fact that much solid data is being added yearly to their understanding by men of science, we are confronted with a vast body of folklore and pseudoscientific practitioners who have taken up "squatters' rights" to management of many of these conditions down through the years. These are often well-meaning midwives, naturopaths, chiropractors, podiatrists, and others (sometimes even osteopaths may be found adhering to this group in various parts of the country). Well meaning though they may be, and usually provided with the most impeccable of "bedside manners," they uniformly are self-deluded and burdened by outmoded training and a highly structured body of inherited language and methodology. No doubt there is a need for "art" in the practice of healing, but real healing demands science. It is true that there exist qualified practitioners of medicine and surgery who have lapsed into just as much art to the exclusion of science as the groups just listed. But the dictum still holds, that for accredited medical and surgical training, a high scientific standard still prevails: many years of graduate training beyond the college degree, including 4 academic years of medical school, trained and taught by established men of science; 1 to 2 years of internship in a nationally accredited hospital; and usually additional years of residency, research, or clinical fellowship, with periodic postgraduate seminars after beginning practice of medicine-surgery.

Promising trends

The foundation of good medicine of yesteryear was simply correct anatomic and histologic observation. Although still important, the old foundation has been strengthened in past decades by physiologic and biochemical understanding not formerly available. With so much new, verified scientific data available yearly, and consequently bringing growing complexity and further specialization, some interesting developments may be seen. For example, it may chance that a certain vascular disorder might pass from the province of a cardiologist to that of the specialist in metabolic disease.

It is fascinating to watch the evolution of

interaction of the traditional, static, and anatomic view of disease with the more recent biochemical and dynamic viewpoint. Traditional lines of communication are sometimes strained when both the old and new approaches are used with the same patient, and much understanding patience is required of all parties. In such a setting, the modern family physician can serve beautifully as "quarterback" and "commentator" on behalf of the medical team on the one hand, and the patient on the other.

One hears and reads much of continuing medical education, superspecialization, and multidisciplinary approaches. These are big words for simple evolution in medical knowledge and its application. Optimal care of the patient is still at the heart of each of these ideas. The more difficult medical problems nowadays require modern training and a cooperative medical team approach involving several physicians. (As indication of this, we may remind ourselves that most patients now have at least three physicians simultaneously by the time they reach maturity.) When the internist, surgeon, clinical biochemist, and pharmacogeneticist join the immunologist and family physician in caring for the patient with a complex problem, we shall see as happy a day as ever was in man's history. But this ideal multidisciplinary approach is very demanding of every one of the parties concerned. Each physician must have a speaking acquaintance with the field of every other team member, or the result will be a Tower of Babel. Mutual respect is no less crucial among specialists than among mankind. Every patient can also do much to keep things on an even keel among all concerned, for ultimately it is the emotional response in a patient that can make or break a satisfactory medical management program.

We ought never grow too old or too busy to take time to learn and understand the new facts as they become available. That sorry state can happen in the life of a student, a funeral home ambulance service director, a physician, or anyone else; it takes careful planning and practice to avoid this universal pitfall.

Disease in its many forms constitutes a continuing impingement on man. Our habits, our likes and dislikes, our jobs, our hobbies, our diet and its timing, and our exercise and its balance are no less important to good health than favorable ancestry and wise physicians. The following examples indicate how physical breakdown can occur, as though "we did it to ourselves," quite unintentionally. In them, look for broader applicability, and draw your own conclusions as you read on.

Diseases caused by nutrient deficiency

Diseases caused by nutrient deficiency may present as disorders of the brain, skin, gastrointestinal tract, or other tissues; and complaints often vary dramatically from one person to the next. For example, one patient with pellagra (caused by mixed vitamin-protein deficiency, with thiamine shortage paramount) might first grow mentally (or emotionally) unstable; another might notice skin irritations; a third, loss of appetite or frequent bowel movements. Every medical student has learned the typical "pellagra triad" of "dermatitis, diarrhea, dementia"; but every practicing physician has missed several early or partial pellagra syndromes (that is, how the disease presents itself in the patient) when his index of suspicion was primed only with the whole picture, full-blown, out of the textbook.

Babies, children, college students, and middle-aged and elderly persons are all subject to disease caused by nutrient deficiency if their diet does not match their needs and capability for digestion-absorption (which is itself variable, determined by genetic and other factors). Many roads may lead to a given state of nutrient deficiency. Failure to ingest, to absorb, or to excrete the proper amount may be probable causes, as may failure of affected tissues to respond properly to a given nutrient. Of course the opposite may also occur: excesses of nutrients can build up at any point along the pathway just given. Too much vitamin A, for example, makes the brain swell: headache, double vision, and personality change may occur. For example, in sarcoidosis, vitamin D is absorbed from the intestine in excess, and hypercalcemia (too much calcium in body fluids) can occur. In someone using oily laxatives, all fat-soluble vitamins may be carried through the intestines unabsorbed, leading to deficiency of vitamins A, E, K, and D.* Too rapid transit through the intestines from any cause (even emotional) may rob the body of required nutrients: vitamins, minerals, water, fat, proteins, carbohydrates. Many drugs taken orally are irritating to the lining of the intestines and cause more rapid transit of intestinal contents; antibiotics, which change intestinal bacterial populations drastically, are especially apt to do this. Intestinal parasites (one in every ten of us is housing some parasite or other right now) compete for nutrients with the host. Loss of a critical part of the intestines (as through surgery or disease) may lead to failure to absorb enough vitamin B_{12}, for example.

Troubles in the upper gastrointestinal tract make it harder on each succeeding portion to function properly. One common train of events through the years (often seen in charity clinics and outpatient veterans' facilities) is for loss of molar teeth to occur (through neglect of dental hygiene, possibly combined with improper diet or chewing tobacco). This loss of chewing ability is not apt to be met with a perfect change in diet (as for example, a food mill to prechew all items on the menu that are not liquid). As a result, there will likely follow in a few years esophagitis, peptic ulcer, bleeding (or perforation or obstruction from scar) within the stomach, surgical removal of part of the upper gastrointestinal tract, rapid transit of nutrients and failure to absorb

them properly, colitis, weight loss, rectal inflammation, or anal disease.

Metabolic considerations

Metabolic disease, like allergy, is truly an ecologic discipline: it represents a meeting ground on heredity and environment; a vast body of solid information relatively independent of distortion by a consuming public has been amassed about it; and it embraces all tissues and organs of the body. We shall not be able to touch base with all of the current developments in this field, partially because one of the problems of a research discipline is that a separate language will evolve for its own communication purposes but will be hard to comprehend outside the field.

We have just seen how there can be either too much or too little of a particular nutrient from the diet at any given point along the gastrointestinal tract and how a secondary disease may result as abnormal physiology in the lower part of the gastrointestinal tract follows some original difficulty in the upper part. If one can see that connection, it will not be hard to think similarly on a molecular level about events too rapid and tiny for detection even by a microscope or blood test: the actual biochemistry inside cells. As at the macroscopic level, here there are several important metabolic sequences in which there must be proper input, proper absorption (by carrier or transport systems), proper digestion and conversion by enzymes, proper reabsorption, excretion, and coordination with related biochemical pathways inside the cell. One can visualize the cell's "assembly line."

If we had time, we might focus on each cell type in turn, noting the organ or tissue where it occurs, how it works, how things can go wrong, and what this means in terms of the health of the rest of the body. There was never a more fascinating or important frontier to explore—and medical research provides us with more new facts daily than many of us can even begin to digest. A quarter century ago it would have been impossible to present this topic; each

---

*Waterfowl have been killed in massive numbers by oil spills; the oil in their intestines deprives them of fat-soluble vitamins (from fish) and is itself a sufficient cause of disease and death in these birds. The oil accumulates in the birds' intestines as they attempt to preen it from their feathers with their bills. Blindness follows as retinal cells are deprived of vitamin A.

of us should plan to take a fresh peek at it every few years from now on.*

Cell integration. Metabolic diseases pose three other considerations besides what is happening along the assembly line. First, each of us, except identical twins, is biochemically unique from the moment of birth; afterward, even identical twins begin to differ. At the level of cell biochemistry, this means that our grandparents and parents gave us variable genetic material; therefore, no two of us handle any given chemical compound in precisely the same way, for each enzyme has at least three kinds of genes determining its (a) presence or absence, (b) activity enhancement, or (c) activity repression. We were certainly not created equal in a physical-chemical sense.

Second, each initial, intermediate, and final compound has its own intrinsic toxicity as well as useful metabolic function. A change of rate somewhere along the assembly line can quickly lead to both a relative lack of one chemical compound and an excess of another. The more steps in the assembly line—the more enzymes involved —the more chance for individual variation according to genetics.

Third, the more we learn in biochemistry, the more we see interrelated among adjacent biochemical pathways. Any given metabolic cycle at any given step can be affected by certain of the body's own chemical products and byproducts from other cycles. Such feedback influences may be positive or negative, direct or indirect, on any given step along the assembly line.

Finally, the living cell does not (save for a very few specialized cells) distinguish between native and foreign chemical compounds. Drugs, hormones, nutrients and body-synthesized molecules are handled impartially according to existing metabolic pathways.

Pharmacogenetics. The discussion of cell integration brings us to the fundamental problems of how our genetic differences affect the way we handle certain chemical compounds (pharmacogenetics). It is very important for the physician to know the metabolic options and the odds before he prescribes even a single drug. Your family history becomes highly significant to the family doctor as he ponders this problem; many good clues can be drawn from an accurate family medical history. Thus, it may become quite clear from review of your relatives' past and present medical history that a few or all of you in the family do not handle normally such common drugs as sedatives, antihistamines, analgesics and sulfonamides, nor such foods as wheat, corn, egg, milk, sugar, the amino acid leucine (richly present in dairy products), and others.

Just as there are foodstuff–metabolic pathway interactions, so also are there drug–food–metabolic interactions and even drug–drug–food–metabolic interactions to plague the physician and his patient. It is enough to make strong men weep in frustration— this is, except for the wonderful probability that in the near future we shall have computer help in predicting troubles before they occur, as well as in explaining existing metabolic diseases. Over five hundred drug–drug interactions are known to medical science that call for adjustment in dosage undreamed of just a few years ago.

Happily for medicine, the careful study of certain drug–host interactions can be used as a tool by which to diagnose and manage, quite early in life, some of the chronic diseases, such as the porphyria group,* before they can result in disease in

---

*Pertinent periodicals that help keep us abreast of such new data include *Science, Scientific American,* and *Today's Health.* For family physicians, *Hospital Practice* has helped greatly.

*Among the first to appreciate such a connection (porphyria in young adult life, degenerative autoimmune disease later on in the same patients) have been Waldenström and Forssman and their colleagues in Sweden. A useful case report and review of the world literature on this subject was published by these authors in the Swiss medical literature in 1967 (in German). This is not the first time North Americans have fallen behind in friendly competition with scientific investigators in other parts of the world. Any scientist should read French and German as well as English, if he would keep current in his field.

many tissues and organs. It may even be that some of the most poorly understood diseases will yield to a pharmacogenetic approach: diabetes, rheumatoid arthritis, systemic sclerosis (stiffening of skin and other tissues), dermatomyositis (skin and muscle inflammation), and lupus erythematosus (a common multiple organ-system disease affecting kidney, skin, bone marrow, and small blood vessels in essentially all parts of the body).

Systematic observation of the whole population of an area, however mixed and transient it may be, is another avenue by which basic clues to disease cause may legitimately be sought. The recent Framingham Study in Massachusetts, by our National Institutes of Health, was highly productive in this way.* Unfortunately, our Federal government could find no way to continue it.

Occupation-caused diseases

Nowhere in our experience have more solid bits of data been gathered about human tolerance for certain common chemical substances than in the fields of occupational medicine and industrial hygiene. Wise management has always looked to the health of its workers, especially while on the job. Even one plant physician alone is often in a good position to evaluate human responses to new materials in the environment, if he has the cooperation of management.

Where management is less than wise, there will be not only trouble between labor and management, but also undue occupational illness. Since small business and small industry cannot usually afford the services of a specialist in industrial hygiene, the vast majority of workers in industry in the United States is not well protected from industrial illness. Those in management often feel that competition with the large organizations requires that corners be cut and worker safety sacrificed. On the other hand, the

same arguments are mustered among large competing corporations in our country. Too seldom has a strong voice been heard in opposition to careless industrial exposures of the more subtle kind: noise, mists, dusts, vapors, powders, and solutions.

Forward-thinking management, like modern medicine, looks elsewhere for examples and advice in most areas of industrial hygiene. Thus we find that British medicine has contributed a vast and useful body of guidelines to the prevention of a disease almost universal in cotton textile mill workers exposed to airborne lint: byssinosis, with its inevitable pulmonary emphysema and fibrosis. And, again, in one small area of the produce-packing industry (in the northwestern United States), we have the example of one lone plant physician and his tenacious, astute judgment: Dr. Quimby, who has helped greatly in reducing respiratory disease in apple packers exposed to dyed dust. Such a person could do much for the plastics and resin industries if able to apply his knowledge of toxicities for organic solvents and catalysts in designing good preventive medical practices in industry. Each new industry, as each old industry, needs enlightened management and "a good Dr. Quimby." There is no substitute for a man on the scene, trained to observe for possible trouble, both expected and unexpected. How many knitting mill employees and executives have succumbed to variations of leukemia? No one knows, if there is no plant physician charged with seeing to the health implications of the operation, and not just available in his office to sew up cuts and set fractures.

In America we also lag behind certain European countries as regards safety in mining and in coal and steel industries. Why should there be any question, any fight, about the magnitude of the problem of "black lung," silicosis, metal fume fever, and other diseases common in these related industries? We see no reason to delay effective legislation that will make management solely responsible for the prevention of these and other industrial diseases. It ought not

---

*Kannel, William B.: The Framingham study and chronic disease prevention, Hospital Practice **5:** 78, March 1970.

require nearly so much time and expense to take the example of other countries with good methods as it does to engage in protracted debate at the expense of all taxpayers (whose voice may fail against those johnny-on-the-spot lobbyists of the wrong approach). How long our country can afford the laissez-faire ethics of various levels of bureaucracy in matters of health is a real question for each of us.

Harmful chemicals and disease

For years western civilization has been dominated by the petroleum age, with its products derived from coal and oil. As long as we have internal combustion engines and production machinery we shall inhale, contact, and ingest repeatedly a variety of petroleum and related products, including such additives as bacteriostatic and fungicidal compounds, rust inhibitors, viscosity regulators, antigummers, antiknocks, dyes, odorants and deodorants, and detergents. Inflammation of skin and mucous membranes, allergic disorders, and poisonings will all be our lot until we take the responsibility of controlling our Pandora's box of environmental insults loosed upon us in the past, present, and future.

Chromates, organic mercurials, halogenated hydrocarbons, benzene and phenolic compounds and their substituents are all active biochemically, though this is usually incidental to their intended industrial uses. Although excellent plant-handling practices may be found, the finished product may receive other treatment and be brought again into contact with human beings or the plants and animals upon which we depend for life. All the compounds listed—and many, many more unlisted—have very real threshold limits for safe human exposure.* Sad to relate, we usually do not bother to learn the limits for safe exposure of critical fellow members of our environment, the plants and animals. Even sadder, the finished

---

*American Conference of Government Industrial Hygienists Committee on Threshold Limit Values, rev. ed., Cincinnati, 1966.

products as used by consumers may not even be fully labelled. Wander through a hardware or paint store sometime, and look at the labels. How many list the complete analysis accurately? How many give detailed instructions as to safe use? Does any tell the tolerance of earthworms, bluebirds, pets, or livestock for that particular product?

If we do not maintain careful watch over our industrial and chemical hazards, which are mostly invisible but mostly predictable in the light of modern knowledge, it will only be by sheerest accident that we avoid a host of diseases resulting from our customary handling of such products. Usually we see only what we look for, whereas we ought always to look for trouble where biologically active substances are concerned. Perhaps what is needed most are laws adequate for ensuring recognition, quantitation, and longitudinal monitoring of chemical exposures caused directly and indirectly by industrial products.

Allergic disease

Earlier we briefly mentioned host immunology, with emphasis on circulating antibodies as protective in the face of infectious disease, especially viral diseases. Not all immune responses are useful in preventing disease, however; quite the contrary may occur. When it does, it is called an allergy.

An allergy is an altered response to familiar substances. For an allergy to develop, one requires the appropriate genetic makeup and past history of exposure to a given allergenic substance, or antigen (anything able to provoke an immune response). Four basic types of allergic responses are currently recognized (Table 7-3). In theory, allergic disease can affect any organ or tissue in any vertebrate animal. The older the animal, the more chance for chronic allergic disease to be present, for with each passing year the host is exposed to new sensitizing antigens and more of the old familiar ones. Antigens from outside sources include those found in drugs; foods; and airborne particles, such as dust, pollen, animal dander, insect matter, other proteins and polysac-

Table 7-3. Types of allergic response in human beings (may be mixed)

	Type I	Type II	Type III	Type IV
Antibody involved	Fixed to mast cell near small blood vessels in skin and membranes; many names: gamma E, IgE, atopic reagin	Circulates; is called: IgG (gamma G) and IgM (gamma M) Activates an enzyme that injures cells	Circulates in complex with its antigens In blood, in lymph and tissue fluids, IgG or IgM; damage as in Type II to cells or membranes	None; small (immune) lymphocytes circulating from blood to tissues to lymph node Response dictated by thymus gland
Antigen site	Portals of entry: skin, mucous membranes	Membrane of any cell fixed or circulating	Circulates in complex with specific antibodies	Tissues outside the circulation in any organ
Typical example	Rayweed Hayfever	Quinidine producing loss of platelets with bleeding	Tetanus antitoxin causing "serum sickness"	Poison ivy
Nature of antigen in example	Pollen Proteins	Drug plus its cell membrane receptor	Horse serum proteins	Plant oleoresin Pentadeca-catechol plus skin receptor
Final common chemical (and source) doing damage	Mast cell Histamine	Antibody-coated cell destroyed by rupture or removal; see Type III	Enzymes of certain leukocytes damage any membrane; as in Type II	Active chemicals secreted by lymphocytes
Permanent damage if any	None, if surviving transient edema in vital areas	Depends on extent of damage and whether cell is replaceable	Tissue loss, healing with scarring, in proportion to vascular membrane injury upstream	Granuloma may calcify or heal with scarring; loss of tissue if cells not replaced
Prevention	Advance use of antihistamine Avoidance	Avoid this and similar drugs in future, if known	Same as for Type II	Preferably, avoid exposure (as for all other types)
Emergency treatment	Epinephrine	Platelet transfusion as needed	Heparin Cortisone	Cortisone

charides. Critical aspects in the development of allergic disease include dose and avenue of exposure, rate and time sequence of exposure, prior allergic state, available levels of histamine and other chemical substances responsible for allergic disease, and the host capacity for repair (in turn dependent upon nutritional state and genetically determined metabolic pathways).

Since the substances producing an allergic reaction must produce lesions via the effects of biologically active chemicals found in all human beings, allergic disease itself produces no unique appearance or symptoms in any given tissue or organ. For example, a particular allergic person's asthma might one time be caused by his allergy (perhaps to house dust), but it could equally well be caused by a nonallergic insult the next time (such as phosgene, liberated when a Freon propellant of some aerosol can is released near a hot electric space heater; phosgene was used as a war gas because it is strongly irritating to respiratory membranes). Strangling on gastric juice, blood clots lodging in the pulmonary arteries, or sudden left-sided

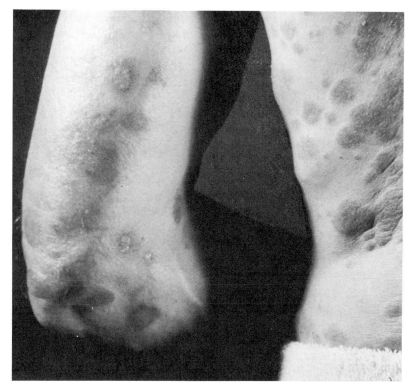

Fig. 7-7. Severe chronic hypersensitivity reaction to an organic diamine—one of the potent chemicals commonly found in household goods.

heart failure can also produce an asthmatic reaction that any observer might believe to be caused by an allergy.

What is peculiar to allergy is that at least one previous exposure to the offending antigen is required beforehand; a latent period is required for production of antibodies or immune lymphocytes; and then further exposure to the identical antigen will result in an allergic reaction.

Many of the body's own proteins, fats, and polysaccharides are antigenic (able to cause allergy). Under certain conditions allergic responses can be provoked to some of the body's own material, but some primary infectious disease agent or chemical exposure is almost always the trigger for such a reaction. Some families are quick to develop such autoallergic aspects in their disease. Though we do not understand why, diabetics are apt to have higher than average levels of antibodies to certain gastric cell antigens; patients with pernicious anemia

have the same, but also have antibodies to the gastric protein secretory product known as the "intrinsic factor," which is required for absorption of vitamin B_{12} in the terminal small bowel. Patients with degenerative thyroid, adrenal, pigment cell, and many other organ diseases also have higher than average antibody levels to antigens produced in those organs and tissues.

Neoplasia (tumors and cancer)

Much research is being conducted on tumors and cancer. Here, too, it appears that genetics is just as important as in other categories of disease. Some tumors are caused by both DNA and RNA viruses (referring to the type of nucleic acid in the virus particle). The genetic susceptibility to infection by both DNA and RNA viruses is variable. As a further complication, in at least one instance the same virus seems to be able to cause two different types of neoplastic response (mononucleosis, Burkitt's lymphoma), depending on the race of the person infected, on the geographic location of the person, and on the existence of other diseases in that person.

Not all tumors or cancers are known to be virus caused; at present most have unknown causes. It may be that any agent that can damage genetic material in cell nuclei in a crippling, but not fatal, way can cause neoplastic change in that cell or its descendants. Many physical and chemical agents might inflict such damage to genes. No doubt there is variable genetic capability for repair of damage to nucleic acid: one victim might make repairs leading to neoplastic change, whereas another might make different repairs. Once a cell has developed into a tumor cell, it may be that host immunology comes into play in determining whether that cell is destroyed immunologically or tolerated. There is some evidence that different tumor antigens evoke different host antibodies, with one type (cytotoxic antibody) able to destroy the cell bearing that antigen, the other antibody (blocking type) more or less protecting the tumor cell from the action of the former antibody.

As with any disease process, causes must be fully understood before dependable treatment and cure may be expected. Nowhere in medicine is there such panic as in anything having to do with cancer. Much time and money are being wasted in trial-and-error clinical research procedures. In the long run, it is foolish to try a shortcut to success when too many of the basic questions remain unanswered because of inadequate training of research personnel and excessive impatience of their backers. Pure research in basic sciences has often produced unexpected benefit. Trained investigators who are free to continue research on basic biologic truths are invaluable to those dealing specifically with cancer.

The patients themselves have much to teach physicians; we were learning fast from the Framingham study when it was discontinued because of impatience in Washington. Systematic study of population groups in relation to their environment—the essence of ecology—is useful epidemiology and can point to the questions we ought to be asking about certain diseases. To answer these questions, in turn, might send us back to the research laboratory.

COMMON DYSFUNCTIONAL SYNDROMES
Heart disease

For many years physicians have been managing patients who have heart trouble, and they have acquired much art and skill at it. A variety of sophisticated tools exists by which the heart's functions may be measured, and additional years of training are required in order to properly operate them with minimal risk to the patients. The importance of these tools is apt to be overemphasized, however, if it distracts us from continued study of basic mechanisms of heart disease. Happily, such basic research is quite active.

Another feature in the evolution of delivery of care to the cardiac patient is that the patient may come to expect certain regimens and to evaluate his physician in terms of which regimen is used, irrespective of its pertinence to his own situation from the medical viewpoint. (This happens in all specialties, not just in cardiology.) It is the rare patient nowadays who will follow orders completely. The physician must give clear, firm instructions, while at the same time he must continually question, evaluate, and remain openminded as new scientific data become available. All things considered, a confident patient lends stability to the health team, and his own condition stands to benefit more surely.

Causes of heart damage. First, hard work does not injure the normal heart; in fact, the heart thrives on regular exertion: it grows, becomes more efficient at using oxygen, delivers more blood per beat, and recovers faster after damaging illnesses (if it has been well exercised regularly in advance of the illness). It is highly useful to reach middle age owning the heart of an active athlete.

Heart function can be compromised by too great an increase in the circulation's volume or in its pressure. A common way to develop the first condition might be to combine excessive sodium intake with fluid intake, as in eating salty cocktail foods while drinking the usual party beverages. In normal people, the blood volume will not rise without the pressure rising also. The reverse can happen, though: fatigue, anger, and fear can all raise the blood pressure. These are causes of increased volume and pressure that the individual himself can partially control; there are others that the physician is better equipped to manage.

Blood vessels that supply the heart can be choked shut by inflammatory diseases, such as allergy or infection, or by metabolic diseases, such as those causing lipid and cholesterol deposits. Naturally, the heart must suffer harmful consequences, including muscle weakened or killed (infarcted). There are many ways to increase deposit-prone fatty material borne in the bloodstream and laid down in heart vessel walls: too much of something wrong in the diet; too little of something essential; failure to clear the bloodstream normally, as when the phagocytes are poisoned, whether by alcohol or by a vascular allergy; or even a critical enzyme missing somewhere in fat metabolism, as in the lipid storage diseases such as Fabry's disease.

The skeleton of the heart is a figure-eight–shaped cartilage; this tissue can be weakened by agents that are able to damage cartilage: certain metabolites that are products of either normal or faulty metabolism, or even substances present in our diet. Rats, for example (resembling human beings in many ways and hence useful for medical research) can be shown to suffer cartilage damage when fed sweet pea seeds. Much further research along these lines is needed.

Also requiring much more study is how atheromas (cholesterol plaques and plugs) are able to accumulate in the blood vessels. What are the normal clearing mechanisms? How may the normal clearance be increased or impaired? Are vegetable fats (unsaturated fats) really better for us than animal fats? After all, they do polymerize (grow larger molecules) more readily, and they do tend to form peroxides sometimes.

Among the more common, better-understood causes of heart damage are infections of the inner lining of the heart, with permanent valve damage and loss of the pump's efficiency, such as endocarditis and valvular stenosis. Endocarditis is common in heroin addicts; otherwise, it is most apt to follow valve damage from syphilis or rheumatic fever. Heart muscle inflammation—myocarditis—can develop from infection, allergy, or metabolic poisoning, such as "beer drinkers' heart." There can also be competition for space either within the heart's covering tissue (pericardium) or between the pericardium and the heart. This can be caused by a bleeding stab wound of the heart, a chronic infection such as tuberculosis, or a tumor; there are other causes as well.

Heart failure. Whether the original problem was coronary vascular disease (that is, diseased heart vessels), myocarditis, high blood pressure (hypertension), or diseased heart valves, the failing heart may lead to death unless the cause is a reversible one. We are fortunate that artificial valves are now being used regularly in open-heart surgery, that so many useful drugs are available by which high blood pressures and blood volumes may be favorably changed, and that simple dietary adjustment can so often turn the tide in favor of a return to good health.

Lung failure

Three general ways exist by which the lung may fail. Lung tissues might be waterlogged from drowning, from breathing irritating gases or smokes, or from a failing heart. This type of failure would create a diffusion impairment, in which inspired air has to travel through thicker tissues to reach the bloodstream and blood-borne gases such as carbon dioxide likewise must travel a longer path en route to the airways for excretion. The second cause of lung failure can be illustrated by emphysema: the air coming in cannot mix well with blood, because the two seldom meet in the lung. There may be stale air trapped in large air sacs (alveoli) and stale blood in scarred, narrowed vessels, but the blood basically detours around the obstructions and returns to the heart without ever having the chance to pick up oxygen and discard carbon dioxide. Finally, the lung may also fail because neither is air being brought to it (ventilatory paralysis) nor blood (clotting in the pulmonary artery).

Causes. We understand considerably more about lung diseases than about heart disease; that is, we have more useful knowledge as to causes and prevention. Even where no cure is possible, palliation almost always is. Some of the causes of lung failure are reversible: clots in the main pulmonary artery, if caught quickly; bronchitis, if infection is eradicated, smoking stopped, allergy brought under control, and occupational air pollutants avoided; pneumonia, careful management of this group of acute inflammatory lung diseases by physicians, including prompt treatment with proper antibiotics when required; space-occupying diseases— large cysts, fluid collections, tumors within the chest are all often correctable surgically.

Modern management of lung failure is best done in or close to a hospital center with a trained team and proper equipment; good management is not cheap. Gas mixtures for ventilating the lung can be varied according to patient needs, delivered under varying pressure, supplied in the proper volume, and even worn and used as a portable pack, in some cases. In a case of sudden respiratory (ventilatory) arrest, the hospital anesthesiologist often takes the leading role; this may then pass to the chest surgeon (who can best relieve major airway obstructions), to the chest physician, and then to the ventilation therapist. But all function as a team together with the family physician and the newest member, the rehabilitation counsellor, who is especially important in chronic disease.

Prevention. Useful life and its enjoyment is far better achieved via prevention of respiratory disease than via treatment. "Of all sad words of tongue or pen, the saddest are these: it might have been" applies to the smoker, the welder, the cotton mill worker, the lacquer sprayer, the miner, the metal grinder, the crop duster, or whoever forgot or did not know to wear an adequate protective mask daily during his working years and had not the good sense to refuse to smoke. Cough, shortness of breath, and chest discomfort are useful warning signs that we ought never to ignore when it comes to ensuring our future health; unfortunately, with many chest diseases they come quite late, after much damage is already established, as is the case with emphysema.

Kidney failure

Metabolic, allergic, and vascular diseases, poisonings, birth defects, and infections can all lead to kidney malfunction and failure. Whereas volatile wastes can be excreted by the lung, nonvolatile waste excretion largely depends on the kidney. In turn, a good kidney needs a good heart, healthy vessels, and a free path to the outside.

Examples of reversible kidney disease include infections managed promptly and well by the physician, obstructions of the lower urinary tract managed promptly by the urologist, and renal stones whose cause is accurately diagnosed and corrected. Chronic, progressive renal disease nowadays can fall back upon the expertise of a fairly new specialty, nephrology, as well as a kidney team, available at every good hospital center and medical school.

All generalized diseases of blood vessels affect the kidney; so do many metabolic diseases such as diabetes, gout, adrenal diseases, and parathyroid diseases. Certain genetically determined conditions are primarily kidney disorders, including many enzyme deficiencies and some storage diseases. Heavy metal poisoning, hydrocarbon poisoning, extensive burns, and excessive drugstore headache remedies such as phenacetin can likewise injure the kidney or be severe enough to cause kidney failure. There are many other causes of renal disease.

The high cost of failure. In hemodialysis a patient with kidney failure, or with no kidneys at all, is connected by way of his blood vessels to a machine through which his blood travels and by which they are cleansed of wastes. This procedure is best done overnight three times weekly; many patients learn how to continue a home program of dialysis, with their own dialysis machines in the bedroom. Wise physicians and obedient patients can achieve much extension of useful life by this means.

Although effective, it is extremely expensive to be trained in one's own dialysis program and to invest in one's own machine. Hopefully, with continued research we can achieve simpler and less expensive equipment; but it is obviously best in the long run to invest in programs by which we may know the causes and prevention of renal diseases. So many useful tools are available for continuing research—physical chemistry, immunopathology, electron microscopy, tissue culture, and animal models of disease—that we can ill-afford to neglect even one such avenue.

When to see the doctor. Blood in the urine, burning on urination, pains in the pelvic area, back pain, too much or too little urine, abnormal discharges all call for immediate medical attention, especially when accompanied by loss of appetite, nausea, fever, or chills. The importance of prompt and careful urine examination (naked eye, chemical, and microscopic tests are routine nowadays) has long been recognized: in ancient Rome, no matter what the patient complained of, it was a capital offense to fail to examine his urine.

Liver failure

As the kidney is our major excretory organ, so the liver is our metabolizer and factory, as well as the body's main detoxification unit. The liver needs continuous perfusion by blood: both portal venous blood, bearing substances absorbed from the gastrointestinal tract, and hepatic artery blood, which carries oxygen. Obstruction of any of the three vessels—two entering, one leaving the liver—can damage liver structure and function. There are many other causes of reversible and irreversible liver damage. Liver cells are closely related to cells that form capillaries; both have tremendous capacity for regeneration. Likewise, both

are subject to many of the same insults (viruses thrive in both, for example).

Dietary toxins (chiefly alcohol), other enzyme poisons, and general protein poisons can cause both temporary and permanent liver damage. Parasitic and infectious agents can invade the liver (bile passages, bloodstream, or liver cells themselves) to cause disease. Amoebae, hepatitis viruses, and malaria parasites are examples of living disease agents adapted for life in the liver, and thus the liver is apt to suffer most when these agents invade. Hepatitis (inflammation of the liver) can be mild, or it can be severe enough to cause jaundice or even massive liver cell necrosis (death), quickly leading to death of the host. Less severe but more chronic damage, combined with scar formation and spotty regeneration of liver cells, is known as cirrhosis (which can be compared with pulmonary emphysema).

Cirrhosis does not always lead to liver failure, but it does distort bile duct and blood vessel anatomy within the liver. Dammed up behind constricting bands of scar tissue, portal blood may follow paths of least resistance via collateral detours, by-passing the liver. This portal blood may now be dumped into the systemic (whole body) circulation just as it came from the intestines, with untold effect upon the host's immune responsiveness and nutrition. Other effects are more apparent, such as massive hemorrhages from engorged collateral vessels never meant to carry this extra blood. Liver tissue deprived of normal blood supplies cannot function well in its usual production of plasma proteins, particularly albumin and several clotting factors. Another measure of diseased liver cells is a fall in urea, which is normally made in the liver, and a rise in ammonia, which is produced in the intestines by the action of bacterial and host enzymes on protein.

Endocrine failure

Glands of internal secretion have also had a separate subspecialty for several years. Endocrinology is linked to metabolism as allergy is to immunology; in each case there is a clinical practice grounded upon a research-level foundation.

Heading the list of endocrine glands is the pituitary gland, nestled beneath the brain, and regulated by the hypothalamus. The posterior lobe of the pituitary gland has to do with the body's water balance and with uterine muscle activity, the anterior lobe with stimulation of the endocrine glands and other tissues.

Infections and vascular diseases at the base of the brain may injure the pituitary gland. Interestingly enough, its function is affected by both nicotine and alcohol. Tumors may arise in any of its several cell types. Some of these tumors are dangerous because of their pressure effects on neighboring structures; others are functional as well, among them being the tumor causing pituitary gigantism, or the giants of our storied past and present. Other pituitary diseases include hereditary metabolic diseases of pituitary tissues, such as pituitary dwarfism. Finally, the pituitary may be damaged in accidental trauma, in shock, and in heatstroke or other high fevers.

Deprived of pituitary stimulation, just as if they were themselves diseased, certain endocrine glands malfunction and reduce their own glandular secretions, including hormones: secretions of the ovary, testis, adrenal, and thyroid glands diminish, and the tissues of these glands shrink. Various other consequences result from reduction in hormone levels: energy declines, hair growth decreases, the body's metabolic rate (and temperature) decrease, appetite drops, muscle action is slowed, more sleep may be required, sex drive is lost, and personality change often occurs.

Isolated endocrine failure and overactivity. Individual endocrine glands may also suffer disease independent of the others. Infections and autoallergic disorders account for many of these, metabolic diseases and tumors for others. It is curious that the body may be made just as ill by too much of a particular hormone as by too little, though not in the same ways. Even more curious is the fact that the natural 24 hour cycle of endocrine activity is attuned to the earth's rotation about the sun (that is, with waking and sleeping hours, daylight and dark); a lunar monthly cycle also exists for adult females. Thus, biologic rhythms, so impotrant in lower animal and in plant life, are still very much with us human beings and also account for the particular evolution of certain parasitic diseases dependent upon man for part of the reproductive cycle, such as malaria and filariasis.*

Diabetes mellitus. Of all the diseases of the endocrine glands, diabetes is by far the most common. Its cause is completely unknown as of this writing, and no single deficiency is yet recognized, which might account for its varied aspects: cataracts; atherosclerosis; disordered metabolism of carbohydrates, fats, and proteins; disease of the walls of small blood vessels, including those of the eye and kidney; and nerve degeneration.

Since no cause is known, there is no cure presently available for diabetes mellitus. Nonetheless, certain features of the disease can be controlled or prevented: high blood glucose levels, overacidity, dehydration, coma, and early death. All these aspects are controllable only under good medical management. Extra insulin can be given by injection to improve the body's faulty metabolism, such as bringing the blood glucose level down and preventing fat breakdown and overacidity. Firm dietary control is the basic requirement of diabetics. They, more than any other group, must have daily regular meal schedules and regular sleeping habits. The better they become creatures of fixed health habit, the longer may they expect to enjoy good health.

Brain damage

Our brains are such specialized tissues that they, more than any others, depend on a fine balance of nutrients provided by other organs. For instance, brain tissue can use only glucose for food. Steady supplies of

*Hawking, Frank: The clock of the malaria parasite, Scientific American **222**:123, June 1970.

oxygen are critical; the brain does not function well anaerobically. Extra physiologic barriers separate the brain from circulating blood; extra time is correspondingly required by the brain and spinal cord to maintain an equilibrium with compounds whose levels are changing in the bloodstream.

Causes of brain damage. Trauma (forceful injury) leads the list of causes of brain damage. Vascular disease is next. Clots deprive brain cells of normal supplies of blood carrying glucose and oxygen; hemorrhage within the skull builds up damaging pressure levels against normal brain tissue. Tumors, infections, metabolic diseases, and poisonings all contribute to the incidence of brain damage. Each category has reversible and irreversible potential; brain tissue destroyed does not grow back. Therefore, viral infections of the brain, such as encephalitis, might be of worse prognosis than a bacterial meningitis treated early and properly, that is, meningitis near enough to the brain to affect it, but not destroying brain tissue unless negligence affords time for extension of the infection through the meninges (covering membranes) to the brain proper.

Irreversible change results when brain tissue is lost. The pattern of disease in the patient will vary according to which tissues are lost, since certain areas of the brain control certain body functions. Depending on the location of the brain injury, the result may be death; permanent coma; loss of sight, hearing, smell, or taste; personality change; loss of sensations in some part of the body; muscle or nerve weakness or spasm; lack of coordination and balance; paralysis; convulsions; loss of temperature control; and a great number of other deficiencies.

Brain death is a highly important medicolegal, as well as medical, point nowadays. We used to think that absence of proof of electrical activity in the cerebral cortex, as reflected by a flat tracing by the electroencephalogram, meant proof of its absence, that is, death of the brain. Now, however, it is clear that in certain cases a person

with a one-time flat EEG, as from drug coma or severe loss of body heat, can return to an apparently normal state of health. The preceding might be called an example of general brain failure; it may be reversed, though rarely. Localized brain damage, such as a contusion (bruise) of the brain, may likewise be reversible.

Gastrointestinal disease

Most of us regard the esophagus as the first part of the gastrointestintal tract; actually, we ought first to think of the mouth and oral cavity, including the tongue, teeth, jaw muscles, taste buds, and salivary glands. Dentition and mastication have been discussed in Chapter 3; their importance to what follows as food traverses the gastrointestinal tract cannot be overemphasized. In the middle-aged and elderly, far more incidences of esophagitis (inflammation of the esophagus), peptic ulcer, diverticulitis (formation and inflammation of bowel pockets), and anorectal disease occur in the toothless portion of the population than in those with teeth.

Each part of the gastrointestintal tract provides essential functions; the body as a whole, not to mention successive portions of the gastrointestinal tract itself, does not function well when deprived of sections of the gastrointestintal tract. It is true that life can be sustained with all but a critical foot or two of small bowel remaining as absorptive and digestive surface; but only at great cost—in dollars, discomfort, and inconvenience.

So important is the gastrointestintal tract that a variety of medical and surgical specialties has evolved to deal with its complaints. With the advent of molecular medicine even more disciplines have entered the picture so that now we have gastroenterologists, abdominal surgeons, proctologists, immunologists, thoracic surgeons, and metabolic disease experts all involved in study and care of the gastrointestintal tract.

Despite the fact that our language is rich in descriptive terms derived from this part of our anatomy ("he's got guts"; "what's eating you"; "never could stomach that"; "she makes me sick to my stomach"), we must agree with Tyor* that it gets slighted in the public eye, as well as the profession's. A really good stool exam is hard to obtain even in otherwise good hospitals. Our ability to diagnose accurately and promptly amebic colitis, for example, has diminished in many quarters. Other parasites likewise are overlooked, yet parasitic disease of the gastrointestinal tract is quite common in all parts of the United States—and it is curable.

Clues to look for. Indications of disease of the gastrointestinal tract include weight loss, loose stool or more than one daily (sustained for many days), nausea, loss of appetite, constipation, vomiting, abdominal pain or swelling, blood or mucus passed from mouth or the rectum (with or without normal stool), very pale or dark, tarry stools, and bulky, frothy, sour, or foul stools.

Harmful habits. Alcohol (ethanol, if over 8%) is damaging to the lining tissues of esophagus and stomach. Strongly basic and/or acid substances are likewise harmful. Aspirin, vinegar, strong (especially if piping hot) coffee and tea, chili peppers, and a variety of irritating spices (such as found in mustard, catsup, steak sauce, luncheon meats, and cola beverages) will take their toll if used often or in large quantity. Protein foods that are subject to considerable enzyme action prior to freezing or that have been stored long at temperatures above freezing are apt to contain degenerative products—polypeptides and amines—that can be absorbed and act as mild poisons. These are apt to present a problem for some people, especially those whose esophagus and stomach are already irritated, when eating seafoods, nuts, cheeses, country ham, smoked fish, canned meats, cold cuts, sausage, and hot dogs. One need not, as a rule, give up all these foods mentioned; all he need do is go easy and mix them with safer foods in the same meal. Dilution with bland items is often a dependable approach.

---

*Tyor, Malcolm P.: The gastroenterologist "gap," Hospital Practice 4:76, December 1969.

Finally, one should beware of pork still pink after cooking (including the bacon wrapping of a rare steak), meatloaf and meat salads in uninspected kitchens, and roadhouse bar fare. Trichinosis and acute food poisonings still occur in these settings.

Bone marrow damage

Many common environmental and dietary substances can reach the bone marrow; those that are fat soluble will stay there for some time (since marrow contains so much fat normally). Whether one eats, breathes, or touches them, many marrow poisons can enter the body and affect important marrow functions. Even small amounts and low exposure rates can cause cells to malfunction or to multiply and work overtime; high doses and rapid exposure rates tend to kill cells or stop some of their functions. This applies to both living and nonliving agents.

Marrow cells at risk include red blood cell factories, certain white cell factories, platelet (thrombocyte, critical in blood clotting) factories, fat cells, fibroblasts (fiber formers), immune cells (lymphocytes, the antibody factories, and plasma cells), capillary blood vessel cells, and macrophages (garbage collectors).

Alcohol, benzene, toluene, phenol, alkylbenzenes, chlorinated hydrocarbons, naphthalene, xylenes, and a host of other everyday compounds are extremely toxic to marrow cells and their functions. Dry cleaning fluids, spot removers, paint thinners, enamel solvents, paint removers, antifreeze, motor fuels, brake fluid, heating oil, chloramphenicol, insecticides, moth crystals, Lysol, spirit-base paints, varnishes, and shellac all can harm the marrow even when used as directed on the label, or in common practice otherwise.

Not only these chemicals, but a variety of living agents and their toxins, and even allergic diseases can cause marrow cell diseases. Marrow disease may be generalized, or one cell type may be singled out for damage; combinations of damage are common. For reasons yet unclear, sometimes one cell type multiplies at the expense of others. At times, the picture in circulating blood can accurately reflect what is going on "back at the oasis," in the marrow; at other times a direct examination of bone marrow tissue is required for diagnosis. Complete failure of all marrow functions can occur; sometimes this has been reversible; sometimes, as when the offending poison or infectious agent is never known or avoidable death is inevitable, despite a succession of transfusions and marrow transplants (quite a new approach).

A PAUSE TO REFLECT

What has been said so far? That disease is easy to understand and to manage; simple to predict and avoid? Not by a long shot! Man himself is too complex for such perfect understanding; his illnesses are not easier to fathom. Most of them have multiple causes: a genetic pattern, a dietary habit, an environmental background, and one or more causal agents. One man's meat may be another's poison—but which man, and which poison? Disease may one time be acute and self-limiting; the next time, the same disorder may be chronic and progressive, as with melanoma, a frequently malignant tumor, sometimes vanishing spontaneously.

Hence we caution against ambitious and ill-defined, vaguely structured health-planning activities. For example, in New Guinea, some time back, DDT was given carte blanche for use as the main thrust against malaria-bearing mosquitos. House lizards ate the poisoned insects, sickened, and grew sluggish, were eaten by cats, which, being more sensitive to DDT, soon died. The rodent population next exploded, and bubonic plague returned to the area. Adding insult to injury was another disaster: since house lizards had been keeping in check the beetles whose larvae ate up frame timbers and roof thatch, the native houses began to fall down, victimized by an unchecked transient spurt in the beetles and larvae populations. The program, designed to eliminate one cause of disease, obviously backfired. It is certainly better to ask advice of the expert (the real one, in terms of human problems, is nothing if not ecologically oriented).

GOOD SENSE IN HEALTH

Most of us feel that, as in religion, law, politics, and education, health care is too important to be left to the experts alone. After all, each of us has as much to teach as to learn. When we consider health care, it sounds peculiar to make an artificial division between a provider class and a consumer class. Every individual is, in the final analysis, a member of both. No expert can help anyone who is unwilling to take the responsibility for accurately making and reporting his own observations or who is reluctant to follow advice given. Each member of society must assume an appropriate measure of responsibility for his own and others' welfare.

Health care is also an issue encompassing our entire society. Its complexity involves more than a patient describing an illness or a physician prescribing treatment. The complications of delivering and financing health care need to be considered often by every individual, physician, and representative of government involved, without losing sight of the final product: health.

The following examples, which have been taken directly from clinical experience, have been chosen to illustrate one or more of the problems that make health care a complex idea. These problems involve health care delivery in varied social and geographic settings, achieving ecologic balance in health care, integration of all disciplines involved in health care, and the need for communication based on mutual interpersonal respect. You may wish to identify the various single problems illustrated in the examples. Questions are provided to stimulate discussion about the elements involved in the examples.

A Mexican migrant fruit picker (who does not speak English) has been arrested "for public drunkenness" after falling from a tree. What are his chances for being understood and receiving appropriate medical attention in time?

A black teenager has been arrested and jailed for belligerent behavior at a time of social unrest. His neglected cold and sore throat turn out to be presymptoms of pneumonia and meningitis. If the diseases remain untreated, they will not only infect others but may lead to the boy's death. What are his chances for prompt and proper care in your community? Can your town give the best care that modern medical bacteriology can offer? At what stages could your town have given effective preventive medicine in this case?

A third example is more complex. In a family group representing three generations, it has been noticed that many males and females have had kidney trouble. The affected males have rarely survived past puberty; they have succumbed to progressive kidney failure. Affected girls have survived to middle age, bearing children, some of whom seem to have inherited the kidney trouble.

The present third generation has already lost one boy to the disease; two others are known to be affected, and there are several girls with protein always present in the urine, as discovered by family physicians and pediatricians. Though economically self-sufficient and substantial members of the community, this family is not financially, emotionally, or intellectually prepared to intervene in the natural course of this kidney disease. Unconsciously, perhaps, they have developed what they feel to be the best course to follow.

They never mention the disease; they accept it and care tenderly for all affected by it as long as life lasts. Death often comes at home, and not after long-term, expensive hospitalization. To receive renal dialysis the children affected would have to leave home, accompanied by one or both parents, who are needed at home and in the community.

Renal dialysis would cost several thousand dollars per year per patient and would postpone the inevitable death only by a few short years. Renal transplant would also mean leaving home for unfamiliar territory, the loss of a breadwinner or a housewife or both for a few weeks (or months), and severe strain upon all personal and family schedules, not to mention the community health budget, or even that of the state.

A new physician, with recent training and new ideas, comes to the community. He mentions to the patient he examines the possibility of visiting a renal disease center for diagnosis and offers to find a program that might be available free of charge in a distant city. He knows that certain basic studies are in progress than can be used to discover the exact nature of the family's kidney disease and possibly suggest more effective ways of managing it. But the effect of his suggestions is to alarm all others concerned and to anger those involved in the family's health care. Discussions rapidly reach an impasse; effective communication is lost. What are the other factors to consider in such a case where the physician knows how to cure or manage the course of a disease? How would you respond to the problem if this were your family?

The spoiled son of a local business and political figure, after infecting his date simultaneouly with two venereal diseases, is seen driving his car into two others and finally into the lake at an old ferry landing. In your town, what are the ways available to ensure that the witnesses will take proper action? If the girl has contacted a physician, what action should he take about the problem, aside from management of the disease? How can each successive step in all these problems be managed or prevented?

PART III

Family health

Whenever a decision or choice is to be made concerning behavior,
the moral decision will be the one which works toward the creation
of trust, confidence, and integrity in relationships. It should increase the
capacity of individuals to cooperate, and enhance the sense of
self-respect in the individual. Acts which create distrust, suspicion, and
misunderstanding, which build barriers and destroy integrity, are immoral.
They decrease the individual's sense of self-respect, and rather than
producing a capacity to work together they separate people and break
down the capacity for communication.

LESTER A. KIRKENDALL

CHAPTER 8

Understanding male-female relationships

One of the most widely discussed and studied topics today is human relationships. In fact, conversations of man landing on the moon, the possibility of nuclear warfare or conquering cancer all seem to take a back seat to the topic of human relationships between nations, families, and individuals. You need only to review the significant attention of the Federal government in recent years to individual rights, antipoverty, wiretapping, and juvenile delinquency. Many of our priority programs and needs have changed, but unfortunately our manner of responding to them has not changed significantly. College students have been accused of many things, but the most significant accusation is that they are basically following the same old line of those before them in attacking traditional human relationship problems. We feel that this conclusion is incorrect and propose that the present generation is too intelligent and much more in tune with the times of the seventies. With this in mind, we hope that they will contribute significantly to more adequate solutions of problems of human relationships.

Our primary concern in this chapter is that of exploring one special phase of human relationships, the relationship of males and females prior to marriage. Most of you are single and interested in understanding how to improve your relationships with the individuals you are dating or contemplating marrying. Some of you may be married and/or a parent and may consider such discussion trivial and unnecessary. But, as has been emphasized throughout the book, attention has to be given not only to those things that exist today but also to those unpredictable problems that may arise at some time in the future. Whether you have children or not, a basic understanding of the aforementioned problems is essential to a good family life as it relates to your marriage.

DEVELOPMENT AND DIFFERENCES OF MALES AND FEMALES
Physical differences

Most people become conscious in early life that males and females differ physically. From the time the little boy discovers that he and his daddy have a penis while his sister and mother do not, to the time when the adolescent becomes acutely conscious of the young girl's developing curves and breasts while he takes pride in his own bulging muscles, most can say, "Viva the difference."

The average girl physically develops to maturity sooner than the average boy. This occurs whether it is in early life when the infant begins to walk, the girl at 9 to 10 months, the boy at 10 to 12 months, or whether it is in later life when the girl at 11 to 13 years develops an interest in the opposite sex. The average boy of that age is still interested in sports and other boys.

Differences in height and weight occur with most boys being taller and heavier than girls. This difference usually lasts throughout life although individual variations occur. However, the greatest physical difference is in the reproductive systems of the female and male.

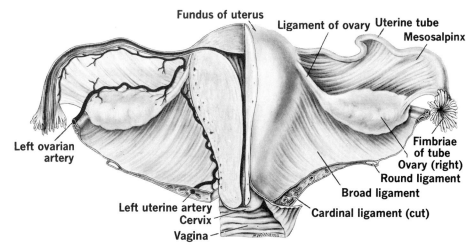

Fundus of uterus

Ligament of ovary Uterine tube

Mesosalpinx

Left ovarian
artery

Fimbriae
of tube
Ovary (right)
Round ligament
Broad ligament

Left uterine artery
Cervix
Vagina

Cardinal ligament (cut)

Fig. 8-1. Posterior view of uterus and associated structures. On the left side of the drawing the posterior portion of the uterus has been removed to show the cavity, and the left uterine tube has been opened longitudinally. (From Francis, C. C: Introduction to human anatomy, ed. 5, St. Louis, 1968, The C. V. Mosby Co.)

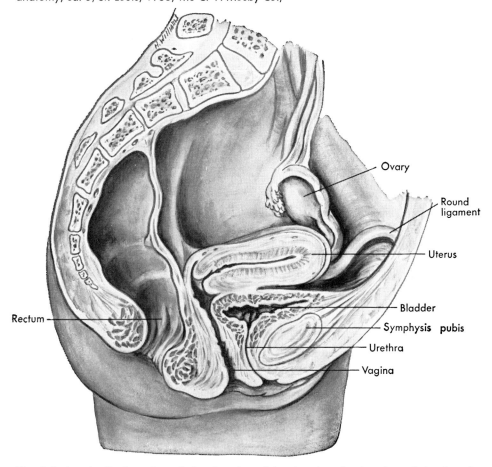

Ovary

Round
ligament

Uterus

Bladder
Symphysis pubis
Urethra
Vagina

Rectum

Fig. 8-2. Longitudinal section of the female pelvis, showing the location of the female reproductive organs. (From Anthony, C. P.: Structure and function of the body, ed. 3, St. Louis, 1968, The C. V. Mosby Co.)

The reproductive systems of the male and female are meant to complement each other. With adolescence, secondary sex characteristics become striking. At this time, the pituitary gland develops hormones that affect sexual development. In the girl of about 10 to 12 years of age, the female follicle-stimulating hormone (FSH) of the anterior pituitary begins to function and is carried by the bloodstream to the girl's ovaries. This hormone helps initiate secondary sex characteristics that change a tomboy, who has not differed much in her bodily development from a boy up to that time, into an appealing woman. To understand these changes one must know something about a girl's reproductive system and the hormones that help produce these changes.

The female's reproductive system includes two ovaries, two fallopian tubes that lead from the ovaries to the uterus, associated glands such as Bartholin's and Skene's glands, the vagina, the vulva, and the clitoris.

The ovaries, about 1 inch wide and 1½ inches long, produce the ova (eggs). The ovaries are estimated to contain about 400,000 immature follicles at birth and to produce one ovum each month from puberty to menopause. The ovary has probably a thousand times more follicles than will be used. When a girl enters puberty, the follicle-stimulating hormone of the anterior pituitary stimulates a follicle each month to ripen and rupture. This occurs about the twelfth to fourteenth day after the first day of the menstrual flow. When the

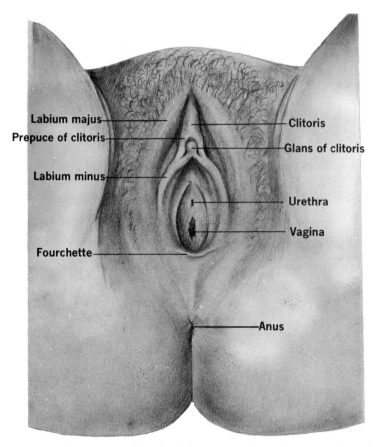

Fig. 8-3. External female genitalia. The labia majora have been parted to show deeper structures. (From Francis, C. C: Introduction to human anatomy, ed. 5, St. Louis, 1968, The C. V. Mosby Co.)

follicle ruptures and an ovum is freed, this ovum is swept into the fallopian tube and by hairlike ciliary action of the tube to the uterus. The uterus is a hollow pear-shaped muscular pouch about 3 inches long by 2 inches wide at its top, narrowing down to a neck (cervix), which is about ½ to 1 inch wide. The uterus is lined by the endometrium, which is a soft tissue supplied with many blood vessels. The lining grows thicker at the beginning of each month in preparation to receive a fertilized ovum. If conception does not take place, the lining is shed as a bleeding discharge and passes from the cervix out the vagina. This bleeding is called the menstrual flow.

The cervix opens into the vagina, a tube 3 to 4 inches long, which permits the erect penis of the male to be introduced during intercourse. The hymen is a thin membrane that stretches across the vaginal opening. It may not always be present in adult females, as it may have been ruptured by strenous activities or masturbation. The external female genitalia consist of the vulva and clitoris. The vulva consists of two pairs of lip-shaped skin, the labia minora and labia majora. Where the labia meet in front is the highly sensitive clitoris. Its tissue fills with blood, and it becomes erect when a woman is sexually excited, as does the penis in the male. Bartholin's and Skene's glands are near the vaginal opening. During sexual stimulation they supply a lubricating fluid. Preintercouse sex play will cause these glands to function better during intercourse.

As a follicle ripens, it also secretes the female sex hormone estrogen. Estrogen causes the breasts to become enlarged and also plays a role in the thickening of the endometrial lining of the uterus.

The ruptured follicle, acted on by another hormone produced from the anterior pituitary, called the luteinizing hormone (LH), transforms the ruptured follicle into the corpus luteum, which then begins to produce a hormone called progesterone.

The ovum may become fertilized by the sperm from the male. This occurs when sperm introduced by the penis into the vagina swim up the uterus and meet the ovum in the fallopian tube where the sperm penetrates the ovum and conception takes place. After conception, the corpus luteum secretes its hormones for 9 months, thus suspending ovulation and menstruation while the pregnancy reaches term. If an ovum is not fertilized, the corpus luteum ceases its function, and the endometrium sloughs off and passes through the vagina as the menstrual flow. This process normally recurs about every 28 days, and menstrual flow may last 3 to 5 days, although in some individuals variation is noted.

Menstruation is a completely normal physiologic phenomenon. It is perfectly safe to bathe or shower while one is menstruating. A woman does not emanate any abnormal vapors during her period and can engage in any normal activity during this time. Occasionally women may have cramps during the time the uterus is attempting to expel the endometrial lining.

The uterus is a wonderfully elastic organ, and if pregnancy takes place, the fertilized ovum becomes firmly embedded in the wall of the uterus, and menstruation ceases for a 9-month period because of the progesterone secretion of the corpus luteum. The uterus progressively enlarges to contain the growing fetus. The uterus, vagina, and uterine ligaments contain much elastic tissue that permits them to stretch to accommodate this growth, and they return to near-normal size after delivery.

The average American woman's menstrual periods cease at 45 to 50 years of age when the menopause, or female climacteric, is reached. Physiologic changes, which include diminished vaginal secretions, some atrophy or shrinkage of the breasts, and some occasional hot flashes, are all normal. Hot flashes may be relieved by estrogen injections. One's attitude toward menopause is important. It is a perfectly normal event that signifies the termination of the child-bearing period, while normal sexual interest and satisfaction continue undiminished. In fact, sexual interest frequently may be increased because there is

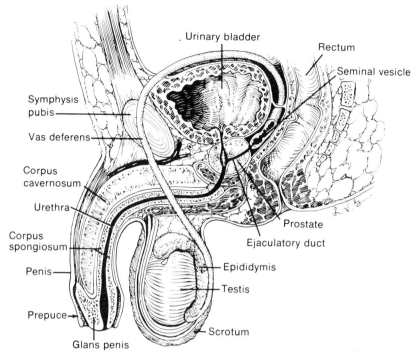

Fig. 8-4. Illustration of male genital organs. (From Tuttle, W. W., and Schottelius, B. A.: Textbook of physiology, ed. 16, St. Louis, 1969, The C. V. Mosby Co.)

no longer a fear of pregnancy from intercourse.

The male reproductive system is designed primarily to complement that of the female and to deliver to it the sperm necessary to impregnate an ovum so that a new life may be conceived. The testes, scrotum, epididymis, vas deferens, seminal vesicles, prostate gland, urethra, and penis make up the male reproductive system.

The testes develop in the abdominal cavity before birth. During fetal life, they gradually descend through the abdominal cavity and reach the scrotum during the seventh month of prenatal life. At puberty the testes begin producing sperm from a series of cells in the seminiferous tubules in the testes. The production of sperm is called spermatogenesis. This process, stimulated to begin around 14 to 15 years of age, starts as a result of stimulation of the testes by the gonadotropic hormone released by the anterior pituitary just as a girl's ovaries are stimulated to produce an ovum.

Interstitial cells of the testes produce the male sex hormone testosterone. Testosterone is responsible for the production of the hair on a man's face and for his deep voice, as well as other secondary male sex characteristics. The penis also increases in size with this anterior pituitary gonadotropic stimulation, while pubic and axillary hair begin to grow along with the appearance of facial hair and the wide broad shoulders of the male adult. In later life, testosterone may be partially responsible for baldness.

Following their production, sperm are stored within the vas deferens, which is a tube running from the epididymis of the testes to the ejaculatory duct. The epididymis is a group of collecting tubules attached directly to the testes. The scrotum contains the testes and aids in protecting and supporting as well as controlling the temperature of the testes by raising the testes in cold weather or perspiring freely in warm weather. The testes cannot produce sperm if they are too warm. Occasionally, the testes fail to descend from the abdomen. Such failure is called cryptorchidism. Testes retained in the abdomen cannot produce sperm because of the higher temperature in the abdominal cavity. During coitus, the ejaculatory duct and most of the male reproductive system undergoes a simultaneous muscular contraction, which results in ejaculation of between four hundred and five hundred million sperm together with supporting fluids through the external opening in the glans penis.

Supporting fluids, or semen, come from the seminal vesicles, the prostate gland, and Cowper's glands, all of which eventually discharge into the urethra. The seminal vesicle fluid discharged into the ejaculatory duct contains considerable fructose, which is thought to serve as nutrition for the sperm.

The prostate gland surrounds the urethra, which is the tube leading from the bladder through the penis. The urethra carries urine from the bladder or semen with sperm from the reproductive organs but never both at the same time, for passage from the bladder automatically closes with erection of the penis. The prostate gland secrets a thin, alkaline, milky fluid that neutralizes the medium in which sperm swim. Without it an acid condition, such as that of the vaginal tract, will kill sperm in a few minutes.

Cowper's glands are about pea size and are located at the base of the penis. They secrete a clear oily lubricant into the urethra at the time of sexual excitement.

The penis is composed of spongy tissue rich in blood vessels, called the corpus cavernosum, which make up the shaft of the penis, while the head is covered by a fold of skin called the prepuce. In order to keep the head of the penis clean, circumcision, removal of this foreskin, is performed. The penis increases in size at puberty. During sexual excitement, it becomes markedly engorged with blood and becomes erect.

The erection of the penis as it becomes engorged with blood in sexual excitement is the first step in transferring sperm to the vagina of the female. This erection is under control of the parasympathetic nerves that dilate the arteries of the penis while constricting the veins. Blood fills the penis, causing it to become erect. Cowper's glands then secrete a lubricating substance into the urethra; and an orgasm begins with a peristaltic action in the testes, which spreads to the seminal vesicles, vas deferens, and prostate gland, which then discharge their secretions. About a teaspoonful of semen is discharged from the penis.

Many men secrete normal amounts of testosterone in old age, whereas in others there is a decline in the 40's and 50's, with a lessening of sexual activity. A male who loses his testes before puberty is a eunuch. He has less muscle mass, smaller genitalia, and less hair both over the body and on the face. If the testes are lost after puberty, other sex traits are not usually changed. Erection and ejaculation are possible, but no sperm are present in both of these conditions.

Emotional differences

Males and females may differ emotionally in degree. Many are well adjusted to their surroundings as individuals; all shades of variations in emotions may be found among both males and females. There are certain basic emotional needs all persons feel in varying degrees: security, affection, the need to feel an accepted member of a congenial group, independence, and certain sexual and physical needs.

In our culture for many centuries man has been the provider and protector. In early civilizations man went forth to battle for his female mate and protected her. This characteristic has continued so that emotionally, man needs to feel that he can adequately provide and care for his female counterpart. The constant exposure to competition and the necessity to provide and protect usually leads to a realistic attitude in a well-adjusted man's life and to independence of thought and action. Man soon learns some reasonable dependence on others; he develops the ability to love others as he matures emotionally. Constant necessity to make daily choices not only for himself but for his family helps him choose to forego immediate pleasure for the sake of more lasting values.

All emotions are accompanied by pleasant or unpleasant feelings, and nearly all emotional responses are associated with some significant physiologic response (see Chapter 2). Most of you are familiar with the emotional responses preceding an important examination or making a speech in class when one gets the "jitters" and is tense. Anxiety reactions are stressful, as if the person were in danger, and if persistent and chronic, can lead to actual organic changes.

The range of stimuli that can arouse emotions is wide and leads to conditioned behavior. Girls are conditioned to find pleasure in playing with dolls, while boys are conditioned to reject dolls. Males are frequently taught that it is not manly to cry, while females are generally excused for their tears. Our emotions and our responses to them gradually make up our personality. We probably inherit some basic elements of our personality, but the major direction of our personality growth—reaction to our surroundings and the people we meet, the experiences we undergo and the way we cope with them—is learned behavior. This leads each individual to construct attitudes, preferences, responses, skills, and values that are unique.

Less stress to make daily decisions leads to a slower development of long-range decision planning in the female. The average female leads a more sheltered life, although women are now becoming much more established in business. Women customarily are thought to be more easily affected by joy, fear, and disaster than are men, although much of this depends on their training and experiences.

Social development

Nearly everyone in our culture goes through childhood and youth as the member of a family unit, which is customarily composed of the wife and mother, the husband and father, perhaps other children, and various relatives or in-laws who all play some part in the development of one's social life as a child. Everyone is influenced by his contact with and imitation of persons with whom he lives. Children can accurately be said to be little mirrors reflecting the attitudes and feelings of their parents. Later they may come to discard or even rebel at some of these attitudes.

Initially, the infant is most affected by his mother. She spends more time with the infant than anyone else. During his first year the infant develops a sense of trust, which usually comes first with the mother and then the father. As his needs are met, his security grows. As he is loved, fondled, and cared for, his mental processes are stimulated by those about him. We now know that an infant who does not have loving attention from those about him will cease to grow and eventually die. We further know that one of the common causes of mental retardation is isolation, in which an infant is placed in a crib or playpen by too busy parents and so is isolated from external human stimulation. The normally reared child learns to love and trust his parents and through these experiences comes to trust friends. Anxieties, tensions, fears, and insecurities of the parent may readily be mirrored in the child. These feelings can be very upsetting to a child, as his self-concept is built largely from his responses to others in his environment.

From 1 to 4 years of age the child develops a sense of free choice. If his choice is helped by a consistency of affection from his parents, his adjustment to his surroundings and playmates will usually be sound. The child tests himself and his skills. Freud discovered that the reactions of the mother and father toward the experiences of the infant and child can greatly influence the developing personality of an older child. Freud also felt that the individual was born with certain biologic drives, which he called the id. The most important of these drives he felt was the sex drive, which he called the libido. The sex drives become fully functional in adolescence, while they are dormant in the child. The libido was thought to be in conflict with social customs, which called for repression of libido. The system of repression Freud called the superego.

A sense of accomplishment and responsibility develops as one leaves kindergarten and goes into the first grade. With the growing sense of accomplishment, the need for status and the competition for it begin. The child learns to adjust to proper limitations without being too greatly disturbed. He develops a sense of justice and fair play through his learned experiences, but his greatest need is still for complete trust in a familiar person. Personal security is dependent upon a close human relationship in the family unit. This can be fulfilled by parents, by brothers and sisters, by close relatives and friends, or a combination of all of these. The child is markedly influenced by group standards but turns more to the family unit for guidance and standards.

The adolescent develops a strong urge toward self-assertion, which brings on a period of many readjustments and difficulties. The adolescent boy and girl now look less to the family unit for personal security, affection, and dependable service, although these are still required. Adolescents' need for understanding and independence of thought and action becomes paramount. They are now biologically mature but recognize the repressions society puts on sexual outlets, which leads to conflicts between their biologic urge and society's definition of what is acceptable behavior.

Personal identity becomes important and is a mixture of what one is, what he likes to think he is, and what he would like to become. The drive for independence is strong and may take the form of rebellion against parental authority. The adolescent tends to associate strongly with a group, class, or gang outside the family unit and to conform to their ideas of behavior and dress. He must begin to develop his own controls and standards of conduct and dependability while becoming conscious of the needs of others.

Insecurity develops as he views his lack of experience as an adult. He tends to cling to a childhood dependence while trying to become independent. Growing up and retaining one's filial love and respect is not always easy. Adolescents are eager for social acceptance and approval of older age groups while they need to be accepted by their own group. The adolescent is going through a readjustment period of reevaluating himself, his family, and his place in his environment; so adolescence is also a period of uncertainty.

Jung, a Swiss psychologist, thought that the entire system of human energies was spread through nutritional, nervous, endocrine, maternal, and sexual expression. How one decides to direct these energies is a willful choice, which may consciously or unconsciously be made; but these energies play an important part in what kind of person one will become. Some characteristics are genetically acquired, whereas others are learned behavior from our experiences with other individuals in our surroundings and how we learn to adjust to them. The infinite combinations possible gives each person a uniqueness that makes life so interesting.

THE FAMILY

The family represents the basic frame of reference for all human relationships. This may be debated in some circles, but nonetheless it is very difficult to find another significantly justified basic unit. All individuals belong to a family unit. As interpreted here, a family consists of a father, mother, and one or more children. Other schools of thought assert that it simply consists of at least a husband and wife. The fact remains that you were born of parents. You may never have seen these parents, but they exist or existed. Until such time as human life can be created without the union of a sperm and an ovum, it will remain so.

Duvall has devised a series of stages possible in a family life cycle, which may assist in identifying your family placement. Her stages are as follows:*

*Duvall, Evelyn: Family development, Philadelphia, 1957, J. B. Lippincott Co., pp. 3-5.

I. Beginning families (married couple without children)
II. Childbearing families (oldest child, birth to 30 months)
III. Families with preschool children (oldest child, 2½ to 6 years)
IV. Families with school children (oldest child 6 to 13 years)
V. Families with teen-agers (oldest child, 13 to 20 years)
VI. Families as launching centers (first child gone to last child's leaving home)
VII. Families in middle years (empty nest to retirement)
VIII. Aging families (retirement to death of one or both spouses)

How are you identified within any of the above stages of the family life cycle? What do Duvall's stages of the family life cycle imply about human relationships? Obviously they identify you as a member of your parents' family and/or of your own family if you are married. They also plot the sequential evolvement of individual family member relationships. As an unmarried individual, you are probably identified anywhere from stage III to stage VIII. As a married person, you may be identified anywhere within the eight different stages.

Your personal life is centered around your family unit. This unit is primarily social and moral. There are those who say that the family is no longer as important as it was in past years, but such an indictment against a unit as salient as the family is difficult to accept.

Zimmerman and Cervantes support the ongoing status of the family by drawing the following conclusions from their extensive study of American families:*

1. The number of good families is rapidly increasing. The average good family now has three or more children. They are reproducing themselves faster than is generally believed.

*Zimmerman, Carle C., and Cervantes, Lucius F.: Successful American families, New York, 1960, Roman Littlefield Co., Inc.

2. The children of good families promise to be even better than their parents. These children are going to school longer than their parents did. They are also displaying greater creativity.
3. The bad families are improving. Deliberate association with good families is helping them to avoid repeating their past errors.

Their interpretation of the good family was that no child dropped out of school before completing high school, no child was arrested as a juvenile, and that there was no divorce or desertion of parents. Using these factors as criteria, it is easy to see that many American families are judged as being good. At the same time, it must be recognized that if families are bad, the couples who formed them may have been lacking in understanding the human relationship of males and females prior to and during the marriages.

Human relationships consist of social, emotional, physical, and spiritual factors. These must be kept in mind in any discussion of good premarriage orientation. The focus must of course be on a firm foundation of stable human relationships, which will be discussed here in a sociosexual context, beginning with the moment boy and girl first become interested in each other.

The way the young child reacts to life establishes a reasonable prediction pattern for later male-female relationships. From the critical moment when a child begins to recognize and understand concepts about persons of the opposite sex, parents are obligated to commence his education on family life and sex. The particulars of this obligation will be discussed in Chapter 9. The remainder of this chapter is devoted to more general, basic considerations.

DATING AND COURTSHIP

Dating and courting represent the significant first steps in sociosexual adjustment. The great majority of college students experience the feeling of total adequacy in the process; nevertheless, varying degrees of uncertainty are often present.

Dating and courtship are possibly trivial

to the majority of you who have had such experiences since junior or senior high school. College life, however, presents some problems that are possibly more serious than those of your high school days. The significance of the various problems depends upon the kind of college you are attending, its location, and your needs and desires. College environments are somewhat atypical of American life in general. You, and to a degree, other persons of your age group, are also atypical of the vast majority of Americans older and younger than you.

A few leading questions serve to point up several of the factors involved in dating during your college years. Is there an equal number of male and female students enrolled in your college? Are you a campus student, or do you live in a boarding house or at home? Have you been supervised rather closely by parents in your dating and courting experiences? Do you have personality problems that make it difficult for you to get dates? If not, what is your primary objective in dating or courting a person of the opposite sex?

College campuses, on occasion, have been branded social dynasties where men and women have been conditioned to place major emphasis on dating and courting rather than on academic education. But it must be recognized that dating and courting occupy an important place in the minds and activities of healthy American college students. If there are problems, chances are that they are the result of excesses or abstinence.

Why do you date?

It is difficult to appraise all of the positive reasons, but it may be proposed that you date for one or more of the following reasons:

1. To satisfy the need for companionship with a member of the opposite sex
2. To make new friends
3. To have wholesome social experiences
4. To improve your human relationships with members of the opposite sex
5. To prepare yourself for courting that favorite man or woman

6. To test your reactions to the problems of sexual desires and impulses
7. To appraise the merits of a possible marriage partner

We can readily see, then, that dating fulfills both a social and an educational function. Many times you will be invited out to social gatherings that require a partner of the opposite sex, such as in dancing or double dating with another couple. You will learn much in your various contacts with the opposite sex, for such contacts usually are a pleasurable, educational experience. Romantic relations between boys and girls begin in various ways at different ages and follow the customs of the time and the social group of which one is a member. We find styles in human relations just as we do in clothes or in other areas. Customs may change, but heterosexual interest is a normal part of young development. In elementary school such interest may be displayed by walking together to or from school. This usually broadens to include parties and dances. Society exercises controls over individual behavior by economic conditions as well as customs, traditions, laws, and standards that govern conduct and enforce behavior. Biologically, young people are ready for mating at adolescence; but each generation learns the rules of sexual behavior from parents, teachers, the church, and friends. Economic forces also condition mating. The structure of our economic and educational life forces young people to spend considerable time in dating, in selecting a mate, and in undergoing a period of engagement.

Le Masters constructed a comprehensive scheme that, in general, illustrates the process and evaluation of dating and courtship.* An adapted form is shown below.

The American courtship system

(1)	(2)	(3)	(4)	(5)	(6)
Group dating	Random dating	Going steady	Pinned	Engagement	Monogamous marriage

*Le Masters, E. E.: Modern courtship and marriage, New York, 1962, The Macmillan Co.

Group dating

Group dating occurs relatively early in life. For the girl it may be classed as pre-debutante dating. The social setting is usually relatively public and supervised by adult chaperones. Church affairs, home parties, and school dances lead the list of the events that provide good settings for group dating. To a degree, most young people begin their dating in this fashion.

If you feel that this discussion is not germaine to the topic of dating as it relates to college men and women, pause to ponder the uncertainties of the early adolescent in terms of interests, needs, impulses, and desires. You may then begin to comprehend the need for a deliberate and careful transition from one-to-group relationships to one-to-one relationships; that is, one fellow, his date, and others, on the one hand, and one fellow and his date, on the other. Whether or not group dating is really necessary depends on two important factors—the emotional maturity of the young couple and the philosophy of early dating held by the parents.

Random dating

Random dating may be referred to as an exploratory type of dating, which serves many purposes. It may also be referred to as "playing the field." Traditionally, the young adults of America have taken the advantage of extending their social relationships to include several persons of the opposite sex as dates at different times. These actions are based on the belief that it is good to relate to several persons, to compare, and finally to make a decision about the individual one likes best. It is a type of dating that is not considered very serious until a pattern of dating occurs with only one person of the opposite sex. As this becomes apparent, the individual launches into the stage of going steady.

Going steady

This stage of courtship seems to be that preferred by college students in general. Reasons for this may be as follows:

1. The college student is generally inter-ested in marriage if not already married.
2. College students are expected to assume a more adult role, and randon dating is not generally considered adult.
3. Except for a few lower-division students living at home, parental supervision of dating is absent.
4. Going steady tends more readily to identify individuals on campus as a social unit.
5. Going steady tends to reduce the overall economic costs of dating.

These statements represent the positive side of the picture. Most college students apparently have few problems, but several harmful problems can arise in such a steady relationship. Most parties see no ending to their dating and courtship, but it sometimes happens that one wants to terminate such a relationship after a long period of time and the other does not. Each year some college students of both sexes are upset with problems of steady dates who have "deserted" them, and they have not been able to make the needed emotional adjustments. In such instances, it is wise for these people repeatedly to remind themselves that the individual of the opposite sex is like a bus—another one is sure to come by sooner or later—and one should not grieve or retreat into a shell over an imagined catastrophe.

Going steady implies that one has taken himself out of circulation, so far as other persons are concerned, for dating. If one wants to break off a steady relationship with a young man or woman, it will take some time getting back into the mainstream of random dating, as he may have been identified as x person's steady date.

Sex impulses and drives also present a serious problem for steady dates. The familiarity and natural closeness of these persons increase the possibility of premarital sex relations. It becomes increasingly more difficult to resist the sexual desires and demands of a person with whom one becomes more intimate over an extended period of time.

Dates arranged by a third party

The arrangement of dates by a third party is generally more novel than it is necessary. The third party is usually a computer used in relation to compatibility research, a mating or dating bureau, or a friend. Dating by computer is a craze that has infiltrated many of our campuses. The original concept was that of determining the compatibility of different individuals. The original purpose was basic research, which often leads to action research or pragmatic implementation.

This kind of program works as follows. Data covering the personality, characteristics, and other individual facts are punched into IBM cards. All of the available cards are scanned, checked, and matched by a computer. A few years ago *Look Magazine* reported on a major computer matching project of Harvard University undergraduate students.* The project was called Operation Match. It was estimated that in a 9-month period, 100,000 college students paid more than $300,000 to acquire the names of five computer-programmed compatible dates.

The arguments for and against computer-programmed dating are many. One of the outstanding ones for is that it reduces the anxiety and possible frustration of a blind date. On the other side, it may be argued that it is too mechanized and diminishes the pleasurable anticipation of meeting an unknown date.

A dating or mating bureau is an old concept. The primary data of dating bureaus are, however, basically the same; only the treatment of the data is different. These bureaus may be commercial, or they may be a voluntary service such as found in a fraternity, sorority, or social club. Data are recorded on standard forms and may include hobbies, vocational interests, social interests, physical characteristics, and, of course, a photograph. The individual seek-

ing the services of the bureau has the opportunity to make the final decision.

Dates arranged by friends may or may not be blind dates, although the great majority are blind dates. If one accepts a blind date, he is basically agreeing to trust the judgment of his friend. When the friends know each other very well, the chances of getting a good date are fairly good. The converse may be true if they do not know each other well. If they do not, anxiety about the date could be very significant.

Pinning

Pinning may be considered a forerunner of engagement, that is, a promise to be engaged. It basically means that the fellow has presented his pin, and the lady has agreed to wear it until an "official" decision can be made about marriage. Of course, the symbol presented may be something other than a pin; the pin generally refers to a fraternity pin. The symbol may be an athletic letter, sweater, or pin, band letter or sweater, class ring, Masonic pin, or any other similar token. It is generally proposed that pinning works best when the couple involved is fairly certain that there is some possibility of becoming engaged. Careless and indiscreet pinning may lead to serious problems for one or both persons. Exploitation for personal and vain reasons can be the result if pinning is not prudently considered.

Engagement

Being engaged represents the first significant step toward marriage. When two persons are certain that they are in love and want to marry, they announce their plans to their friends. Traditionally, this is the time when couples plan the pattern of their future life together.

Ideally, the decision to become engaged is made objectively by the couple, probably over many hours of talking and being together. Prior relationships are important if engagements are to lead to successful marriage. The fellow usually seeks the approval of the girl's parents or guardian, thus

---

*Boy-girl computer, Look Magazine, February 22, 1966, pp. 30-35.

enlisting their interest and cooperation in this joint endeavor. This can go a long way in building up respect and solidifying in-law relationships so that they will be harmonious in the future.

The announcement of the engagement is traditionally made by the young woman's parents, although customs may vary. At times, the marriage date may be announced, although at other times the exact date may be uncertain. Occasionally, there are secret engagements because of special reasons. Engagement is an important step between dating and marriage; today, it is generally considered a testing period.

It has been proposed that the following are advantages of engagement:

1. It may save a man from being dazzled by the supposed glamour of his fiancée, since it gives him opportunities to see her in everyday clothes over a period of time.
2. It enables both to become much better acquainted with the other's family and to become accepted by them.
3. It provides the opportunity to create an amorous monopoly in which "old flames" and rivals are eliminated as love objects.
4. It provides insight into the relative responsiveness of the other.
5. It gives full opportunity to discuss children, whether the wife will work, handling of money, child discipline, extramartial friendships, and other vital issues that often do not seem appropriate in the dating and courtship stages.
6. It provides time to arrange financial affairs and gradually to get ready for the economic burden of marriage, sharing business and professional interests, and discovering similarities and differences in attitudes about marriage.
7. It gives both participants a chance occasionally to slip into the role of husband and wife and to learn what might be expected, while still in the engagement period.

Pressing questions that usually should be answered before marriage are: (1) Can you live on the husband's earnings? (2) Shall the wife work? If so, for how long? (3) Who will manage the family finances? (4) How many children should you have, and when? (5) Where will you, as a couple, live?

UNDERSTANDING SEX IMPULSES AND DRIVES

Differences between males and females are generally obvious. The differences are often described in terms of secondary sex characteristics. It is commonly accepted that the bodies differ, that the pitch of the voice differs, that the amount of hair present differs, and that the sex organs differ. In spite of these overt factors, they do not represent the primary difference between the sexes. The primary difference is not the body itself but the egg and sperm cells, which are carried and matured by the respective bodies. Proof of this concept of the difference between the sexes is readily depicted by the influence of these cells on the body in which they are contained.

The sex of individuals is determined before the body actually commences to take the form of male or female. Early in life the sex cells may be removed and the actual secondary sex characteristics of the individual may be prevented from developing. A castrated male may have the ovaries from a female implanted in his body, and his body can be conditioned to display distinct female features.

Sex impulses in the female correspond to the following:

1. The production of the ova is periodical or seasonal. Ova are not produced during pregnancy, menstruation, and immediately following menstruation.
2. The sexual impulses and appetites of the average female harmonize with the times of ova production.
3. As contrasted to those of the male, the female's sex appetites and impulses are, on the average, less keen and more periodical.

Sex impulses and appetites of the male generally conform to the following:

1. The sperm are produced continually.
2. It is assumed that the peak periods of sexual appetites for the average male are ever present.
3. The male, therefore, is more sexually active than the female. Generally, males can be stimulated to a peak state of sexual intensity at any time because of a very ardent state of consciousness.

Stimulation of sex impulses and drives

The stimulation of impulses and drives is frequently misunderstood. Since sexual fulfillment is considered one of the basic drives of men and women, an understanding of the things that stimulate individuals for the mating process may go a long way in reducing possible frustrations and conflicts. There are any number of classes of stimuli, but generally they may be classified as intrinsic or extrinsic.

Intrinsic:

1. The presence of abnormal formations and irritations of the sex organs
2. A distended bladder
3. Secretions of hormones from the gonads
4. The effects of drugs
5. The filling of the seminal cavities

Extrinsic

1. Masturbation or similar mechanical forms
2. Sensual response to the appeal of pictures
3. Contacts with or exposure to parts of the male or female body
4. Keen psychologic states of mind—extreme curiosity, consciousness, and imagination

General sex attitudes and behavior

Since individuals are naturally stimulated both intrinsically and extrinsically, it is obviously normal for mature individuals to experience sex impulses, drives, and needs. The pronounced lack of knowledge and understanding among the general popula-

tion about matters related to sex makes the problem too important to be taken lightly.

Obtaining sexual satisfaction outside marriage is not always easy, for our social code of conduct presents many stumbling blocks that can cause significant frustrations and emotional problems. Sex appeal is everywhere. You are confronted with it in advertising. Movies and television shows have capitalized on sex appeal by making it pay at the box office and in the ratings. Our dress, epecially that of women, has succeeded in being sexually appealing. One of the authors, in a conversation with a fellow professor, asked him what he considerd the most distracting thing in his classes. He responded, "the lovely young ladies who invariably sit in the front row of the classroom and intentionally or unintentionally test my resistance to sex appeal."

Attitudes toward sex vary according to the times or to the philosophy of life of the individual. When the times are good, purposeful, and free of serious anxieties, tensions, and frustration, sex assumes a less important role in the lives of people.

Your range of interest in sex is as wide as that of the general population. The attention that you, as a college student, have received in countless publications is no accident. Many words have been written to explain the complications that have influenced you at a time when the possibilities of choice are astronomical. When attitudes are not wholesome and healthy, the consequences of responding to uncontrolled stimuli can be hazardous.

Healthy attitudes place sex in its proper perspective. They assist individuals in establishing good values, making proper judgments, and understanding consequences of all acts.

The manner in which college students manage their sex impulses varies with the individual. The variables that influence the individual are family background, social class, personal values, religious influences, and general attitude toward the social moral code. Table 8-1 summarizes the sexual outlets of unmarried college students. Kinsey

Table 8-1. Frequency of five sex outlets for 16- to 20-year-old single college men and women

Sex behavior	Percentage of total sex outlet	
	Men	Women
Masturbation	66%	65%
Orgasm in sleep	16	4
Premarital intercourse	10	10
Petting	5	18
Homosexual activities	3	3
Total sex outlet	100%	100%

Adapted from Kinsey, Alfred C., and others: Sexual behavior in the human male, Philadelphia, 1953, W. B. Saunders Co.

and his co-workers found that the vast majority of college students used some means other than premarital sexual intercourse to satisfy sex impulses.

MASTURBATION

Masturbation is the voluntary means of creating an orgasm without engaging in sexual intercourse. Other terms used to describe it include self-abuse, onanism, playing with oneself, and autoerotism. It is most often practiced in secret but may sometimes be practiced in the presence of one or more persons of the same or different sexes. It is generally thought to be physically, mentally, and morally wrong. Traditionally, it has been reported to lead to feeblemindedness, to render persons incapable of having satisfactory sex relations with persons of the opposite sex, to lead to insanity, and to cause acne. Medical opinion, however, supports the fact that it produces none of the physical effects and few of the mental and emotional effects that were once thought true.

Most individuals, by adulthood, will have masturbated to orgasm at least once: for males a conservative estimate is 90%, and for females it is about 70%. With these factors in mind, it may reasonably be concluded that the practice of masturbation is more typical than atypical of American sexual habits.

Sound evidence that masturbation is physically or emotionally harmful does not exist. But the evidence does not negate the fact that the practice may be a sign of more deep-seated emotional problems. When practiced solely for the physical results, the act becomes one of simple fantasy. When it is used as a means to compensate for the inability to get along with members of the opposite sex or a means of escaping marriage, it represents "abnormal behavior." Even in these instances it is not the cause of social or emotional problems but a sign of them.

When practice of masturbation takes on addiction proportions, that is, if practiced every day or so, the act demands the advice of a physician or counselor. McKinney's suggestions for those who have not become addicted to masturbation but practice it regularly are also useful. They are summarized as follows:*

1. Understand that masturbation is practiced by normal persons who will overcome it, that it is not limited to abnormal persons, that its physical consequences are negligible, and that its undeceivable effects on personality are worry, disgust, feelings of guilt, and undue self-attention.

2. Understand that a habit or attitude so strong as one related to the sex urge cannot be changed in a short period of time and also that some regression may take place.

3. Participate in social and physical activities with your own and the opposite sex.

4. Participate in extracurricular activities, since they satisfy most of the dominant human motives and distract attention from one's self.

5. Understand that masturbation may be a sign of insecurity and that such realization and participation in social activities may relieve anxiety and help

---

*McKinney, Fred: Psychology of personal adjustment, New York, 1960, John Wiley & Sons, Inc., pp. 509-513.

one gain self-assurance and acceptance by others.

A few suggestions for parents dealing with the problem as it relates to adolescents are as follows:

1. Do not get excited.
2. Do not label your child as evil or as a future patient of a mental hospital.
3. Try to find plausible reasons for the behavior.
4. Discuss the problem with him calmly and with a nonjudgmental attitude.
5. Accept the fact that punishment or threats of punishment will be of little value.
6. Do not expect the child to drop the habit overnight.
7. Develop such a relationship with your child that he will feel free to come to you and talk to you about masturbation, petting, or any problems that bother him.

ORGASM IN SLEEP

Most people experience fantasies of the sex act. These fantasies or dreams basically represent a natural means of relieving sexual stresses that are not relieved by other means. The nocturnal emission, or "wet dream," occurs during sleep. Although it was assumed to be experienced only by the male, it is also experienced by the female, but with much less frequency, and it rarely provides the female with the degree of relief of sexual tensions as it does with the male. Serious aftereffects do not exist. The soiled sheets or bedclothes may cause a negligible degree of frustration.

The process of nocturnal emission helps to refute the belief held by some men that the normal physiologic sex stimuli create a biologic necessity for satisfying the sexual appetite. If the sex appetite is unrelieved voluntarily, the seminal vesicles will void themselves by natural emissions.

PETTING

Petting occurs in various forms but is considered a voluntary or spontaneous means of stimulating the sexual desires of oneself or of another person. It may range from kissing to the stimulation of the sex organs. The primary purpose or interest in kissing is generally directed love or affection. The primary purpose in stimulation of the sex organs is to cause the other person to respond through sexual intercourse.

Young people, however, often use petting as an attempt to avoid sexual intercourse. They are generally capable of petting and stopping short of the point of climax, or orgasm. Petting represents a pleasant experience for most of those who are able to control the boundaries.

Males and females differ in their concepts of who should do the petting and of the desirability of petting. In most instances, the petting is executed by the male, who also finds it more desirable and pleasant than the female.

What would you do to restrain the extent of petting if it were offensive to you? No one knows the specific answer to every situation, but suggestions can be made for restraint, if one desires it. Since it has been assumed that the responsibility is primarily that of the female, a proper frame of reference for suggestions should be that adhered to by the female.

Judson and Mary Landis conducted a study to establish the manner in which young women attempted to solve this problem.* A sample of 200 girls indicated the manner in which they attempted to control the extent of petting. Their techniques were ranked according to frequency of use. The nine most frequently used techniques were ranked as follows:

1. Be honest, say "no" sincerely.
2. Keep talking, make interesting conversation.
3. Avoid circumstances in which it is likely to happen.
4. Plan dates thoroughly.
5. Double—or group—date.

---

*Landis, Judson, T., and Landis, Mary G.: Youth and marriage: a student manual, ed. 2, Englewood Cliffs, N. J., © 1957, Prentice-Hall, Inc., p. 40.

Table 8-2. Relationship involvement and erotic intimacy level at which offensiveness occurs in petting

	Necking and petting above the waist		Petting below the waist		Attempted intercourse or attempted intercourse with violence		
	No.	Percent	No.	Percent	No.	Percent	Total
Ride home, first date, or occasional date	411	55.0	60	31.4	25	30.1	496 (48.5%)
Regular or steady date	295	39.4	104	54.5	43	51.8	442 (43.3%)
Pinned or engaged	42	5.6	27	14.1	15	18.1	84 (8.2%)
Totals	748	100	191	100	83	100	1,022 (100%)

Data from Kirkpatrick, Clifford: Male sex aggression on a university campus, Amer. Soc. Rev. **22**:55, February 1957.

6. Let the boy know your attitude from the start.
7. Set an early curfew.
8. Plan afterdate activities.
9. Use reason.

As a sexual outlet, petting is assumed to be an acceptable medium as long as its purpose is not that of a basic stimulus for sexual intercourse. "Light" petting as a means of love and affection represents a wholesome activity within our social code of relationships.

HOMOSEXUALITY

As a means of sexual outlet, homosexuality is considered a deviant form of behavior. In the female homosexuality is referred to as lesbianism, and in the male it is uranism. It is a condition in which persons form significant emotional or sexual associations with someone of their own sex. Although it is generally accepted that sex experiences represent the key identifier, this may not be true. The disorder is basically psychologic in origin, stemming from the individual's improper identification with the sexes.

In tracing the general growth and development of a child, it is found that from birth to adolescence the significant relationships are between individuals of the same sex. Little boys enjoy playing most with other little boys, and little girls enjoy playing most with other little girls; but when they reach adolescence, the relationships are often directed to members of the opposite sex. If this transition of attention does not occur then, homosexuality may be present.

Homosexuals do not always have the characteristics and personalities that they are often presumed to have. All lesbians do not possess outstanding male secondary sex characteristics. Lesbians have been identified as beautiful, feminine persons and/or mothers of several children. Likewise, all uranians do not possess outstanding female secondary sex characteristics. Uranians have been identified as outstanding athletes or fathers of several children. Marriage, however, may often serve as an acceptable shield to cover up homosexual tendencies.

The low tolerance level of the public toward homosexuality is often unwarranted. Homosexuality is a serious health problem that should be dealt with as any other health disorder or illness. But frequently in many sections of the United States state legislatures or city councils overreact to the problem by enacting harsh legislation that treats the practice of homosexuality as a minor or major crime.

PREMARITAL INTERCOURSE

Petting may be excessively heavy but may never be classified as sexual intercourse. Intercourse is experienced only when the penis of the male penetrates the vagina of the female.

A 1969 survey to determine in depth students' sexual attitudes and behavior differentiated between men's and women's attitudes and conduct at San Francisco State University, Pembroke, Bryn Mawr, the University of Illinois, and the University of Alabama. It concentrated on sophomores, juniors, and seniors. The report does not give actual numbers interviewed, only percentages. At the two extremes, 57% of the women at San Francisco State University and 19% of the women at the University of Alabama said they had engaged in sexual intercourse, while the rates for men were 62% at San Francisco State and 47% at the University of Alabama. Most women began sexual intercourse from 18 to 20 years of age, as did the men. Most women, over 80%, felt that a girl would not lose the respect of a boy with whom she had intercourse before she married him; most girls, 60% to 90%, felt that it was not permissible for a girl to have intercourse with someone she did not love; and most girls, 82% to 93%, thought it was possible for a woman to be satisfied with one man for her entire life.

In the 1930's and 1940's sociologic studies were said to show that women who engaged in premarital intercourse had more emotional conflicts and underwent more psychologic stress than those who remained virgins until marriage. This was thought to be because of their conflict with social and religious standards, with anxiety and guilt resulting. In sharp contrast, in the study reported above about 76% to 93% of those who had engaged in intercourse were emotionally contented. Of the women students who were interviewed, over half dated twice a week or more, and most had dated 10 to 20 or more times since entering college. The University of Alabama, where sexual activity was low, had a high degree of social dating.

Just what conclusions one may draw from these figures suggesting increased premarital activity is speculative. Determining how many people who have had premarital intercourse will have an enjoyable, long-lasting,

and fulfilling sex life during marriage would, of course, demand a follow-up of their sexual life after 5 or 10 years of marriage. College is a short interval from which to draw long-lasting conclusions regarding premarital activities. Unquestionably, there is more sexual permissiveness in colleges than there used to be.

College men and women experience premarital intercourse less frequently than do noncollege persons of the same age. This conclusion does not eliminate the possibility of several significant problems affecting those involved.

Although sexual intercourse out of wedlock has long been considered a cardinal violation of our social code, contemporary attitudes have relaxed somewhat. The code is still fairly rigid when applied to young women but is highly flexible as it relates to the male. Prior to marriage, as well as during marriage, the female rarely determines the frequency of sexual activity. The sex impulses of the male, as earlier discussed, are so much more pronounced that he is the primary activator.

Mature men and women have to weigh all factors in deciding about premarital sexual intercourse. Although logic and rational thinking go a long way in providing plausible answers, the solution must include consideration of what is outside the realm of the rational.

What factors might be considered?

1. There is no absolute physiologic need for participating in the sex act. Thousands of people are celibates and display no clinical anomalies. Our wonderful bodies have a way of relieving whatever tensions are created by the sex urge.

2. Physical and emotional hazards may seriously affect one or both individuals. Maturity, knowledge, and healthful attitudes generally dictate the seriousness of the aftereffects of the act.

3. The purpose of engaging in premarital sexual intercourse must be well defined and accepted by both persons. Confusion of purpose frequently leads to feelings of anxiety or guilt, which could seriously affect

one's subsequent sexual experiences in marriage.

4. Acceptance of unforeseen obligations has to be a basic consideration. If the woman becomes pregnant, the socially accepted thing is that she and the man involved marry. At this point, one's sexual conduct definitely becomes someone else's business. If the persons involved decide not to marry, the care of the child still remains to be considered.

Premarital intercourse is more widespread now than ever before in our history; it seems reasonable to assume that the attitude of permissiveness will continue to expand. How you respond to this changing climate will be a reflection of the type of individual you are as well as a reflection of the society in which you live.

INTERCOURSE AND CONTRACEPTION

The population explosion is much talked about. It has led to increased interest in methods of contraception and to increased demand for more widespread knowledge regarding contraceptive devices. The unwed mother who is on relief drawing welfare checks and supposedly increasing her monthly allowance by creating new children whom she cannot support has been repeatedly denounced in the press and nearly every study conducted. There is no doubt that a worldwide plan for population control is needed, when we repeatedly read that two-thirds of the people of the world go to bed hungry every night. Unless we quickly learn and disseminate some effective method of birth control, our world will face misery and famine. This is well recognized by nearly all sociologists who have studied the problem.

Rhythm method

The Roman Catholic church has long recognized the need for birth control and advocates use of the rhythm method. This method is based upon a careful study of the individual woman's time of ovulation. A woman ovulates only once during her menstrual cycle, and pregnancy may occur only during an approximate 24- to 48-hour period following ovulation. In 28-day cycles ovulation occurs the twelfth to fourteenth day after the first day of the previous menstrual cycle, although there may be some individual variations. The ovum lives only 24 to 48 hours. The sperm is said to be able to fertilize the ovum only within 48 hours after it is injected into the vagina, although it may remain alive and in motion in the uterus several days after intercourse. Thus, the basis for the rhythm method is to avoid intercourse at the time of ovulation.

In general, the couple may consider the first third of a menstrual cycle a relatively safe period, the middle third an unsafe or fertile time, and the last third a safe period. This method requires that a woman have a regular menstrual cycle, which most women do not, and requires that the male keep track of his wife's periods accurately and avoid intercourse during the unsafe periods of 1 to 3 days before and 1 to 3 days after the presumed time of ovulation. Since women often forget when their last period began and since most women do not have regular cycles, the rhythm method may not always work.

The advantages of the rhythm method are that it requires no device or medical preparation; it does not usually require medical supervision after the regularity of the cycle is established; and it involves no cost.

Charting a woman's basal temperature rectally in bed before she gets up each morning and assumes activity has shown that at the time of ovulation there is a slight elevation (from 0.3 to 0.8 of a degree) of the basal body temperature, which persists until the next menstrual period begins. The rhythm method should not be used until the woman has charted her basal temperature for 3 months to determine the average time of ovulation. Many factors other than ovulation may also cause a rise in body temperature, so the charting method is not always reliable.

Another method of charting is to keep a calendar of the menstrual cycle for a period of 12 consecutive months. Day one of the

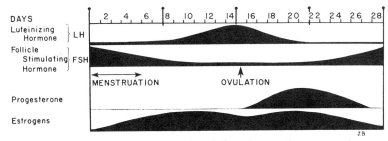

Fig. 8-5. Diagram to show varying levels of female sex hormones during a 28-day menstrual cycle. (From Francis, C. C, and Farrell, G. L.: Integrated anatomy and physiology, ed. 3, St. Louis, 1957, The C. V. Mosby Co.)

menstrual cycle is the first day of menstruation, and the day before menstruation starts is the last day of the cycle. The number of days in the longest cycle and the number of days in the shortest cycle should be determined for 12 months. The number of days in the shortest cycle minus 18 days is the first fertile day. In a 28-day cycle, this will be the tenth day. Subtracting 11 days from the number of days in the longest cycle in the 12 months establishes the last fertile day. In a 31-day schedule, this will be the twentieth day. The fertile time thus would be from the tenth to the twentieth day. The calendar should be marked indefinitely if this method of charting is used.

Diaphragm and spermicidal creams

The diaphragm with spermicidal jelly has been a frequently used method in the United States. Most physicians considered it the best method after the condom until the development of oral contraceptives. A diaphragm is made of soft rubber stretched about a circular spring coil. The diaphragm lies diagonally across the vagina and prevents the sperm from entering the uterus. It comes in various sizes, so a physician must fit it to the size of the woman's cervix. It is easy to insert and cannot be felt by the penis. A special spermicidal contraceptive jelly or cream must be used with the diaphragm to increase its reliability. The diaphragm may be inserted any time before sexual intercourse and must be left in place at least 6 hours after intercourse.

Intrauterine devices

Intrauterine devices (spiral, loop, saf-t-coil) to prevent implantation of the ovum in the uterus have long been used; but some have caused bleeding, pain, or both. New synthetic materials, such as silicone, better tolerated by the uterus, are allowing more frequent use of intrauterine devices. They may be left in the uterus for months or years and seem to be very effective. They are inexpensive, simple, and among the most effective birth control devices, currently ranking next to the pill in effectiveness. Complications occur fairly often, however, as with the pill.

The doctor inserts the proper size I.U.D. in the female's uterus. The process takes only a few seconds, and once inserted there is usually no pain. The best time to have it inserted is after a menstrual period. It has no effect on the regularity of the menstrual periods, although there may be a heavier flow during the first period following insertion of the I.U.D. A little bleeding may occur between periods.

Contraceptive pill

The birth control pill is the most recent and most popular contraceptive device used in this country. A great deal has been written about the safety of the pill. It has been argued that it may cause blood clots in some women or produce or speed up the growth of cancer in others, but after a 10-year study the Federal government has concluded that its use is safe.

The pill works by preventing ovulation

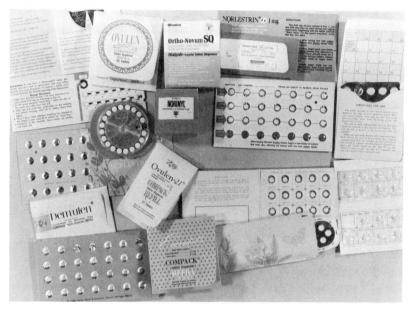

Fig. 8-6. The birth control pill is packaged attractively and in a variety of ways to reinforce the habit for regularity, which the woman must develop to ensure maximum effectiveness.

so that no ovum is available to be fertilized. It contains synthetic progesterone, which suppresses the pituitary's follicle-stimulating hormone and the luteinizing hormone. The pill is taken by mouth starting the fifth day of the menstrual cycle and continued daily for 20 days and then stopped until the fifth day of the next cycle.

The pill has produced side effects such as nausea, fluid retention, growth of fibroids, and blurring vision. It should be prescribed only by a physician, and its use is not recommended if the woman has a history of liver disease; thrombophlebitis (clotting of veins); cancer, either present or suspected, of the breast or genital organs; or undiagnosed vaginal bleeding. When taken as directed, it appears to be practically 100% effective. When it is stopped, normal ovulation appears to be resumed. Whether other untoward results will appear after a number of years, as its opponents claim, is not yet known.

Condom

For men, the condom, a thin, soft rubber tube that fits over the penis, has long been an effective contraceptive device if it is reliably made and used. As was recommended in the case of the diaphragm, spermicidal creams or jellies should be used with the condom.

Withdrawal

Coitus interruptus, or withdrawal of the penis just prior to ejaculation, has been practiced for centuries. It is not reliable, and the sudden interruption of the sex act at its climax is not advised because of the traumatic mental and emotional responses of either person engaged in the sex act.

Table 8-3 summarizes the limitations of the various birth control methods and their effectiveness.

THE SEXUAL BALANCE

One thing that bothers me about WLU—which I'm *for* in so many respects—is that it's so man-hating. Surely, it can't be *all* their fault that we're the way we are. There *is* such a thing as self-determination, you know (and God knows we have *never* been discriminated against the way Negroes have). I've found, as have many women I know, that you *can* make it (money, success) if you work your fanny off and align yourself with

Table 8-3. Limitations and effectiveness of birth control methods

Method	Effectiveness if used correctly	Need for sustained motivation	Need for action at time of coitus	Need to replenish supplies	Need for medical services	Need for careful instruction	Reduced opportunity for coitus	Unsuitable for menstrually irregular women	Early side effects (common, not serious)	Early side effects (rare, serious)	Late side effects
Pills	****	1		1	3	1			1	1	?
IUD	***				3				1	1	?
Diaphragm with jelly or cream	***	1	1	1	2	2					
Condom	***	1	2	1							
Temperature rhythm	***	1				3	2	1			
Calendar rhythm	**	1				3	2	1			
Chemicals (foams, etc.)	**	1	2	1							
Withdrawal	**	2	3								
Douche	*	1	3								

*Indicates level of effectiveness; 1-3 indicates degree of limitation compared with other methods (1—low, 2—medium, 3—high; ? indicates undetermined status).

some *enlightened* men who are smart enough to realize they need you to be good as you need *yourself* to be. Every day I see girls in jobs who never turn in an idea, stay home two days a week with cramps *(cramps?!),* conveniently get "snowbound" on Monday after a Saturday and Sunday skiing—and these are *not* secretaries and file girls but women who are already in junior editor and copywriting jobs. Nobody's brainwashing *them* to be "feminine," passive—and lazy. I know wives you couldn't *drive* out of the house with a poisoned, pointed stick (except to go shopping, lunching, bridging, or maybe fashion-showing) even though a man is encouraging them as hard as he can to *do* something and *be* something. No it *isn't* too late just because you've been roosting for awhile. Stores need stock clerks, yes? A stock clerk can become a salesgirl; a salegirl can make junior buyer; a junior buyer can make (—well whatever she *wants*). Yes, I know this is a simplistic approach and better we should start from babyhood with a whole new set of attitudes about what women ought to do and achieve, but when that happens, there probably are going to be a lot of unhappy (lazy) women griping about something *else,* I daresay. (And don't get me started on alimony and how women exploit *men!*) (Helen Gurley Brown)*

Male-female relations are more democratic today. Each sex is expected to know, understand, and respect the other. Our double standards are beginning to be shaken by many forces, and we now have what is basically a single standard. The traditional concept of the woman in the house and the man on the job is no longer as true as it once was. This change has been caused by several developing trends. Some are as follows:

1. More and more young women are graduating from college with salable skills.
2. Women are competing with men for many positions originally reserved for men.
3. The use of birth control measures has assisted in liberating the female, to a degree, from the sex restrictions cited earlier in the chapter.

*Komisar, Lucy: The new feminism, Saturday Review, February 21, 1970, p. 29. Copyright 1970, Saturday Review, Inc.

4. Indications are that men are beginning to accept sex on a common basis with women. For example, dating and courtship practices involve going "dutch" more frequently.

Only through improvement in male-female relationships is there a basis for building a life-affirming social, religious, and moral code.

CHAPTER 9

Responsibilities in marriage

Never before in the history of America has the institution of marriage been under the observation it is today. The American marriages of the 1970's are entering an unparalleled era of change and transition, with a major reappraisal of the institution in the balance.

Most people in this country have been affected, directly or indirectly, by a divorce. For every four marriages there is one divorce. It is estimated that about 25% of all first-born American children are born out of wedlock. The above are only two of the major problems that receive much attention. Added to these, however, is a multitude of responsibilities of both persons in a marriage, which if not met will result in marital disaster.

CONCEPTS OF MARRIAGE

Marriage is both a serious and natural extension of premarital male-female relationships. It represents a solidification of commitment to the aspirations shared by individuals who want to be together as husband and wife for the rest of their lives. It is a contract of binding significance, which contains certain agreements about concepts that are, unfortunately, frequently misunderstood or not commonly accepted.

To love, honor, and obey presupposes a great many obligations of one partner to the other. How many couples, during the blissful marriage ceremony, really comprehend the significance of these three words?

In 1968 there were 2,059,000 marriages, which was a rate of 10.3 marriages per 1,000 population in the United States and the highest since 1951. Preliminary data since 1968 indicate that the trend is still upward.

In 1968 an estimated 573,000 divorces and annulments were granted in the United States. The rate was 11.2 per 1,000 population. The divorce rate does not seem to be increasing significantly. This, of course, does not eliminate the need for directing attention to solving the problem of approximately one-half million divorces and annulments each year.

The relationship of marriage partners has changed. In times past the woman was considered the servant of the man. Today, she works right along with him and he with her. She helps fill the financial coffers, and he helps change the diapers and wash the clothes. With the advent of more acceptance of reliable contraceptives and the acquisition of economic power, women have more freedom for self-determination. The concept of equal responsibility is thus becoming a serious consideration for persons who anticipate marriage.

Men die earlier than women, thereby adding to an ever growing number of widows. Women make up three-fourths of the widowed population.

The 1968 estimate of the marital status of Americans 15 years old and older is quite revealing. A summary of this status is presented in Table 9-1.

The age of 15 years can be misleading, however, for in most states throughout the country the minimum ages for marrying is higher. With specific conditions, the states of Alabama, New Hampshire, South Carolina, Texas, and Utah will allow legal

Table 9-1. Marital status of United States population—1968 (15 years and over)

	Percent of males	Percent of females
Single	18.2	13.4
Married	75.6	70.6
Widowed or divorced	6.2	16.0
Total	100.0	100.0

Data from Health resources statistics, Washington, D. C., 1970, National Center for Health Statistics.

marriages for females of less than fifteen years of age. New Hampshire is the only state that allows a male of less than 15 years of age to marry.

QUALIFYING FOR MARRIAGE

Do you qualify for marriage? Are you ready? How do you know? These three elementary questions require serious answers, which only you are in a position to provide. A comprehensive treatment of the problems could only occur in a complete course on courtship and marriage. The treatment of the problem here is directed toward the basic factors that are intended to provoke study of the general health issues as they may relate to you and your approach to the solution of problems in marriage.

The basic frame of reference must, naturally, be a description of happily married couples in terms of mental, emotional, and social aspects. It is our own impression that happily married men as a group

1. Show evidence of a stable emotional tone
2. React to others cooperatively, as reflected in their attitudes toward business superiors, with whom they work well; their attitudes toward women, which reflect equalitarian ideals; and their benevolent attitudes toward the inferior and underprivileged
3. Tend to be unself-conscious and somewhat extroverted in a gathering of people
4. Compared with unhappy husbands show superior initiative, a greater

tendency to take responsibility, and greater willingness to give close attention to details in their daily work
5. Like methodical procedures and methodical people
6. In money matters are conservative and cautious
7. Are active politically and socially
8. Have a favorable attitude toward religion

Happily married women as a group

1. Demonstrate kindly attitudes toward others and expect kindly attitudes in return
2. Do not take offense and are not unduly concerned about the impression they make upon others
3. Do not look upon social relationships as a rivalry situation
4. Are cooperative
5. Do not often object to a subordinate role to their husband
6. Are not annoyed by advice from others
7. Enjoy activities that bring education or pleasurable opportunities to others and like to do things for the dependent or underprivileged
8. Are methodical and painstaking in their work, attentive to detail, and careful in regard to money
9. Tend to be moderate in religion, morals, and politics
10. Demonstrate a quiet self-assurance and an optimistic outlook upon life

The basic key is stability, ability to foresee potential problems, and harmony of interpersonal relationships between husband and wife.

To marry or not to marry

Our society generally expects most persons to marry. There are, however, individuals whose constitutional and personal characteristics make them poor marriage risks. These will be discussed later.

There are several factors that sustain the preference of marrying rather than not:

1. There are fewer incidents of psychoses and crime among married individuals.

2. The death rate among married men is half that of single men.
3. Married individuals are generally happier than single ones.
4. The social outlets of married individuals are generally more numerous than those of single persons.
5. The Internal Revenue Service provides a significant financial credit to married couples who file joint returns in most cases of tax reporting.

The need for companionship may be the basic reason. Men and women often deplore the idea of being alone without intimate mates, and our society has approved of such intimacy only in marriage. What happens to one when one grows old alone? Who really cares for the person who is mateless and/or childless?

Sexual gratification and physical attraction are sometimes underlying reasons for marriage. Unless one is extremely cautious about marriage for this reason, the chances are that there will be subsequent, serious marital problems. A young man who marries a young lady simply because marriage is the only way to get her into bed needs serious counseling. Sexual appeal in marriages of this type may soon wane and leave a relationship void of any genuine sharing.

Economic motives are the reason for some marriages. Though rarely admitted by individuals, couples do marry to merge financial interests, such as that cited in relation to income tax reporting. A young female college student revealed that she and her husband were conditioned to marry because of the alleged benefits of two independent incomes to support economic obligations and the benefit of tax credits. In some rare instances relatives have been known to marry in order to keep their wealth within the family.

The reasons for marrying may be as defined as the number of individuals who attempt to define the reasons. The basic factor that remains relatively constant is that most people marry because they have fallen in love with a special person. Love remains the common denominator, but it cannot be relied upon as the panacea of other possible shortcomings.

Age and marriage

The young woman marries at about 20 years of age and the young man at about 23 years. What is the best age to marry? No one knows. The only logical time is when the persons are mature enough, physically, emotionally, and financially. Some people are ready before their twentieth year, whereas others are never really old enough. There are certain risks involved in marrying one who is well into the middle years of life. A woman or man who marries for the first time at 30 or 40 probably brings to the marriage many years of independent living and thinking, which may be difficult to vary in order to complement a good marital relationship. The relative ages of the man and woman are rarely debated unless the difference happens to be extremely great. It is commonly accepted that the man should be older than the woman. Eight percent of all men marry women who are several years younger than themselves. The reasons for this practice are obvious.

It has been found that the happiest couples were those in which the husband was 4 or 5 years older than the wife. The happier group of wives were 5 to 6 years older than their husbands. The happiest group of husbands had wives who were 12 or more years younger than themselves.

Age differences, when not too extreme, offer only minor problems to a happy marriage. Interest and attitude differences present more serious problems. If one marries an older person as a substitute parent or simply because the other individual has already achieved a stable position in life, one may be entering marriage on an unstable basis.

Contemporary times emphasize the need for comprehensive education. Emerging from the straits of conventional attitudes, women are excelling in practically every professional area. A graduate student once revealed that he had been engaged to a young woman who was completing a medical degree. He became obsessed with the alleged negative implications of her being ultimately more educated than he could ever hope to be and broke the engagement. The student was preoccupied with his concept of society's traditional attitude toward the superior educational role of the male. For some individuals differences have very little negative impact on the marriage. If there is a serious question of difference, the greater degree of formal education should be in favor of the male.

MARRIAGE LAWS

Many references have been made to the contractual significance of marriage. Each person agrees to a transition in legal status. However, the newly formed relationship is more than a simple contract. The marriage may be entered into by mutual consent, but it cannot be terminated as simply. Each state has many laws to regulate marriage, including regulations of age, health status, kinship, interracial marriages, relations between parents and children, and legal means of dissolving marriage. Summaries of some marriage and divorce laws are presented in Tables 9-2 and 9-3.

Prohibited marriages

As mentioned above, persons may enter into marriage by mutual consent. This consent, however, must be aproved by each state. Some states have laws that rule out certain combinations of people thought to be unsuitable for marriage.

Interracial marriages. Marriage between certain races is forbidden by many state laws. Twenty-two states prohibit marriages between blacks and whites, and in addition eight of these states forbid marriages between orientals and whites.

Kinship. Prohibition of marriages between close relatives are old and quite prevalent. Persons of an immediate family related by blood may not marry. First cousins are prohibited from marrying each other in more than half of the states. A few states prohibit the marriage of even more distant relatives. The reasons forbidding such mar-

riages are based on genetic factors. A defective family strain might be carried by both cousins and thus increase the probability that their offspring might inherit the defect. Many on the grounds for divorce covered in Table 9-3 are also grounds for prohibiting marriage.

Medical examination

About 90% of the states require a medical examination prior to marriage. The primary purpose of this examination, in most states, is to ascertain whether the person has a venereal disease (Table 9-2). Some states also require the person to be examined for feeblemindedness, mental incompetence, imbecility, insanity, chronic alcoholism, drug addiction, and infectious tuberculosis. North Dakota and Oregon require the most comprehensive medical examinations.

Obtaining the license

All states require that a couple secure a license from an official state officer, usually a county judge or a clerk. Most of the states also require a marriage ceremony and that the marriage be witnessed and officially recorded.

Waiting period

Most of the states require a waiting period ranging from 1 to 7 days. The majority of the waiting periods are between the time of applying for a license and the issuance of the license, although one may also exist between the time of issuing the license and the marriage. The waiting period is designed to reduce elopements or impulsive decisions to marry.

Terminating the marriage

There are two ways in which a marriage may be legally terminated: divorce and annulment. As a result of either one of these actions, the husband and wife are legally free to go their own ways or to marry someone else.

Divorce. The only ground for divorce recognized by all states is adultery. Legal grounds for divorce are not necessarily the real reasons for obtaining the terminating

Table 9-2. Marriage laws: 1967

State	Age at which marriage can be contracted with parental consent		Age below which parental consent is required		Physical examination and blood test for male and female		Waiting period	
					Period between examination and issuance of license	Scope of medical examination	Before issuance of license	After issuance of license
	Male	Female	Male	Female				
Alabama	17(a)	14(a)	21	18	30 da.	(b)	—	—
Alaska	18(c)	16(c)	21	18	30 da.	(b)	3 da.	—
Arizona	18(c)	16(c)	21	18	30 da.	(b)	—	—
Arkansas	18(c)	16(c)	21	18	30 da.	(b)	3 da.	—
California	18(a, d)	16(a, d)	21	18	30 da.	(b)	—	—
Colorado	16(d)	16(d)	21	18	30 da.	(b)	—	—
Connecticut	16(d)	16(d)	21	21	40 da.	(b)	4 da.	—
Delaware	18(c)	16(c)	21	18	30 da.	(b)	—	(e)
Florida	18(a, c)	16(a, c)	21	21	30 da.	(b)	3 da.	—
Georgia	18(c, f)	16(c, f)	19(f)	19(f)	30 da.	(b)	3 da.(g)	—
Hawaii	18	16(d)	20	20	30 da.	(b)	3 da.	—
Idaho	18	16(d)	21	18	30 da.	(b)	—	—
Illinois	18	16	21	18	15 da.	(b)	—	—
Indiana	18(c)	16(c)	21	18	30 da.	(b)	3 da.	—
Iowa	18(c)	16(c)	21	18	20 da.	(b)	3 da.	—
Kansas	18(d)	18(d)	21	18	30 da.	(b, h)	3 da.	—
Kentucky	18(a, c)	16(a, c)	21	21	15 da.	(b)	3 da.	—
Louisiana	18(d)	16(d)	21	21	10 da.	(b)	—	72 hrs.
Maine	16(d)	16(d)	21	18	30 da.	(b)	5 da.	—
Maryland	18(c)	16(c)	21	18	—	—	48 hrs.	—
Massachusetts	18(d)	16(d)	21	18	30 da.	(b)	3 da.	—
Michigan	(i)	16(c)	18	18	30 da.	(b)	3 da.	—
Minnesota	18(a)	16(j)	21	18	—	—	5 da.	—
Mississippi	17(d)	15(d)	21	21	30 da.	(b)	3 da.	—
Missouri	15(d)	15(d)	21	18	15 da.	(b)	3 da.	—
Montana	18(d)	16(d)	21	18	20 da.	(b)	5 da.	—
Nebraska	18(c)	16(c)	21	21	30 da.	(b)	—	—
Nevada	18(a, d)	16(a, d)	21	18	—	—	—	—
New Hampshire	14(k)	13(k)	20	18	30 da.	(b)	5 da.	—
New Jersey	18(d)	16(d)	21	18	30 da.	(b)	72 hrs.	—
New Mexico	18(c)	16(c)	21	18	30 da.	(b)	3 da.	—
New York	16	16(d)	21	18	30 da.	(b)	—	24 hrs.(l)
North Carolina	16	16(c)	18	18	30 da.	(m)	(n)	—

Note: Common law marriage is recognized in Alabama, Colorado, Florida, Georgia, Idaho, Iowa, Kansas, Montana, Ohio, Oklahoma, Pennsylvania, Rhode Island, South Carolina, Texas, and the District of Columbia. (a) Parental consent not required if minor was previously married. (b) Venereal diseases. (c) Statute establishes procedure whereby younger parties may obtain license in case of pregnancy or birth of a child. (d) Statute establishes procedure whereby younger parties may obtain license in special circumstances. (e) Residents, 24 hours; nonresidents, 96 hours. (f) If parties are under 19 years of age, proof of age and the consent of parents in person required. If a parent is ill, an affidavit by the incapacitated parent and a physician's affidavit to that effect required. (g) Unless parties are 21 years of age or older, or female is pregnant, or applicants are the parents of a living child born out of wedlock. (h) Feeblemindedness. (i) No provision in law for parental consent for males. (j) Parental consent and permission of judge required. In Oregon, permission of judge required for male under 19 years of age or female under 17. (k) Below age of consent parties need parental consent and permission of judge. (l) Marriage may not be solemnized within three days from date on which specimen for serological test was taken. (m) Venereal diseases and mental incompetence. (n) Forty-eight hours if both are nonresidents. (o) Feeblemindedness, imbecility, insanity, chronic alcoholism, and venereal diseases. In Washington, also advanced tuberculosis and, if male, contagious venereal diseases. (p) If one or both parties are below the age for marriage without parental consent. (q) Time limit between date of examination and expiration of marriage license. (r) Venereal diseases, feeblemindedness, mental illness, drug addiction, and chronic alcoholism. (s) Infectious tuberculosis and venereal diseases. (t) If female is nonresident, must complete license five days prior to marriage. (u) Unless parties are 21 years of age or older.

Table 9-2. Marriage laws: 1967—cont'd

| State | Age at which marriage can be contracted with parental consent | | Age below which parental consent is required | | Physical examination and blood test for male and female | | | |
	Male	Female	Male	Female	Period between examination and issuance of license	Scope of medical examination	Waiting period Before issuance of license	Waiting period After issuance of license
North Dakota	18	15	21	18	30 da.	(o)	—	—
Ohio	18(c)	16(c)	21	21	30 da.	(b)	5 da.	—
Oklahoma	18(c)	15(c)	21	18	30 da.	(b)	72 hr.(p)	—
Oregon	18(j)	15(j)	21	18	30 da.(q)	(r)	7 da.	—
Pennsylvania	16(d)	16(d)	21	21	30 da.	(b)	3 da.	—
Rhode Island	18(d)	16(d)	21	21	40 da.	(s)	—	(t)
South Carolina	16(c)	14(c)	18	18	—	—	24 hrs.	—
South Dakota	18(c)	16(c)	21	18	20 da.	(b)	—	—
Tennessee	16(d)	16(d)	21	21	30 da.	(b)	3 da.(u)	—
Texas	16	14	21	18	15 da.	(b)	3 da.(p)	—
Utah	16(a)	14(a)	21	18	30 da.	(b)	—	—
Vermont	18(d)	16(d)	21	18	30 da.	(b)	—	5 da.
Virginia	18(a, c)	16(a, c)	21	21	30 da.	(b)	—	—
Washington	17(d)	17(d)	21	18	—	(o)	3 da.	—
West Virginia	18(a)	16(a)	21	21	30 da.	(b)	3 da.	—
Wisconsin	18	16	21	18	20 da.	(b)	5 da.	—
Wyoming	18	16	21	21	30 da.	(b)	—	—

decree. They mirror only in part the marital problems that preceded the divorce; they also depend upon the statutory provisions in each state as outlined in Table 9-3. A large amount of evidence points to the conclusion that a great number of divorces are obtained on grounds least unpleasant to advance under the various state laws and easiest to establish in legislation.

Annulment. Practically every state has some legal provision for annulment of a marriage. The annulment is most frequently granted when the marriage violated a law that prohibited marriage or when it was against some other established legal policy. Some of the more common grounds for annulment are illegal age, fraud or misrepresentation, interracial marriage, degree of kinship, one person is legally married to a third, use of force or threats, and mental incapacity.

Other laws

There are many additional laws that regulate marriage, but the limits of this book

do not allow the treatment of all areas. It is, however, recommended that you study other publications that discuss laws in which you may be especially interested. There are laws that cover common-law marriages, property rights of couples, personal relations, legal separations, and other factors.

SEX CONSIDERATIONS

A premarital health examination by a licensed physician may yield benefits above the legal requirements. A man and woman both may obtain detailed advice about their role in sexual intercourse, together with advice about family planning and contraception. In the woman's case, a simple pelvic examination will usually disclose any pelvic abnormality, such as a tough and intact hymen that may interfere with satisfactory sexual relations. Rarely does a physician talk over sex and emotional problems with the bride-to-be. Most physicians give counseling only when asked specifically.

An exceptionally indiscreet physician might feel that such an examination is

Table 9-3. Grounds for divorce: 1968

	Pregnancy at marriage*	Impotence	Sexual malformation†	Desertion	Abandonment	Nonsupport	Mental cruelty	Physical cruelty
Alabama	Yes	Yes	Yes	2 years#	1 year	2 years#	No	Yes
Alaska	No	Yes**	No	1 year	No	1 year	Yes	Yes
Arizona	Yes	Yes**	Yes**	1 year	No	1 year	Yes	Yes
Arkansas	No	Yes**	No	1 year	1 year	Yes	Yes	Yes
California	No	No	No	1 year	1 year	1 year	Yes	Yes
Colorado	No	Yes	No	1 year	No	1 year	Yes	Yes
Connecticut	Yes[8]	Yes[8]	Yes[8]	3 years	Yes[9]	Yes[9]	Yes[9]	Yes[9]
Delaware	No	No	No	2 years	No	Yes	Yes	Yes
District of Columbia	No	No	No	1 year	1 year	No	No	Yes
Florida	No	Yes	Yes	1 year	No	No	Yes	Yes
Georgia	Yes	Yes**	No	1 year	No	No	Yes	Yes
Hawaii	No	No	No	6 mo.	No	60 days	60 days	Yes
Idaho	No	No	No	1 year	Yes	1 year	Yes	Yes
Illinois	No	Yes	No	1 year	No	No	Yes[15]	Yes[15]
Indiana	No	Yes**	No	2 years	2 years	2 years	Yes	Yes
Iowa	Yes	No	No	2 years	No	No	Yes	Yes
Kansas	No	No	No	Yes[18]	1 year	Yes[18]	Yes	Yes
Kentucky	Yes	Yes	Yes	No	1 year	No	6 mos.	Yes
Louisiana	No	No	No	No	No	No	No	No
Maine	No	Yes	No	3 years	3 years	Yes	Yes	Yes
Maryland	No	Yes**	No	18 mos.	18 mos.	No	No	No
Massachusetts	No	Yes	No	2 years	No	Yes	No	Yes
Michigan	No	Yes**	Yes**	2 years	No	Yes	Yes	Yes
Minnesota	No	Yes	No	1 year	No	No	Yes	Yes
Mississippi	Yes	Yes	No	1 year	No	No	Yes[24]	Yes[24]
Missouri	Yes	Yes**	No	1 year	No	Yes	Yes[25]	Yes[25]
Montana	No	No	No	1 year	1 year	1 year	1 year	Yes
Nebraska	Yes	Yes**	No	2 years	2 years	Yes	Yes	Yes
Nevada	No	Yes**	No	1 year	No	1 year	Yes	Yes
New Hampshire	No	Yes	Yes	2 years	2 years	2 years	Yes	Yes
New Jersey	No	No	No	2 years	No	No	Yes[24]	Yes[24]
New Mexico	Yes	Yes	No	No	Yes	Yes	Yes[24]	Yes[24]
New York	No	No	No	No	2 years	No	Yes	Yes
North Carolina	Yes	Yes**	No	No	No	No	No	No
North Dakota	No	No	No	1 year	1 year	1 year	Yes	Yes
Ohio	No	Yes	No	1 year	1 year	Yes	Yes	Yes
Oklahoma	Yes	Yes	No	1 year	1 year	Yes	Yes	Yes
Oregon	No	Yes**	No	1 year	No	No	Yes	Yes

*By another man, pregnancy unknown to husband. †Preventing intercourse. **Existing at inception of marriage. ‡Without [1]Imprisonment for two years of seven-year sentence. [2]Crime against nature. [3]Divorce after period of four years of decree of divorce from bed and board or decree of separate maintenance: Colorado (after three years), Minnesota (after two years), Utah (after three years). [4]Incompatibility. [5]Personal indignities. (In Tennessee, available as a ground only to a wife.) [6]Unsound mind. [7]When not on testimony of spouse, or if before marriage without knowledge of spouse. [8]Assuming concealed from spouse, may be grounds under fraudulent contract. [9]Intolerable cruelty: together with other difficulty such may be grounds under intolerable cruelty; legal separation. [10]Violent and ungovernable temper. [11]Attempt to obtain divorce outside state of domicile if divorce obtained. [12]Involving moral turpitude and two-year sentence. [13]Where sentence is of life or imprisonment for seven years or more (Hawaii); of at least three years, 18 months of which must be served before filing suit (applies also to conviction of misdemeanor) (Maryland); of five years or more (Massachusetts); commitment to prison for three years (Wisconsin); to penitentiary (Mississippi); for not less than two years (District of Columbia). [14]Hansen's disease; expiration of term in decree of separate maintenance and no reconciliation. [15]Extreme and repeated. [16]If communicated. [17]Attempt to take life of spouse. [18]Gross neglect of duty. [19]Confinement at hard labor. [20]Public defamation of spouse; attempt on life of spouse; being fugitive from justice. [21]Sentence dissolves marriage. [22]May be grounds under allegation of cruelty. [23]Sentenced to imprisonment of three years or more. [24]Habitual cruelty (Indiana), habitual cruel and in-

Habitual drunkenness	Habitual use of drugs	Venereal disease	Mental incapacity**	Post-marital insanity	Conviction of felony	Life imprisonment	Fraud	Living apart‡	Refuse to cohabit	Prior marriage existing	Other grounds
Yes	Yes	No	No	5 years	Yes[1]	No	No	No	No	No	2, 3
1 year	Yes	No	No	18 mos.	Yes	No	No	No	No	No	4, 5, 6
Yes	Yes	Yes**	No	No	Yes[7]	No	No	5 years	No	No	None
1 year	1 year	Yes	No	3 years	Yes	Yes	No	3 years	Yes	Yes	None
1 year	Yes	No	No	3 years	Yes	Yes	No	No	Yes	No	None
1 year	1 year	No	No	3 years	Yes	No	No	No	No	No	3
Yes	Yes[9]	Yes[9]	Yes[9]	5 years	Yes[9]	Yes	Yes	No	Yes[9]	No	9
2 years**	Yes**	No	No	5 years	Yes	Yes	No	3 years	No	Yes	None
No	No	No	No	No	Yes	Yes	No	1 year	1 year	No	None
Yes	Yes	No	No	No	No	No	No	No	No	Yes	10, 11
Yes	No	No	Yes	2 years	Yes[12]	Yes	Yes	No	No	Yes	None
1 year	1 year	No	No	3 years	Yes[13]	Yes	No	3 years	No	No	14
1 year	Yes	Yes	No	3 years	Yes	Yes	No	5 years	Yes	No	None
2 years	2 years	Yes[16]	No	No	Yes	No	No	No	No	Yes	17
Yes	No	No	No	5 years	Yes	No	No	No	No	No	None
Yes	No	No	No	No	Yes	No	No	No	No	No	None
Yes	Yes[18]	Yes[18]	No	3 years	Yes	Yes	Yes	No	No	Yes	18
1 year	No	Yes	No	5 years	Yes	No	Yes	5 years	No	No	None
No	No	No	No	No	Yes[19]	Yes	No	2 years	No	No	20
Yes	Yes	No	No	No	21	21	No	3 years	3 years	No	None
No	No	No	Yes	3 years	Yes[13]	Yes	No	18 mos.	Yes	Yes	None
Yes	Yes	Yes**	No	No	Yes[13]	Yes	No	No	No	No	None
Yes	Yes[22]	Yes[22]	No	No	Yes[23]	Yes	No	No	Yes[22]	No	11
1 year	Yes[22]	No	No	5 years	Yes	Yes	No	No	Yes[22]	No	3
Yes	Yes	No	Yes	3 years	Yes[13]	No	No	No	No	Yes	24
1 year	No	No	No	No	Yes	Yes	Yes	No	No	Yes	5, 26
1 year	No	No	No	5 years	Yes	No	No	No	No	No	None
Yes	Yes	Yes	No	5 years	Yes[23]	Yes	No	No	No	No	None
Yes	No	No	No	2 years	Yes	Yes	No	1 year	No	No	4
2 years	No	No	No	No	Yes[27]	Yes	No	2 years	2 years[28]	No	28
No	No	No	No	No	No	No	No	No	No	No	None
Yes	No	No	No	5 years	Yes	No	No	No	No	No	4, 24
No	No	No	No	5 years	Yes[29]	No	No	No	No	No	30
No	No	No	No	5 years	No	No	No	1 year	No	No	2
1 year	1 year	No	No	5 years	Yes	No	No	3 years	1 year	No	31
Yes	No	No	No	No	Yes[27]	Yes	Yes	No	1 year	Yes	11
Yes	No	No	No	5 years	Yes[27]	No	Yes	No	No	No	4, 11
1 year	No	No	No	2 years	Yes	No	No	No	No	No	5

cohabitation. #In favor of wife only.

human treatment (Mississippi), cruel and inhuman treatment (New Mexico), and extreme cruelty (New Jersey). [25]Cruel or barbarous treatment so as to endanger life. [26]Vagrancy of husband. [27]If imprisoned. [28]Absent and unheard of for two years; absence of wife beyond state for 10 years without consent of husband; joining religious sect that believes marriage unlawful and refusing to cohabit for six months. [29]Confinement of defendant to prison for three or more consecutive years. [30]Living apart for two years after a decree of separation, or after the execution of a separation agreement properly filed and executed. [31]Willful neglect. [32]May be possible under allegation of fraud. [33]For certain enumerated crimes resulting in sentence of two years or more. [34]Five years or less at discretion of judge. [35]If party imprisoned is considered legally dead. [36]Divorce or separation for gross misbehavior of either party. [37]Attempted murder of spouse; refusal of wife to live with husband in this state. [38]If undisclosed at time of marriage. [39]A year after conviction, provided spouse did not testify against other. [40]Imprisonment for three years if confined at time of libel. [41]Intolerable severity. [42]Other grounds for divorce are sodomy or buggery; where either party prior to marriage without knowledge of other had been convicted of infamous offense; where prior to marriage without knowledge of husband, wife had been prostitute. [43]Only within two years from marriage.

Table 9-3. Grounds for divorce: 1968—cont'd

	Pregnancy at marriage*	Impotence	Sexual malformation†	Desertion	Abandonment	Non-support	Mental cruelty	Physical cruelty
Pennsylvania	Yes[32]	Yes**	Yes**	2 years	No	No	No	Yes
Rhode Island	Yes	Yes**	Yes	Yes[34]	Yes[34]	1 year	No	Yes
South Carolina	No	No	No	1 year	No	No	No	Yes
South Dakota	No	No	No	1 year	No	1 year	Yes	Yes
Tennessee	Yes	Yes**	No	1 year	Yes	Yes	Yes	Yes
Texas	No	No	No	3 years	3 years	Yes	Yes[22]	Yes[22]
Utah	Yes**	Yes**	Yes**	1 year	Yes[22]	Yes	Yes	Yes
Vermont	No	No	No	3 years	No	Yes	No	No
Virginia	Yes**	Yes**	No	1 year	1 year	No	No	No
Washington	No	No	No	1 year	1 year	Yes	Yes	Yes
West Virginia	No	No	No	1 year	1 year	No	Yes	Yes
Wisconsin	No	No	No	1 year	No	Yes	Yes	Yes
Wyoming	Yes	Yes[43]	Yes[43]	1 year	1 year	1 year	Yes	Yes

carried out without embarrassment if a nurse is not present, but most desire the presence of a nurse if for no other reason than to chaperone the examination. The patency of the vagina should be estimated by the physician during his pelvic examination of the bride-to-be. Some physicians may use a plastic model of the reproductive system for the patient to observe during the pelvic examination. The model will help identify to the bride-to-be the labia and the clitoris with its sensitive nerve endings and ability to engorge with blood when she is sexually excited. The physician then estimates the patency of the vagina. If a tight hymen or an intact one is present, the patient may be instructed how to smooth out and enlarge the hymenal ring with the finger by stretching it gently but firmly toward the rectum. An anesthetic ointment may be worked into the skin prior to this stretching several times a day. Usually 8 to 10 days of such stretching will suffice. Occasionally minor surgery may be required to dilate or sever a tough hymen.

Further explanations about the new life with new sex habits should be based on trying to satisfy the desires and needs of one's marriage partner. A male may have a more frequent and a greater sex drive at first than his female marriage partner. A woman has many inhibitions to overcome, as she may have had to avoid sex activity and sexual conversation. Young men have been described as sexual predators to the woman, whereas she biologically is feeling the sex urge or drive and psychologically may have many inhibitions. In the manner of habits she has generally been taught to keep her legs together, but to engage in the sex act she must spread her legs wide. She must recognize that the many years of conditioning will take time, patience, and conscious effort to overcome. It is important that the person understand that sex can be discussed just as are other problems of food, entertainment, or habitation between the marriage partners.

It is vital in a marriage to do one's utmost to see that the other's needs and feelings are met. Most of us are self-directed before marriage, but in marriage no 50-50 proportion will work. One must be willing to do much more than seems their share if the marriage is to work.

In any new physical endeavor there is apt to be awkwardness, fumblings, and various attempts at different techniques. Those thinking of marriage should read some

Habitual drunkenness	Habitual use of drugs	Venereal disease	Mental incapacity**	Postmarital insanity	Conviction of felony	Life imprisonment	Fraud	Living apart‡	Refuse to cohabit	Prior marriage existing	Other grounds
No	No	No	No	No	Yes[33]	No	Yes	No	No	Yes	5
Yes	Yes	No	Yes	No	No	35	Yes	10 years	Yes[22]	Yes	36
Yes	Yes	No	No	No	No	No	No	No	No	No	None
1 year	No	No	No	5 years	Yes	No	No	No	No	No	None
Yes	No	No	No	No	Yes	No	No	No	No	Yes	5, 37
Yes[22]	Yes	Yes[38]	No	5 years	Yes[39]	Yes[39]	No	3 years	Yes[22]	No	None
Yes	Yes[22]	No	No	Yes	Yes	Yes	No	No	No	No	3
No	No	No	No	5 years	Yes[40]	No	No	3 years	No	No	41
Yes[22]	Yes[22]	Yes[22]	No	No	Yes	Yes	No	2 years	No	No	42
Yes	No	No	Yes	2 years	Yes[27]	Yes	Yes	2 years	No	No	None
Yes	Yes	No	No	No	Yes	No	No	No	No	No	None
1 year	No	No	No	No	Yes[13]	No	No	5 years	No	No	None
Yes	Yes	No	No	2 years	Yes	No	No	2 years	Yes	No	5

instructional books together. Most brides will have had some experience with sex play to a limited extent prior to marriage. This is also true of the male.

Frequent intercourse on a honeymoon may produce an irritated or abraded penis. If natural secretions do not overcome friction, the use of a lubricating jelly may avoid such trauma. Urethral bruising of the male or female may produce burning on urination with unusual frequency after the third or fourth day of continuous intercourse. Prompt treatment from a physician should be sought, as inflammation of the urethra may extend into the bladder to produce cystitis. Normally a small amount of vaginal discharge in the wife is present and is increased by sexual activity. If the amount is obviously excessive with a yellowish or whitish, frothy, foamy discharge with an odor, vaginitis may be present.

Men usually are reluctant to have a physical examination before marriage. Men may talk about sex in general but do not like to talk about it as a personal matter. Most young males of today have been circumcised, which aids in keeping the penis clean. If the male has not been circumcised and phimosis (a condition in which the prepuce cannot be pulled back over the glans)

occurs, circumcision should be performed. This usually requires 3 to 4 weeks to heal. The testicles are examined for any unilateral enlargement or failure of descent. Hernia should be ruled out by examination of the inguinale canal. A general physical examination should usually accompany these detailed examinations. Occasionally (if there has been a history of urethral discharge) semen ejaculated through masturbation may be collected for examination to determine if the duct system is open.

The premarital examination may disclose minor abnormalities whose surgical correction will leave the genitalia tender while healing. This examination should be scheduled well in advance of the wedding and honeymoon. Three months prior to the wedding is ample time to ensure no subsequent embarrassment, physical discomfort, or interference with plans.

HEREDITY

Heredity is the inborn capacity of the organism to develop parental characteristics and is dependent upon the genetic biochemistry of the cells that form the starting point of the new individual. Offspring resemble their parents in various physical and mental characteristics to the extent that a particular code or message of nucleic acid from both mother and father is found in the single fertilized egg that is their beginning, the zygote. The smallest effective part of any hereditary code is the gene, and the phase of biology concerned with the study of the mechanism of inheritance is genetics.

Long before there was any scientific basis to heredity and therefore a field of genetics as we know it today, man had benefited from the observation of similarity in successive generations. The Egyptians and other Mediterranean peoples, centuries before the birth of Christ, practiced controlled breeding of domesticated animals and developed superior plants (date palms) through controlled breeding procedures. The writings of Aristotle (384-322 B.C.) contain descriptions and interpretations of genetic phenomena. Why better plants and animals resulted was little understood. It was not until Anton Van Leeuwenhoek (1632-1723) developed a simple but efficient microscope through which he could view microorganisms that scientists had the tools to understand and begin to explain this similarity. During the next 100 years, many scientists, experimenting with both plants and animals, added to the available fund of knowledge but failed to make the fundamental breakthrough necessary. It was recognized, for instance, that spermatozoa are necessary for fertilization; but not until the end of the nineteenth century was it known that fertilization was the fusing of the nuclei of a sperm and an ovum. As late as one hundred years ago, a workable theory about the structure and function of the cell nucleus was still lacking.

Gregor J. Mendel (1822-1884), an Augustinian monk and botanist, is known as the founder of the science of genetics. Following 8 years of exhaustive experimentation with the ordinary garden pea at his monastery at Bruna, Moravia (Austria), he published in 1866 a resumé of his findings that have since been called Mendel's law. Others, such as the German botanist Kolreuter, had attempted to solve the same problem; but in Mendel's own words, "no

one experiment has been carried out to such an extent and in such a way as to make it possible to determine the number of different forms with certainty according to their separate generations, or definitely to ascertain their statistical relations." He had two points in his favor; he was, first, a careful scientist and, second, he was both wise and fortunate in selecting for his major work seven plant characteristics that were "constantly differentiating and which occurred in pairs." A brief review of his work will explain this.

Mendel's law may be generalized under the following three points:

1. The characteristics that we inherit are produced by genes (Mendel called them "factors") passed from one generation to the next.
2. These genes are found in paired chromosomes. If there is a difference in the degrees to which each gene in a given pair affects a particular characteristic, the gene that is able to express itself is said to be dominant, and the one that does not express itself is said to be recessive.
3. At germ cell formation the members of each pair of chromosomes separate independently from the other pairs. Each parent then contributes to each offspring only one of every two paired chromosomes. This is a random process.

A description of eye color in the human being is similar to the yellow and green of Mendel's peas. Eye color is determined primarily by a single pair of genes wherein the gene for brown eyes is dominant and the gene for blue eyes is recessive (Fig. 9-1). In the first generation there is a parent who would always "breed true" for brown eyes and one who would always "breed true" for blue eyes. In germ cell formation each chromosome pair would separate, and in any mature sperm or ovum only one gene for eye color would be found. In this example, let us assume that the male present had the only brown-eye genes and the female present had the only blue. All of the male sperm would

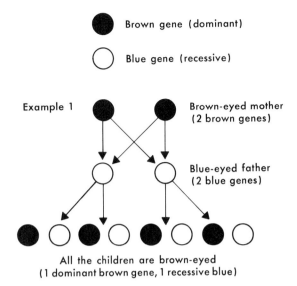

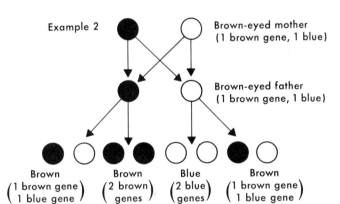

Fig. 9-1. The inheritance of eye color.

carry a gene for brown eyes and all of the female ova would carry a gene for blue eyes. All children then would receive a gene for brown and a gene for blue, and since brown is dominant and blue recessive, they would all be brown eyed.

In the next generation additional mathematical possibilities occur. Notice in Fig. 9-1 that of the four combinations three offspring are brown eyed (that which appears is referred to as phenotype) and one blue eyed; and although there are only two phenotypes, there are three distinctly different genetic combinations (genotypes). One received two genes for brown, two re-

ceived a gene for brown and a gene for blue, and one received two genes for blue.

Genetic basis of heredity

The basic tenets of modern genetics may be summarized as follows:

1. The continuity of living things from one generation to the next is provided for through the formation of new individuals, or reproduction.
2. The study of this continuity is called heredity, whereas the differences between individuals in the same or successive generations is the study of variation.

3. The basic elements that form the living link between generations are found in the nucleus of the cell; in sexual reproduction the gametic nuclei with unpaired chromosomes join to form the zygotic nucleus with paired chromosomes.

4. There are several major constituents of the cell nucleus:

   a. Chromosomes may be thought of as long chains. Each link in the chain is a gene; each gene is responsible either in whole or in part for some characteristic. The normal human being possesses 23 pairs of chromosomes, and the best estimates indicate that each will be made up of something close to 1,000 genes. During the resting stage of cell division, the chromosomes are not seen; but as the cell prepares to divide, the genes appear to group themselves and become thickly coated with additional material.

   b. The nucleoplasm is the gellike substance that surrounds the chromosomes.

   c. There may be more than one nucleolus. These are spherical bodies that act as storage units for material necessary in the cell duplication process.

5. The sum total of genes represents an organization or pattern that carries in condensed form instructions transmitted from parents to offspring. This transmitted code, as well as the environment of each developing cell, determines the appearance of specific characteristics in the newly created individual.

The genetic code

On March 14, 1969, a California Institute of Technology graduate student, Jack Griffith, succeeded in photographing a molecule of deoxyribonucleic acid (DNA), the chemical determining all characteristics in all organisms. The event was notable for the contribution it made to genetics. Although

this substance had been discovered about 100 years ago, its biologic importance was explained by Francis Crick and James Watson only in 1953.

DNA is a large molecule consisting of five chemical elements: carbon, hydrogen, nitrogen, oxygen, and phosphorus. These elements are arranged in two long chains of

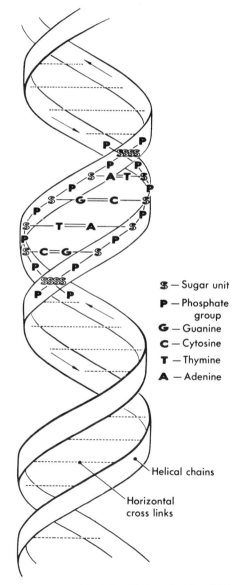

Fig. 9-2. The double helix DNA molecule of Crick is diagrammatically represented as he assumes it exists. (From Braungart, D. C., and Buddeke, R.: An introduction to animal biology, ed. 7, St. Louis, 1968, The C. V. Mosby Co.)

alternating sugar and phosphate molecules and nitrogen bases. They are held together by cross links called hydrogen bonds. Adenine, cytosine, guanine, and thymine are the nitrogen bases. One molecule of DNA contains thousands of these elements.

Chromosomes are made up of three kinds of chemicals. DNA is only one of the chemicals; the other two are proteins and ribonucleic acid (RNA). DNA appears to be the most concerned with heredity, although many geneticists believe that elements in the cytoplasm, or outer layer of the cell, may exert some influence. DNA apparently has the ability to reproduce itself down to the final atom.

Every time a cell divides, it duplicates itself, producing two new identical cells. The DNA in each cell untwines itself and splits lengthwise. Two single chains are produced whose backbones are alternating sugar and phosphate groups with bases projecting. Each of the units, mentioned earlier, finds its proper place on each of the single chains, adenine always joining with thymine and cytosine with guanine. Each half thus builds onto its opposite, forming two new molecules. The order of the bases is the same; therefore, the code that transmits characteristics remains the same (Figs. 9-2 and 9-3).

Inherited characteristics

The normal pattern of sex determination is centered in a pair of chromosomes. The female carries a pair that appear identical in size and symbolically are designated as XX.

The Lyen hypothesis has recently suggested that women have one functioning X chromosome in a somatic cell. The males of the human species have an XY chromosome combination. In the human species it has been found that certain parts of the X and Y chromosomes are genetically identical and that the Y chromosome determines maleness. The Y chromosome is smaller than the X chromosome, and it is apparently this combination of the longer X and the short Y that triggers the conception of a male.

The sex ratio at birth is 1.06 : 1 in favor of males. The younger the parents, the greater the possibility of conceiving a male. At conception there is an even greater imbalance in favor of males, but this advantage is counterbalanced by the greater death rate of males before and after birth.

Many traits are determined, not by the complete dominance and recessiveness of genes, but more often by a combining known as incomplete dominance. The classic example used here is skin color, which is determined by the interaction of two pairs of genes located on four different chromosomes. Since this is the case, the Mendelian law of independent assortment would apply.

Mendel showed that when several pairs of alternative characteristics are observed, the several pairs of genes enter into all possible combinations in the progeny. In the pea varieties at his disposal he observed that the seven pairs of differentiating characteristics (such as lightness or darkness of color or wrinkles or lack of wrinkles) recombined

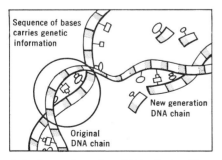
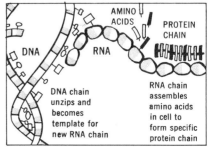

Fig. 9-3. Formation of a DNA chain. (From Public Health Service Publication No. 1546, Washington, D. C., 1967, U. S. Government Printing Office.)

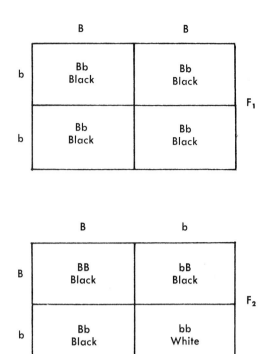

Fig. 9-4. Checkerboard showing the interaction of independent factors affecting skin color, as in matings of blacks (B) and whites (b); F_1, F_2, first and second generations.

at random. Mendel called this process independent assortment. The principle applies only to genes located on mutually exclusive chromosomes.

In the example of skin color all of the offspring in a marriage between a pure black person and a pure white person would have the same genotype, and their skin color would be in between the two extremes of that of the parents. These would be mulattos. When two mulattos marry, the skin color of resulting offspring, on the basis of all mathematical considerations, will range from very light to very dark.

There is a rather vaguely understood concept that longevity is inherited. Evidence abounds to indicate that if one is blessed with long-lived parents, he also will live a long life. Without a doubt heredity plays a large and responsible part, but the blessing of an environment that is also conducive to long life should not be overlooked. The best inheritance will do little good if the recipient is raised in an environment of

disease, malnourishment, and hazards. Growing, however, in a satisfactory environment, the individual certainly has a greater opportunity to live up to whatever his inherited potential may be. The following of wise health practices is, after all, a means whereby we may realize as much of this potential as possible.

As the field of genetics expands, scientists are placing more stress on the effect of the interaction of all genes with each other. This was first thought of as important within the chromosome, but more recent work indicates that the nucleoplasm (the environment surrounding the genes and chromosomes) is also of vital importance. The nucleus is a vast factory, and each molecule within affects and is affected by all the other molecules. No gene actually functions in a void but is influenced by the one above it, the one below it, all the others in the same chromosome, by genes on other chromosomes, and by the nucleoplasm inbetween.

Human traits will serve as examples to

show the complexity of genetics and may indicate why man will perhaps never understand all there is to know about genetics.

The genetics involved in body stature, including total height, width of shoulders, length of extremities, shape of skull, and contour of face, is exceedingly complex. Height alone, for instance, is determined by possibly ten or more pairs of genes. Since tallness is recessive, a person we would define as tall inherits more recessive genes for tallness than dominant genes for shortness. The interaction of the many inherited genes for height and the influence of other inherited body stature characteristics plus the modifying effect of environment will determine the absolute height of any one person. A large sampling of people from any population would include some quite short, some quite tall, and the majority clustered around an average.

The inheritance of intelligence is a much more complex consideration for the geneticist. A good yardstick will allow quite accurate measurements of height; on the other hand, intelligence tests are difficult to construct, often difficult to administer objectively, and so subject to criticism by many investigators. Despite this, it is obvious, because of the wide range of I.Q. (intelligence quotient) scores revealed in any sample, that intelligence is determined by many pairs of genes, which in turn are modified favorably or unfavorably by the environment. Many freshmen with relatively high I.Q.'s have failed along the way because of poor application and self-discipline.

Inherited disorders

We now know that some diseases are genetically inherited. This is the case in mongolism in which an extra chromosome is found. It is now also known that the presence of an extra chromosome is almost always associated with congenital malformations.

In some instances, genes may become altered, or mutant. This is one of the reasons for concern about radioactive fallout, because such irradiation may alter genes. Such mutations are then passed on by the father or mother. If a large number of hereditary factors that produce susceptibility to a given disease are present in a person, then that person may later develop the disease.

As our knowledge increases, we will no doubt learn about more diseases that have a genetic basis. It is now known that hemophilia, diabetes, feeblemindedness, epilepsy, erythroblastosis fetalis, allergies, gout, difficulty in metabolizing milk sugar, and perhaps some cancers and peptic ulcers are among those to which we may inherit a susceptibility. Whether this susceptibility is inherent in the genes or is caused by the uterine environment of the genes (as occurs in German measles, or when emotional upsets by the mother, with increased hydrocortisone circulating, produces cleft palates as in 90% of experimental animals), we can only say our knowledge is still incomplete.

It is well known that the external environment may also produce marked changes; a mother's love is necessary, for instance, or the newborn infant may cease to grow. We also know that if infants are placed in a playpen and not stimulated by contact with people who handle and fondle them, they may become mentally defective.

As our knowledge increases, some see the time when family backgrounds will be sought out in special clinics to determine whether their genetic inheritance will lead to good offspring, although the complexities of genetics are so great that this process will be difficult.

Over the years, the success of man in improving both plants and animals has been based on selective mating and environmental enrichment. If the race is to be improved, many believe that more attention must be given to reproduction of our "good stock" and decrease in the reproduction of our defective stock.

Feeblemindedness is a general term used to describe all mental conditions that permit an I.Q. no higher than 70. Early hereditary work tried to show that feeblemindedness was caused by the presence of a single recessive gene, but scientists today believe it to be operative much as normal levels of intelligence; that is, a condition caused by multiple genes. Evidence continues to indicate that it is a recessive condition, as seen in a marriage between a woman of normal intelligence and a man of inferior intelligence, which he has inherited. All the children from this marriage may be of normal to perhaps superior intelligence. Feeblemindedness may also be caused by certain diseases, such as meningitis or syphilis, or by injuries during or following birth. This is known as acquired feeblemindedness and is not an inherited condition.

Amaurotic familial idiocy is a general type of hereditary mental disorder that is characterized by a widespread derangement of lipid (one group of fats) metabolism and the subsequent buildup of lipid material in nerve cells and other parts of the body. The inheritance involved is the apparent inability to produce the enzyme necessary to metabolize these lipids. Although it occasionally develops in adults, it is most common in children and is identified in rapidly progressive dementia, retinal changes and blindness, generalized convulsive seizures, and eventual death. It passes from generation to generation as a recessive gene.

Phenylketonuria was discovered in 1934. It is an inherited metabolic disorder probably

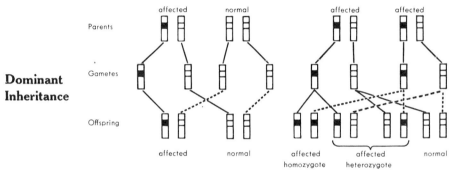

Dominant Inheritance

In dominant inheritance, most of the affected individuals are heterozygous for the abnormality; that is, the chromosomes contain one normal gene and one abnormal gene, and the trait is carried through each successive generation. Diseases transmitted by dominant inheritance include hereditary spherocytosis, achondroplasia, Huntington's chorea, and renal glycosuria.

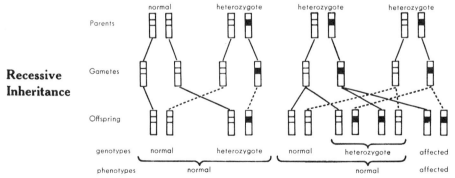

Recessive Inheritance

For a recessive trait to become manifest, the individual must be homozygous for the abnormal gene. Among the numerous conditions transmitted by simple recessive inheritance are sickle cell anemia, phenylketonuria, fructosuria, galactosemia, glycogen storage disease, familial cretinism with goiter, erythropoietic porphyria, and ceruloplasmin deficiency, or Wilson's disease.

Fig. 9-5. Inheritance of disease in man. (From Therapeutic notes, Parke, Davis & Co., September-October 1962.)

caused by a defect in a liver enzyme so that the liver is unable to metabolize an essential amino acid, phenylalanine, into tyrosine. This chemical abnormality leads to gradual mental derangement, associated with a dry, rough skin and abnormal, jerky movements. Putting a drop of ferric chloride on a baby's wet diaper produces a blue-green color, indicating a positive test reaction for phenylketonuria. Since this test is not reliable until the baby is several weeks old, Guthrie's test, in which a few drops of blood from the baby's heel are analyzed, is supplanting it. Early dietary restriction of phenylalanine may prevent brain damage.

Blood groups provide interesting evidence of inheritance at work. Major blood groups of human beings have been divided into groups A, B, AB, and O. About 40% have type A, while type B occurs in about 15%. Type AB is found in about 5% of all people, while type O is found in about 40%. People having type O blood are called universal donors, but cross matching should always be done before type O blood is given to someone having a different blood type.

A factor called the Rh factor is found in the blood of 85% of all people; they are Rh positive, while 15% are Rh negative, as they lack the factor. If a mother is Rh negative and the father Rh positive, a baby has a 50% chance of being Rh positive, as was the father. The mother reacts to this Rh positive substance in the baby's blood to produce substances called antibodies. After one or two pregnancies, the concentration of these mother-produced antibodies become high enough to destroy the blood cells of the baby. If jaundice, caused by excessive blood cell destruction, develops in such a baby, the baby may be treated by almost completely replacing its blood.

Huntington's chorea, or chronic progressive hereditary chorea, shows itself as various grimacing, twisting motions and mental changes associated with gradual atrophy (wasting away) of brain cells of the cortex and basal ganglia. It appears in early to middle adult life. There is no definite cure as yet. Prophylaxis, through the application of

eugenics, offers the best hope until we can identify and manipulate favorably the exact metabolic-genetic lesion.

The study of heredity is fascinating, and the scientific frontier in this area is still a great challenge for those who wish to accept it. The fruits of the study, however, do not belong solely to the scientist. A basic understanding of the mechanics of inheritance and an acceptance of the responsibilities that go with parenthood are important educational elements for everyone.

Most children are born normal and healthy. However, it is estimated that in the United States 1 out of 16 children will have a significant physical or mental abnormality at birth. Some of the more familiar abnormalities, such as clubfoot and cleft palate, are readily detectable at birth; some of the rarer types of abnormalities, such as phenylketonuria, mentioned earlier, remain hidden unless diagnosed by laboratory tests.

Mass screening procedures for child-oriented diseases caused by chromosome malfunctions are limited to a very few research programs. The one disease, however, for which screening is available throughout most of the country is phenylketonuria. In 38 states the law requires that all infants be tested at birth for the disease. Yet for other important maladies, for example homocystinuria, no routine tests are required. A baby born with the defect does not display any gross observable abnormality; homocystinuria can be definitely diagnosed only by laboratory tests. Yet unless this disorder is diagnosed and treated within the first 2 months of life, dislocation of the optic lens, leading to failing vision, and mental retardation may manifest themselves in later childhood.

The law today states that every couple who marry must have a blood test for syphilis, but it states nothing about the couples who have traits for metabolic diseases, any one of which may be as detrimental as syphilis to a baby's health. A case in point is sickle cell anemia, a disease that affects the red blood cells. One in about five hundred American Negroes is afflicted with this disease; 8% to 10% are carriers; that is, they can transmit the disease but do not have the symptoms or signs of it themselves. A simple test can spot this disease, as well as its carriers, but it is questionable how many ever receive the test. If each parent has a recessive gene for sickle cell anemia, the mathematical chances of each of their children having the disease is one in four. For those who are born with the disease, sickle cell anemia is usually fatal before age 30, prior to which there is a long history of hospitalization for blood clots in the spleen, lungs, liver, and other organs. There is currently no satisfactory treatment and no cure.

PARENTHOOD

Once married, most couples consider the desirability of when and why they should become parents. Some enter this period of life unprepared and by accident, whereas others become parents by choice and have a willingness to learn. Although a few have a wisdom beyond their years, most people have had little education for parenthood. The parental urge is felt by some to be second only to the sexual urge in promoting matrimony.

Dating, courtship, working with the problems of young people's interpersonal relationships, and the challenge of adjustment to marriage are preliminary steps on the way to creating a new family. In almost all cultures known, no matter how primitive or advanced or varied, a family structure has existed as a common unit. Creation means exactly that—creating a new life through the union of two people in love. The first step toward parenthood is the unity of desire of both husband and wife sincerely to plan for and want a child. This grows out of mutual love for each other, which includes the satisfaction of the desires of the marriage partner.

In the early months or years of marriage it may be wise to postpone the first child because of educational requirements or economic or health reasons. The child is a dependent and a financial liability until he or she is able to become self-supporting. Medi-

cal and dental care are expensive as well as necessary, and sustaining a good school system is essential if our children are not to be placed at a disadvantage. These simple facts must be recognized, and couples must plan a family that will be appropriate with their ability to sustain it. Some believe now that countries must do likewise. The varied implications of planned parenthood will be discussed later in the chapter.

A child is born

Couples contemplating the creation of a new life must understand certain basic factors concerning the birth process. During sexual intercourse millions of sperm are deposited high in the female vagina close to the cervix, or lower end of the uterus. Although a female orgasm, similar to that which occurs in the male, is not necessary for fertilization to take place, it will facilitate fertilization. Such an orgasm for the female is felt, among other reactions, as pleasurable contractions of the cervix and lower muscular walls of the uterus. This serves to draw the sperm upward toward the fallopian tubes at a faster rate. The sperm, highly mobile now with tail whipping and the small head always oriented to the normal downward flow of the uterine currents, gradually work their way up to the oviducts, where they enter and continue their swim. Many, of course, travel to an oviduct where there is no egg; but if ovulation has recently occurred, at least half will be traveling to the oviduct where there is an egg.

One sperm eventually comes in contact with the ovum and through a chemical dissolution is able to invade the cell membrane. From the moment the head of the sperm is within the membrane, all other sperm, although attracted to the ovum, are unable to pass into it. The exact explanation here is not currently known. The invading sperm still must migrate to the center of the ovum where the male chromosomal material joins with the corresponding female material. Fertilization does not take place until the analogous chromosomes pair up; this joining of nuclear material forms the zygote, a single-celled, fertilized ovum, and marks the creation of a new life. Immediately after fertilization the single-celled zygote divides into two cells, then four, eight, sixteen, and so on. This small ball of cells, still no larger than the 1/100 inch in diameter of the original ovum, gradually moves down the oviduct, and in 3 to 5 days after fertilization it reaches the uterus. About this time it is a hollow sphere filled with fluid and enclosed by a single layer of many hundreds of cells. This stage in embryonic development is called the blastula, and the organism is referred to as an embryo.

During the embryo's journey to the uterus it receives a small amount of nutritive material through absorption from the immediate environment, but most of its food supply comes from the tremendous amount the ovum stored during its development. It is fortunate that the ovum becomes the largest of all body cells, because otherwise the embryo would never survive this period when a direct food supply is lacking. On reaching the uterus the embryo nestles against the inside upper lining in the thick, velvetlike, capillary network prepared during the earlier part of the menstrual cycle. This nestling is called implantation, a term and process not to be confused with fertilization. The embryo in a sense burrows into this lining as it secretes a substance that dissolves some of the endometrium and allows the embryo to move below the immediate surface. At the same time, uterine cells in the immediate region are stimulated to growth and division, and they actually surround the embryo.

Menstruation can no longer occur if the embryo is to develop. Suppression of menstruation is caused by implantation. From the tissue surrounding the embryo a new hormone is produced that stimulates the anterior pituitary to produce increased quantities of luteinizing hormone. Increasing luteinizing hormone in turn increases the quantity of progesterone from the corpus luteum, which does not dry up as in a normal nonfertilized cycle but grows larger. Nature's interest now is to preserve and increase the capillary network in the uterus, and so the need for maintaining progesterone. The corpus luteum and increased progesterone level are maintained for about 7 months.

Division within the embryo continues. At a point on the inside surface a second layer of cells appear, and as these divide, the hollow area within the sphere is gradually filled. Only these few rapidly dividing cells are destined to become the new human being. The other cells, also through division, form into two protective surrounding membranes called the chorion and the amnion and two other membranes called the yolk sac and the allantois. In reptiles and birds these last two are more directly functional, but in man they fold together along with the infolding of the amnion to form the umbilical cord. This cord contains large blood vessels, which serve to carry food to the embryo from the uterus and waste materials to the uterus from the embryo.

The outermost membrane is the chorion, which is the most responsible for the formation of the placenta. Small fingerlike growths on the chorion project into the maternal blood supply and branch into hundreds of smaller fingerlike projections. The uterine blood supply thus is brought to extremely close association with the chorion. The mother's circulatory system transports nutritive material and oxygen to this complex region of chorion membrane projection, now called the placenta, into the uterus. Food and oxygen pass from the mother's blood supply across the chorion, then across the allantois, and through the umbilical vein they are transported to the embryo. Waste materials leave the embryo via the umbilical artery and move across these same two membranes to the mother. The two blood supplies are quite distinct. Materials move by dialysis (diffusion through a membrane) from areas of greater concentration to areas of lesser concentration.

The limits of this text do not allow for an extensive discussion of embryology. In outline form, however, there follow a few of the developmental stages that the embryo

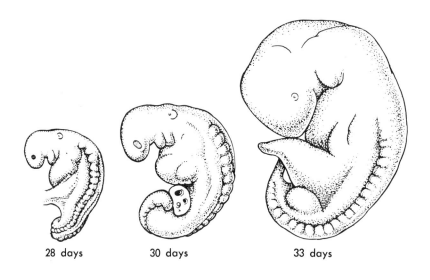

28 days   30 days   33 days

TEN TIMES ACTUAL SIZE

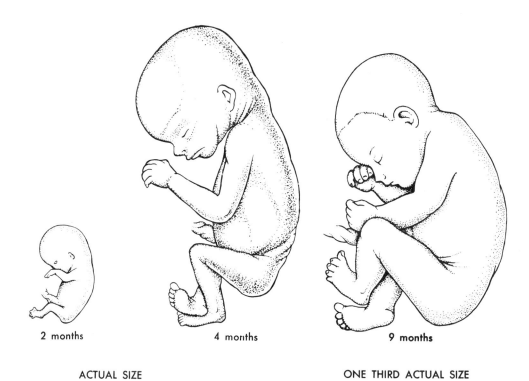

2 months   4 months   9 months

ACTUAL SIZE   ONE THIRD ACTUAL SIZE

Fig. 9-6. Development of the human embryo. (Adapted from Iorio, J.: Principles of obstetrics and gynecology for nurses, ed. 2, St. Louis, 1971, The C. V. Mosby Co.)

attains at 1 month, 3 months, and 6 months of growth within the uterus. Such information represents only approximations both of time and development (see also Fig. 9-6).

I. One month growth in uterus
  A. Form and size
    1. One-fourth inch long and can be identified as a vertebrate
    2. Head and tail evident, but no facial features as yet
    3. Large, beating heart
    4. Four small bulges present, which will later become arms and legs
  B. Nervous system
    1. Group of cells appear on outermost layer of embryo, called neural plate
    2. Neural plate folds on itself to form tube running length of embryo
    3. Brain begins to form at one end of neural tube
  C. Digestive system
    1. Primitive canal present in two sections, foregut and hindgut
    2. Inpocketing appears at head end and tail end

II. Three months growth in uterus
  A. Form and size
    1. Three inches long and weighs about one ounce
    2. Can now be identified as a human and thus is now called a fetus instead of an embryo
    3. Sex differentiation appears
    4. Arms, legs, hands, and feet are evident
    5. Ears present
    6. Small buds that will later become the deciduous (baby) teeth are present
  B. Nervous system
    1. Hindbrain and midbrain quite prominent
    2. Forebrain, where the human capacity for higher thinking takes place, still small and undeveloped
  C. Digestive system
    1. Continuous alimentary canal formed
    2. Stomach commences early functioning, such as the secretion of mucous
    3. Liver begins production of bile and manufacture of red blood cells (This largest of all internal organs will soon take on more than 100 different functions. It is probably the most important single body organ, if such a distinction can be made.)

III. Six months growth in uterus
  A. Form and size
    1. Ten to twelve inches long and weighs about two pounds
    2. Body has soft covering of hair
    3. Eyebrows and eyelashes appear
    4. Skin appears red and wrinkled
    5. Fingernails and toenails present
    6. Skin structure will be formed including nerve endings and the sweat and sebaceous glands
    7. Baby opens its eyes in uterus
    8. Fetal heart beats strong and loud
  B. Other features
    1. Mother experiences some movement as fetus's muscular, skeletal, and nervous systems continue development
    2. Kidneys, which go through three distinct developmental stages, are complete in human form and functioning
    3. Head is still proportionally large, as are heart and liver
    4. Convolutions appear on cerebral hemispheres as forebrain commences its most rapid growth

The human fetus will average 280 days in the uterus from the start of the last menstrual flow prior to fertilization until birth. This is known as the period of gestaton. During this time the most normal position for growth is with the head down, although this position is not necessary for normal growth and delivery. Its movements within the uterus as time passes become more and more violent. At birth the average baby is 20 inches long; the average male baby weighs 7 to 7½ pounds and the average female baby 6½ to 7 pounds.

Family planning

By family planning, we refer to the voluntary control not only of the number of children but also of the spacing of children. Despite disagreements as to what methods of fertility control are regarded as socially acceptable by different cultures, in most of them the principle of family planning is not controversial. Accordingly, with advances in the methods to control fertility, many men and women can exercise greater autonomy with respect to the crucial issues of childbearing and family formation.

The bearing and rearing of offspring fulfill some of the deepest human needs, but the psychic cost from unwanted pregnancies to parents who lack any choice about child spacing and family size is phenomenal. The problem may be expressed in many ways, ranging, for instance, from reinforcement of prior psychopathology, impaired parental competence, to general family destruction. Unwanted pregnancies are a major cause of marriage maladjustment and tension and account for an estimated million or more illegal abortions each year in America.

The quality of early parental nurture is a vitally important determinant of healthy or disturbed childhood development and is itself greatly influenced by the degree to which a pregnancy is desired or unwanted by the mother, since it is she who bears the child and is primarily responsible for its early care. The development of effective contraceptive methods is making it increasingly feasible, at least technically, for individuals to control reproduction.

We have discussed several of the most common forms of contraception in Chapter

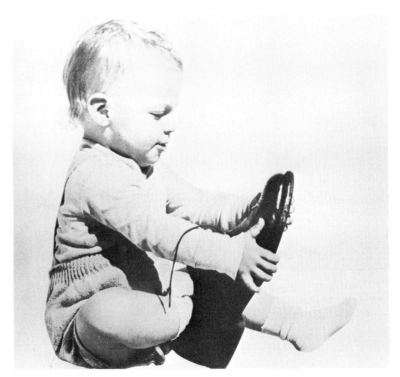

Fig. 9-7. The population problems of our globe today make family planning a dire responsibility of each young married couple. Parents, and those soon to be, must listen to the muted appeal of the next and subsequent generations.

8. At this point, more permanent forms of birth control—sterilization and legal abortion—are of importance.

Sterilization. This is the process by which one is rendered incapable of producing fertile sperm or ova. Sterilization is usually achieved by surgical closure of a pair of small tubes in either the man or woman so that the ovum and sperm cannot meet.

These methods of sterilization do not involve the removal of any gland or organ and should not have any negative effect on the individual's sex life.

The vasectomy is a simple operation that can be performed in a physician's office. A small section is clipped out of each vas deferens and the ends tied with a fine silk suture so that no more sperm pass through.

The statutes in Massachusetts, New Jersey, and Pennsylvania do not indicate legal circumstances for abortion. However, case law in Massachusetts[1] and New Jersey[2] has sanctioned abortion in certain instances.

Statutory Provisions: By States

To Save Woman's Life: Every state except Massachusetts[1], New Jersey[2], and Pennsylvania.

To Preserve Woman's Physical or Mental Health: Alabama, Arkansas, California, Colorado, Delaware, District of Columbia, Georgia, Kansas[3], Maryland, New Mexico, North Carolina, and Oregon[4]. (Washington[5]).

If There Is Indication of Fetal Malformation: Arkansas, Colorado, Delaware, Georgia, Kansas[3], Maryland, New Mexico, North Carolina, and Oregon.

In Case of Rape: Arkansas[6], California, Colorado, Delaware[6], Georgia, Kansas[3], Maryland[6], Mississippi, New Mexico, North Carolina[6], and Oregon[7].

In Case of Incest: Arkansas, California, Colorado, Delaware, Kansas[3], Maryland, New Mexico, North Carolina, and Oregon[7].

Restrictions:

Time Limit for Performing Abortion (From Time of Conception): California (20 weeks), Colorado (16 weeks in case of rape or incest), Delaware (20 weeks)[8],

Maryland (26 weeks)[8], and Oregon (150 days)[9].

Residency Requirements: Arkansas (4 months), Delaware (4 months)[10], Georgia (must be state resident), North Carolina (4 months), and Oregon (must be state resident).

Authority for Decision on Whether to Perform Abortion:

Therapeutic Abortion Board: California, Colorado, Delaware[11, 12], Georgia[11], Maryland[12], and New Mexico.

Consultation of Physicians: Arkansas, Delaware[11], Georgia[11], Kansas[3], Louisiana, Mississippi, North Carolina, Oregon and Wisconsin.

Hospital Policy: In the following states, permission of either the Therapeutic Abortion Board or Consultation is not required, but authority for decision rests with local hospital policy: Alabama, Alaska, Arizona, Connecticut, District of Columbia, Florida, Hawaii, Idaho, Illinois, Indiana, Iowa, Kentucky, Maine, Michigan, Minnesota, Missouri, Montana, Nebraska, Nevada, New Hampshire, New York, North Dakota, Ohio, Oklahoma, Rhode Island, South Carolina, South Dakota, Tennessee, Texas, Utah, Vermont, Virginia, Washington, West Virginia, Wyoming.

---

[1]Commonwealth v. Wheeler (1944): The court held that an assumed danger to physical or mental health would justify abortion. [2]State v. Siciliano (1956): The court held that abortion "is authorized when necessary for avoidance of death or permanent serious injury to the mother." [3]Effective July 1, 1970. [4]In determining whether there is risk to woman's physical or mental health, account may be taken of her total environment—actual or reasonably foreseeable. [5]Case law sanctions abortion to preserve woman's physical or mental health. [6]Forcible. [7]"Felonious intercourse." [8]Not applicable when woman's life is in danger or fetus is dead. [9]Not applicable when woman's life is in danger. [10]Not applicable if woman or husband work in Delaware, if woman has previously been a patient of a Delaware physician, or if woman's life is in danger. [11]Both Board review and Consultation required. [12]Hospital Review Authority.

Usually this process in no way affects the male's normal sexual activities. He is still capable of a normal orgasm, which ejaculates seminal fluid that is free of sperm. It is thought that this is the best method of birth control for men of families where no more children are wanted. One of the major advantages of the vasectomy over other measures is that it eliminates the problems connected with dates of periods, calendars, medical supplies, and remembering routines.

Tubular ligation consists of cutting the fallopian tubes and suturing the ends of the tubes. Once the fallopian tubes have been tied, sperm are prevented from reaching the ovum, and the ovum can no longer enter the uterus. The operation requires a short hospital stay and is frequently performed following the delivery of a baby.

Sterilization is often indicated when:

1. Parents choose to limit their family to the number of children they have. It is frequently difficult to get a doctor to perform surgery when there are not at least two children in the family.
2. There is a threat that a pregnancy will endanger the health or life of the wife or the baby.
3. There is the likelihood of transmitting a hereditary defect.
4. Physical, financial, or emotional factors reduce the possibility of fulfilling the responsibilities of parenthood.

Abortion. An abortion is the process of removing a growing embryo or fetus from the wall of the uterus. There are several medically accepted techniques in use throughout the country.

The most frequently performed type of abortion is dilation and curettage, or D and C. The opening of the lower portion of the uterus is dilated with a series of instruments in graduated sizes to allow the insertion of a curette, or scraping instrument, into the uterus. The contents are then scraped from the wall of the uterus. This procedure is carried out during the first 10 to 12 weeks of pregnancy. Another method for abortion in the early part of a pregnancy

is uterine aspiration. The cervix is dilated, and the uterus is cleaned by means of a vacuum suction machine. For very late pregnancies, a gestation period of up to 20 weeks, a caesarean is indicated. A somewhat newer method is referred to as "salting out." In this procedure, a hypodermic needle is inserted through the abdomen and uterine wall into the amniotic sac. The saline solution kills the embryo or fetus and induces labor.

During 1970 the New York Legislature amended that state's penal law to provide the most liberal abortion statute in the United States. A portion of the decree is as follows:

An abortion act is justifiable when committed upon a female with her consent by a duly licensed physician acting, (a) under a reasonable belief that such an act is necessary to preserve her life, or (b) within 24 weeks from the commencement of her pregnancy. . . .

This portion of the New York State statute becomes clear when seen in the light of the information given in the statutory provisions and restrictions cited in the summary of abortions noted above.

MATERNAL AND CHILD HEALTH

In guarding the unborn, advice is usually directed to the expectant mother, but it should also interest expectant fathers. Much remains to be learned about prevention of defects, but there is much the mother can do, particularly during the first few weeks to 3 months of the pregnancy, to help.

She should choose a good doctor, who is on a reputable hospital staff, as soon as she thinks she is pregnant, and she should follow his advice. She will need medical advice and supervision throughout the pregnancy, whether this is the first or fifth pregnancy. The earliest part of the pregnancy is most important for preventing defects.

If possible, she should plan to have her children before the age of 40, since significantly more birth defects occur as maternal age increases.

The pregnant woman should do everything she can to keep herself well and should avoid all contagious diseases. The most common of these contagious diseases presently known to affect the fetus is German measles (rubella). This disease was thought to be a minor mild disease of childhood, with sore throat, fever, swollen glands of the neck, and a mild rash, until in 1941 Dr. Norman M. Gregg, an Australian eye specialist, found a sudden increase in babies brought to him with cataracts, deafness, and other malformations. He learned that almost all the mothers had had German measles early in pregnancy. Further work has shown that 22% of babies whose mothers have had rubella in the second month of pregnancy will suffer defects, whereas 7% will have defects if rubella occurs in the third month. Babies carried while the disease affects the mother may continue to be actively infected and may infect others. Rubella seems to occur in 7-year cycles. As discussed in Chapter 7, a vaccine against rubella has recently been made available. Prospective mothers may be tested to see if they have had rubella by a simple, reliable test for antibodies. Gamma globulin has been given in the past in the hope of minimizing the effects of the disease, but its effect on protecting the fetus has not been proved.

The pregnant woman should avoid drugs —any medicines, even aspirin—unless they are prescribed by a physician who knows she is pregnant. The most crucial weeks of the baby's existence probably occur before the woman sees a doctor—in the first 2 to 5 weeks of pregnancy—so the responsibility for safeguarding the unborn infant in its most formative and sensitive stage is the mother's. In 1961 and 1962 thalidomide, a sedative so mild that it did not require a prescription, caused thousands of infants in Germany, Great Britian, and Australia to be born with limb defects. Many questions are raised about drugs and their use in pregnancy that cannot yet be answered, despite the fact that most drugs are checked very thoroughly on animals prior to their use on human beings.

Smoking and drinking both may affect the fetus. Cigarette-smoking mothers' babies are found to be smaller in weight and are more apt to be premature. A premature baby is one weighing less than 5½ pounds. Such babies require extra care and more frequent feedings. The temperature and humidity surrounding them require special control, and they have more medical problems than full-term, full-size infants. They are more susceptible to complications resulting from medication. Seventy percent of those weighing less than 3 pounds 5 ounces have been found by the American Medical Association to suffer from mental retardation, speech and hearing difficulties, spastic diplegia, or behavioral problems.

The pregnant woman should avoid x-rays, either for examination or treatment, during the first 3 months of pregnancy. From the second to the sixth week of pregnancy, she should particularly avoid x-rays of the abdomen or pelvic areas. In 1929 it was first noted that some women who had been exposed to x-rays in early pregnancy had brain-damaged babies at birth.

The doctor should manage the baby's birth. His first concern must be the safety of the baby's brain, so the woman should not insist on an excessive amount of pain-relieving drugs or medication that produce deep sleep during the delivery.

To determine the condition of the newborn baby, the Apgar test, devised by Dr. Virginia Apgar in 1953, is used. Close observations of the infant are made at several intervals during the first few minutes after its birth. Each observation consists of five steps:

1. The heart rate is checked either by feeling the heartbeat on the baby's chest or by a stethoscope. A rate of over one hundred gives a top score of two.
2. The respiratory rate is observed. A crying baby has a top score of two; slow or irregular breathing counts one.
3. The muscle tone is observed. Active motion gives a score of two; some flexion of extremities, a score of one; no action or flexion, zero.

4. Reflex irritability shows when the baby's soles are stroked or a catheter is put in its nose. A cry gives a score of two; a grimace, one.
5. The baby's color is best observed on the lips, palms, and soles of the feet. All pink gives a score of two; a pink body with blue extremities, a score of one.

Fifteen percent of all babies may score ten; a score of four calls for resuscitation efforts, although zero-rated babies have more than a 50% chance of survival. This test has been adopted in many countries.

The hazards of being born are real and can be serious. Learning about these hazards might be depressing or uncomfortable, but one can learn much from a study of these processes. The chances are markedly increased that a skilled physician will deliver the baby in good condition. Ninety-three percent of all babies are normal at birth,* so the odds are greatly in both the mother's and the baby's favor. Childbirth is a natural physiologic process, and mothers now get excellent care, as do their newborn babies.

Infant health

Infancy is generally thought of as the first year of a baby's life. The general trend of infant mortality has been progressively downward from 135 per 1,000 live births in 1900 to about 18 per 1,000 live births today. Care of the infant starts from the first minute of life, with the Apgar test.

Food

Of first importance to the infant, after the Apgar test has determined its normal condition, is food. No better food than a mother's milk from the breast has yet been devised; so breast feeding is usually best for the baby, both psychologically and physiologically, providing the mother is properly nourished and otherwise healthy, can provide enough milk, and is willing to nurse the baby. There are many substitutes for

*Beck, Joan: How to raise a brighter child, New York, 1967, Simon & Schuster, Inc.

breast milk, made of cow's milk, goat's milk, and others that have been scientifically altered to make them suit certain needs, but it is beyond the scope of this work to describe an infant's diet. Human milk contains less fat (about 3.3%) as compared with cow's milk (about 4%) or a goat's (about 4.5%); human milk is higher in carbohydrates and lower in proteins. In bottle feedings, great care is necessary in keeping bottles and equipment sterilized.

A pediatrician or a child health clinic should be consulted in problem-feeding cases, although in most instances a licensed doctor of medicine in general practice can provide adequate guides for proper infant feeding. Usually, foods high in vitamin content are first added to the diet, followed by cereals, eggs, and finally fruits, vegetables, and meats. Considerable argument has taken place over whether strained or pureed vegetables and scraped or pureed meats are necessary, but most physicians recommend pureed vegetables and meats. By one year of age, most children can take all the foods of an adequate diet. Besides food, the infant's physical needs are proper rest and cleanliness. Again, a physician or child health clinic should be consulted for detailed instructions.

Protection against infection

Cleanliness has been said to be next to godliness. The infant is likely to be healthier if given a daily bath, although many survive under filthy conditions. If the baby is breast fed, he will acquire some antibody protection from the mother's milk, which will help prevent some infections. Through immunization, diphtheria, whooping cough, tetanus, smallpox, and polio should be rare. Immunizations change as new discoveries make new immunization available. The family physician, pediatrician, or well-baby clinic should be consulted as to what immunizations are currently available and desirable.

The preschool child

The preschool child is one who is 1 to 6 years of age. From the age of 1 to 3 he tends to be an explorer as he begins to walk and to talk. Increased activities multiply his opportunities for accidents and exposure to contagious diseases. Upper respiratory infections are not uncommon in this age group, and people with a cold should avoid contacts with young children. Continued medical and dental supervision by a physician and dentist or through public health clinics are desirable. This will enable the parent to know whether the child's health needs, as regards proper foods, are being met and whether any abnormality is developing that needs attention. A visit to both a physician and dentist or public health clinic every 6 months will give a fairly adequate check on the physical health and development of the child.

Children should have the opportunity to develop in a mental, emotional, and spiritual atmosphere that will give them a happy, loving childhood and lead to responsible citizenship. Child health centers are now available in most areas to make such advice and supervision available to even the most needy. The preschool child needs attention given to sleep, play, and exercise while he is guided into good habits of cleanliness and elimination.

FAMILY INTEGRATION

The raising of a happy family is vital to the individual and to the nation. The social well-being of both the individual in a family and the family as a group depends on many factors.

Security

One of the most important feelings in a family is that of security. An insecure family is a fearful family. We all must expect some trials and tribulations in life. It is necessary to teach children that although the family can provide some security, life will require that they themselves learn to solve the problems they will encounter. This type of security can be provided through personality development.

Throughout the ages philosophers have agreed that material things alone do not provide security. People must learn to de-

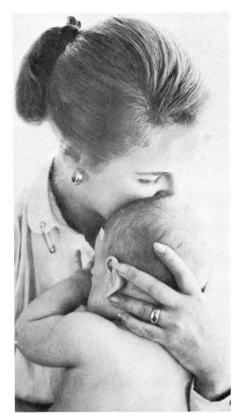

Fig. 9-8. The presence or absence of family security is perceived early in life by the developing child.

velop their personal resources mentally, socially, physically, and spiritually. Insecurity in childhood can provide a groundwork for emotional problems in adult life, whereas a sense of security at any age helps to reinforce emotional balance and the ability to adjust. One needs to balance the need for security with achieving worthwhile goals in life. The child needs to feel that he has understanding and loving parents to whom he can go with his problems and receive a sympathetic, fair hearing.

Economics

Although philosophers have pointed out for over 2,000 years that there is no security in material things alone, we all need adequate finances to carry on a normal life. This means that a family should not generally be started until it is able to manage financial obligations. To meet this requirement the so-called head of the family, which custom has regarded as the male, should have a good job so that he can offer his family the adequate financial resources to meet the family's needs. This is easily said but is difficult to do in today's society. Increasing numbers of married women are working to meet the rising cost of maintaining a family. Today, the child in a family is not only a dependent, as many have pointed out, but is also expensive.

It is wise for the family to work out a budget corresponding to its income. With wives working and supplying part of the income, they will and should have a greater share in deciding how money will be budgeted. No one can tell each family how their financial matters should be handled, but cooperation among all the members of the family is essential. Finances are further discussed in Chapters 11 and 12.

Cooperation

Making a successful marriage will require the greatest degree of cooperation that all members of a family can demonstrate. Various unforseeable, as well as forseeable, problems have to be solved by every new couple. If the problems can be discussed frankly and a successful solution found, the whole family will become closer as a result. The family council idea, in which problems are discussed with the children when they are old enough to participate, will teach cooperation. It is wise to start with simple problems and to make some fun out of the process. Understanding each other's feelings in these matters and avoiding meaningless arguments will eliminate possible tension. Everyone in a family should willingly and cheerfully do much more than his share to increase family cooperation.

House-home

Any new family will have to decide where they will live. There is no way this problem can be solved for a family other than on its own initiative. Most families will do well to have a house or apartment of their own, although sometimes a relative

may have to live with a family or the new couple may have to live with one of their families. This can be made comfortable if everyone does his best to make the situation work. Too often, one hears remarks that a home has become only a house, a place to eat and sleep, with few other activities involving the total family. Parents will have to work out between them how much and what activities should be provided to make a house a home for the whole family.

Family dining

Dining should not only be a time for meals together but should be an energizer for family enthusiasm and a time for sharing. Conversation in which everyone can be included can do much to make family meals a joyous occasion. A family should have regular hours when all members gather at the table for meals. Parents can add much to their family's solidarity by regular meals held at regular hours. Hurried snacks may be taken at school or work at noon, but a good morning breakfast and a regular evening meal together will add much joy to both parents and children, giving them a feeling of togetherness. Most families will not only partake of food together but will want to thank whatever God they believe in for the many blessings of life and food.

Religion

We all believe in something: ourselves, a spirit, a God, or a power greater than our own that exists in the world, call it what we may. No culture has ever been found in which this was not true, and contemporary time is no exception.

Parents who agree on religious principles and teach them to their children have much stronger families and family ties than those who do not agree with each other on these matters. Couples who have the same religious belief and customs can more easily cooperate, not only in their wish to have a blessing before each family meal, but in being able to agree more easily on what kind of religious instruction they wish to give their children in the home and have them get at their church, synagogue, temple, or wherever their religion may require them to meet. Religion is an active, vital force in any family's structure and a necessary force if our world is to become better. Some kind of religious instruction is essential to a maturing family if it is to succeed. Each person is involved in his family and his faith, and his well-being depends on them. If the whole of man is spiritually the master over hatred, fear, anxiety, resentment, and guilt, he will give his family an example that generates a closer and stronger family.

Recreation

We all need recreation at times, to get away from the daily grind, from the fears that daily beset us. We need fellowship with other people. We usually think of recreation as doing something for fun, something we enjoy. The family needs to plan recreation together as much as each individual may find recreation in a class at school, Boy or Girl Scouts, or other social groups. Some activities we can immediately recognize as constructive in nature, that is, as giving a feeling of relief and pleasure, whereas others we recognize as destructive and erosive to the family. No specific guidelines can be given for any family's recreation except to say that it should be an essential part of family life.

Allowances

Young people today soon find they need some money for school lunches and for various recreational purposes. The needs of the infant and young child are looked after by the parents, but monetary allowances should be an early part of a child's life. As children grow older, they need to feel an increasing responsibility for providing some of their own spending money through their own efforts, to help them learn and practice a certain independence. What one works out for an allowance will be influenced by the family's economic status. Other factors will cause great variations, with some young people being forced at an early age to be-

come responsible for themselves and others being protected and provided for all their lives.

Work demands

Work demands should not be tied to a child's allowances. The tasks that need to be done each day as part of daily living should be assigned to children because these tasks have to be done, and children need to be taught they can and must contribute their part. The jobs well done should carry praise; those poorly done or undone should carry a penalty. The penalty should be made to fit the child. For instance, if Johnny is a miser, he may profit by having to pay cash for his carelessness. It is not easy to find jobs for high school and other youth, but daily responsibilities should be assigned about the home and should be done well and promptly.

FAMILY DISINTEGRATION

Family disintegration includes any sort of inharmonious functioning of the family. It may include not only problems between wife and husband but also those between children and parents, other family members, and in-laws. Family disintegration is a varied and complex process. If husbands and wives are unwilling to sacrifice part of their egoistic desires in order to achieve a more effective marital relation, the marriages will likely fail. So long as husbands and wives insist upon viewing their marriage problems outside the context of the other person's involvement, there can be no reasonable chance of integrating their purposes into a marriage that might yield more socially significant values.

Much of the breakdown in family life is objectively evidenced in current problems of separation, desertion, and divorce, as well as in the more subtle phases of domestic discord. One must recognize that many of these disintegrating factors may be ascribed to the complications of change and disruption in today's world. Out of the stress of familial change and the revolt against a vigorous monogamy, two schools of thought on the family exist. One school holds that the traditional norms of the family must be maintained or restored. The other school points the finger of scorn at attempts to maintain a tradition that is all but dead. More and more it appears that people are not certain that they want to face up to the responsibilities of a good marriage. Otto, in his treatment of monogamy, comments:

> There is no question that sex-role and parental role rigidities are in the process of diminishing, and new dimensions of flexibility are making their appearance in marriage and the family.*

Personality clashes

It is indeed impossible to find a family whose members have not experienced problems because of personality differences. Even in the most successful marriages there are irritating personality mannerisms and habits by each of which the other was not aware during courtship and at the time of marriage. If these differences can be accepted without any major adjustment of personal values, in the temper of tolerant give and take, they may present no serious trouble.

According to generalized patterns of personality response, the husband is inclined to be frank, direct, and impulsive and will often be frustrated by the evasive, indirect, and passively resistant behavior of his wife. If, however, the wife insists upon dominating every decision, aways leading the conversation, treating her husband like a servant in the midst of guests, he may acquiesce under such duress; but sooner or later he will give vent to his dislike for such conduct— perhaps explosively.

Many a marriage is dissolved because of incompatibility. Incompatibility may be expressed in many superficial terms, but in the final analysis most couples are incompatible because of unresolved personality differences. No man or woman is truly an island

unto himself or herself. A successful marriage is predicated upon the ability to resolve personality differences and to avoid the irreversible results of serious clashes.

Financial factors

Financial problems may be caused by overextension of budgets, sheer poverty, or business reverses. Despite the romantic model of love, which suffers all, even lack of finances, there is meaningful evidence that long-continued worry and concern over fiscal matters is not conducive to family integration. The varying spending habits of a couple in relation to their financial resources is a common problem. Debt limits in relation to family income are too often exceeded—as, for example, the couple who has monthly debts totalling $800 on a take-home family income of $600.

For all American families the median family income (purchasing power) rose from about $6,000 in 1960 to over $8,000 in 1970. During the 1970's income will be higher for nonfarm families than for those families living on farms, and it will be higher for white than for nonwhite families. The 1970's will show a significant increase in family income, both in dollars earned and in purchasing power, and will also show, hopefully, a reduction in family poverty.

Despite the increase in income and the reduction of poverty, families will continue to be faced with the problems of inflation and recessionary trends. The typical American family will always be faced with the debt-limit problems discussed above.

The desire for affluence has prompted more wives to work. Approximately 50% of all American women work in any single month. About 60% of these women are married and living with their husbands, and almost all contribute to family income. It is frequently the wife's income that raises the family income above poverty levels. The likelihood of a family's escaping poverty is greater if the wife is an earner. Nearly 5 million families have incomes of less than $3,000 each year. Only 5% of all families with working wives fall into this category.

---

*Otto, Herbert A.: Has monogamy failed? Saturday Review, April 25, 1970, p. 23. Copyright 1970 Saturday Review, Inc.

In order to stem the tide of family disintegration caused by financial problems, it is essential to study all the factors that contribute to these problems. The lack of income is a real issue for poverty-stricken families, but in any family many factors must be considered. Much tension may arise because of the wife's working, but it will be minor if the couple has common goals and handles the budget together. Several problems may grow out of the family's economic situation. There may be an unexpected loss of job or a reduction in income. The mate's job may involve a great deal of traveling. The family may adopt measures for financial retrenchment until such time as more income is available; those involved may use personal or other resources to tide them over; they may take steps to find other satisfactory jobs, or if the latter is not acceptable, they may adapt themselves to the reality of the limitations and work out plausible compromises within these limitations.

The hostile, immature, or generally unhappy person confronted by financial problems is indeed hard pressed to devise a workable solution or adjustment to the situation. If that person's mate is immature or overdemanding as well, the differing feelings will serve to exaggerate the negative aspects of the marriage and build irreversible discord.

Parent-child conflicts

It is not easy to be a parent today. The alleged generation gap between parents and children is unprecedented; those over 30 are just out of a youth's set. The power of the peer group, so it is said, is phenomenal. Children now have their own culture, with its own norms, language, dress, and mores. The only real competitor with the child's peer group is the more global aspects of a technologic culture, communicated through the powerful agencies of advertising, the schools, radio, and television. No well-meaning parents should fail to recognize their competition.

Reflect upon relations with your parents when you were very young, and compare your experiences with those of the little boys and girls of today. In these reflections and in your tendency to identify yourselves with them, you might discover the alienation all can feel, both old and young. The young are often used to represent despair, violence, or in many cases the hopes for a better world. All of these tell us something about the young; they tell us even more about parenthood since these are the parents' projections and fantasies of childhood.

The demands of children upon parents are unending. Children demand not only the material necessities of life, but also the love, concern, and companionship that far too few parents are willing to give. Far too many parents are so wrapped up in making a living that little continued attention is given to the social and emotional well-being of their children. Every day some "good" parent is shocked to learn that a son or daughter is a drug addict, pregnant, or has caused a pregnancy, or has in some way "embarrassed" the family. These events establish cause for the famous response, "How could he? I did all any parent could do." Space does not allow the exploration of other examples of conflicts. The tone of the examples given should suffice to illustrate the need for parents to study and respond to the needs of their children in order to reduce the possibilities for family disintegration.

PART IV

The PPBS of personal health

The principal objective of PPBS is to improve the basis for major program decisions. Program objectives are identified and alternative methods of meeting those objectives are subjected to systematic analysis comparing costs and benefits. Cost and benefit data reflect future as well as current implications of program decisions. The budget is the financial expression of the underlying program plan and translates program decisions into appropriation requests.*

PPBS is a new but popular system. Large and small units in government, industry, education, and public and private institutions are adopting and adapting aspects of this most recent management technique for the purpose of improving the decision-making process. A new jargon has been spawned: accountability, objective, evaluation, and cost-benefit are only four from a long list of terms that now accompany any conversation about a planning-programming-budgeting system.

Few will deny the importance of PPBS to large organizations. Even these institutions, however, are having difficulty in applying its theory to operational, everyday activities. It is because of this difficulty that PPBS has not been more universally

accepted. But the system will gain wider acceptance in the immediate years ahead as organizations learn how to apply it to their own individual needs.

There is a lesson in the spread of PPBS that we should grasp and apply at the personal health level. The living, breathing system we each know as "me" is the functioning consequence of millions of stimulus-response activities. To maintain equilibrium at a desired level of productivity is no small challenge even when our environment is immediately and sufficiently responsive to our needs—a condition seldom achieved in real life. Unfortunately, we have inherited a health care system that is sometimes inefficient and insufficient, expensive and variable, inaccessible and mysterious. Many people, when they seek a solution to a personal or family health problem, find the system too complex or expensive for them to deal with. Defensively, they draw back, adjust to their physical, social, emotional, or mental disability, and continue on.

*From the report of the Subcommittee on Economy in Government of the Joint Economic Committee of the United States Congress: The Planning-Programming-Budgeting System: progress and potentials, December 1967.

261

We assume that you are not a passive, unquestioning person, but that you are active, inquiring, and perceptive. As complex as the system is (and it does need improvement), you are capable of understanding it, of analyzing it, and of seeking and receiving whatever medical assistance you need.

But you do need to understand the system and to incorporate the necessary health costs into your total budget. All the activities in which you engage are in competition for your available financial resources. How you apportion these resources will depend on the values you hold and your knowledge of the alternatives. Chapter 10 is an overview of the health care system in the United States today; it is concerned with the planning and programming of your personal health care. Chapter 11 is organized to assist you in coping financially with this system, that is, in the budgeting for your personal health care.

There is meaning in PPBS for individuals as well as organizations. (There is hardly any man-conceived organization more complex than man himself.) We wish you well as you utilize its relevant aspects in the maintenance and improvement of your personal health status.

CHAPTER 10

Health resources in the modern community

As we begin this discussion of health resources in the modern community, consider the following selected facts. In 1969:

1. More than 47 billion dollars was spent on health.
2. Hospitals admitted nearly 31 million patients.
3. An average of nearly 1,300,000 persons were inpatients each day in hospitals.
4. More than 3,900,000 persons were employed in the health field.
5. About 375 primary and secondary health occupations, requiring special education or training, had been described.

These facts make clear that: (1) health care is a major aspect of our total economy, and (2) it constitutes a major problem. It is also obviously complex both to those who function within it (an unfortunate word coinage describes those in this category as the purveyors of health services) but even more so to those who must function through it (the consumers of health services, who of course are not mutually exclusive from the purveyors).

In order to plan a program one must first be able to identify its constituents. By *programming* we mean the organization or structure of the health care system. What are its parts? What kinds of services are received where? By *planning* we mean the coordination of these services into a single functioning system. What mechanisms relate one component, such as hospitals, to another, such as nursing homes or private physicians' offices? What checks are there

to prevent overlap and duplication of services? Do we successfully anticipate professional gaps and fill these before the shortages become acute?

Figures 10-1, 10-2, and 10-3 present in blueprint manner the levels of health organization. You might examine these now, and then return to them as you cover the material that follows. We do not intend to be all-inclusive but rather to cover the major aspects of health programming and planning. Occasional referral back to these diagrams will aid in your understanding.

Both programming and planning of health services are complex. We have made and continue to make many mistakes. For example, the current physician shortage apparently will be met only by changing our traditional image of professional preparation and competencies needed for the tasks prescribed. To help bring about such changes, each person needs some knowledge of the system. So, like Alice in Wonderland, as she gazed into the mirror ("Why, it's turning into a sort of mist now, I declare! It'll be easy enough to get through . . ."), we shall try to make this complex system understandable and traversable.

THE HEALTH SERVICE DELIVERY SYSTEM

In simplified form, there are six types of subsystems in the overall health service delivery system. Although these tend to be intertwined in many ways, they nonetheless are distinct enough to be presented separately.

First, there is the direct, private office

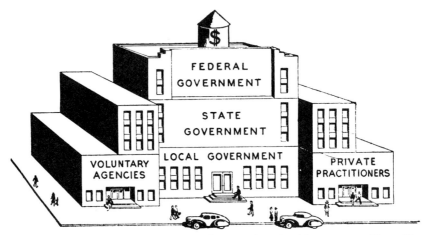

Fig. 10-1. Levels of health organization. The complete health structure. (From Mountin, J. W., and Flook, E.: Guide to health organization in the United States, Public Health Service Publication No. 196, Washington, D. C., 1953, U. S. Government Printing Office.)

practice of the qualified health professionals. This category includes physicians of all types, dentists, clinical psychologists, and many others. A patient either makes personal contact for an appointment or, depending on the nature of the medical problem, is referred by another health professional. This also includes small clinics and physician-controlled group practices where specialists work in proximity to take advantage of laboratories, x-ray equipment, and joint consultation when desirable. This subsystem also includes home visits by private professionals. These, however, are discouraged by the professionals and tend to be decreasing.

The second subsystem is that of group health care. By virtue of employment or membership rights, many people have access to medical and other health services in facilities organized, financed, and managed by factories, stores, business or government agencies, schools, labor unions, and the like.

The third is the very large subsystem of hospitals. We include within this, besides inpatient care, all the services conducted by hospitals, such as outpatient clinics and emergency services. We also include organizations of a similar but not the same nature, such as nursing home care and related

homes and other facilities for several distinctly different groups: the deaf or the blind, unwed mothers, the physically handicapped, the mentally retarded, and halfway homes for alcoholics and drug addicts.

Another subsystem is public health. Personnel functioning in this system do not "practice" in the sense that a private physician does. They detect but rarely treat, refer but generally do not diagnose; they immunize and inspect to reduce and prevent epidemics; they educate to improve the patient's understanding of himself and his family; they make home visits to check on suspected health problems; and they inspect work sites for health and safety hazards. In recent times public health officials have been in the forefront of organized health planning efforts (p. 271).

The fifth subsystem is composed of the vast network of voluntary health agencies. Although direct health services by those in this category are minimal, their impact on the total system is nonetheless impressive.

Sixth, but quite important, is the subsystem represented by the pharmacist and others who sell materials and appliances required by and usually purchased directly by the consumer. Our culture places varying degrees of responsibility on the pharma-

VOLUNTARY
AGENCIES

OFFICIAL AGENCIES

PRIVATE
PRACTITIONERS

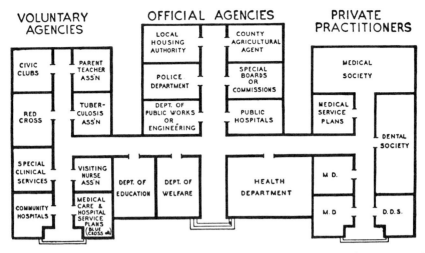

Fig. 10-2. Levels of health organization. The ground floor of the health structure—local official and voluntary agencies and private practitioners. (From Mountin, J. W., and Flook, E.: Guide to health organization in the United States, Public Health Service Publication No. 196, Washington, D. C., 1953, U. S. Government Printing Office.)

VOLUNTARY
AGENCIES

OFFICIAL AGENCIES

PROFESSIONAL
SOCIETIES

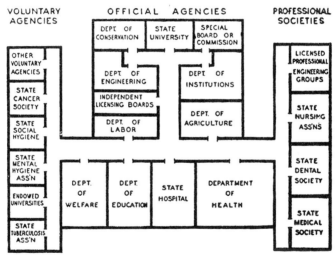

Fig. 10-3. Levels of health organization. The second floor of the health structure—state, official, and voluntary agencies and professional societies. (From Mountin, J. W., and Flook, E.: Guide to health organization in the United States, Public Health Service Publication No. 196, Washington, D. C., 1953, U. S. Government Printing Office.)

cist, as do the health professionals who refer prescriptive needs to him. In many communities he performs in nearly a medical sense; in others he is careful to refer persons to their family physician for the desired advice. The extent of his privilege is legally limited, but he often goes beyond this.

DIRECT PERSONAL HEALTH SERVICES

Many persons with varying skills deliver health services to other persons in a face-to-face relationship. Physicians, by virtue of their number, qualifications, and prestige, do this more regularly than any other professional category. For this reason we will focus on the physician in this section.

Table 10-1. Type of practice and category of physician: 1969

Category	Total active	Number of physicians (M.D.)				Number of D.O.'s in private practice
			Patient care			
			Hospital-based practice			
		Office-based practice	Training programs	Full-time physician staff	Other professional activity	
All specialties	302,966	188,166	51,816	30,755	32,229	11,381
General practice	80,894	56,562	11,740	5,616	6,976	8,651
Medical specialty	71,886	42,449	12,825	7,318	9,294	354
Surgical specialty	93,346	63,878	17,326	7,544	4,598	841
Psychiatry and neurology	25,076	11,975	4,427	4,820	3,854	31
Other specialty*	31,764	13,302	5,498	5,457	7,507	190

Data from Health resources statistics, Washington, D. C., 1970, National Center for Health Statistics.

*Includes aviation medicine, general preventive medicine, occupational medicine, pathology, physical medicine and rehabilitation, public health, and radiology.

Number and type of physicians

The science and art of dealing with the prevention, cure, and alleviation of disease is the province of both doctors of medicine and doctors of osteopathy. In 1969 there were 324,942 physicians holding the degree of Doctor of Medicine (M.D.) and 14,000 with the degree of Doctor of Osteopathy (D.O.). Both kinds of physicians diagnose diseases, treat people who are ill, and in most states, use surgery, drugs, and all other accepted methods of medical care.

The number of physicians providing patient care in single, partnership, group, or other office-based practice per 100,000 population has remained consistent at 100 over the past few years. The ratio of the total number of physicians providing patient care per 100,000 population has increased slightly in recent years to a level of about 148 in 1969.

Specialties outnumber general practitioners about three to one among the active physicians. Medical practice is classified both by physician category and by type of practice. Table 10-1 summarizes these data. A further discussion of specialties within categories, licensure, and other considerations is included in Chapter 11.

The upswing in physician prestige

Through the centuries physicians have been held in varying degrees of repute, mostly poor, as they struggled to expand their knowledge and develop techniques. One writer, L. J. Henderson, has described the physician's grasp of his subject in a manner that falls well short of unqualified confidence: "It was not until about the year 1910 or 1912 in the United States that a random patient with a random disease consulting a doctor chosen at random stood better than a 50-50 chance of benefiting from the encounter."

Through the late years of the nineteenth century and during the early part of the twentieth, the medical profession strove mightily to expand its own scientific and technical know-how; to establish licensing laws for the practice of medicine; to offset, in professional, ethical ways, the malpractice of charlatans, quacks, and the patent medicine industry; and slowly to build a solid image of competence and accomplishment. Gradually the authority sought, with its resulting prestige, was gained.

Specialty fragmentation

As seen in Table 10-1 and again on pp. 292-294, specialties in medicine are the rule today. This was not always so. In earlier times when medical knowledge was limited, the physician could learn most of what he needed during his training period. During his practice he could stay abreast of the stuttering advances by reading the few medical journals available and observing more recently trained physicians with whom he occasionally came in contact. His skill, as good as it could be, did not extend much beyond the black bag he carried everywhere. But the general practitioner gave the medical profession prestige. His humanitarian concerns and selflessness gained the confidence of the lay public to a degree never granted folk practitioners.

Nonetheless, even as the family physician practiced his skills, the development of medical science led to the training of specialized men who seized fragments of his domain. Folk practitioners had earlier travelled a similar developmental path, as reflected in the specialties of bone setters, blood stoppers, baruchers, wart doctors, and others. But the difference soon came to lie in the refinement of knowledge and technique underlying medical specialization and its growth within the control of a single profession.

Specialization, however, created logistic limitations. The radiologist could not carry the "tools of his trade" in the time-honored black bag. No single physician could support a multipurpose diagnostic laboratory. Whereas solo practice once was the rule, physicians now often find it in their own and in the public's interest to join with other physician and professional categories in various symbiotic relationships. With your budget as its focus, group medical practice is discussed on p. 287. It would be well to read that section now before proceeding in this chapter.

The quality of care

However physicians organize themselves, whether in solo practice with referral or in one of several forms of group practice, the choice to utilize their services still remains with the patient. Because the freedom of

choice is there, it is relevant that you should ask where you may receive the best quality of personal medical care. Unfortunately, there is little data to answer this question, but there are some clues.

For example, it is clear that the solo practitioner who fails to avail himself of modern diagnostic and therapeutic facilities cannot, unaided, practice the best possible medicine. Also, when a physician practices in isolation from others of his profession, it is difficult for him to stay abreast of advances in scientific and medical knowledge. Although his technical journals are better and more numerous than they once were, doctors today cannot rely on this medium alone to remain informed. The medical society, organized and strong in nearly every county in the United States, provides both a formal and informal network of practitioners that enhances the professional interaction so vital for an improving quality of care.

Solo practice permits simplified communications between patient and physician and has the fastest "response time" to patient needs and wants. The solo practitioner, however, has sometimes gravitated into relative isolation, losing currency in scientific aspects of the practice of medicine. Group practices, with new physicians added every few years, are somewhat protected against this danger.

When you enter the health care system in search of a personal physician you should consider the pros and cons discussed here. We sometimes view specialization as more costly than beneficial, but this attitude is shortsighted. Group practice (described by Hunt and Goldstein as "a formal association of three or more physicians providing services in more than one medical field or specialty . . ."*) has some of the advantages of solo practice and offsets some of its disadvantages. If you do select a solo prac-

*Hunt, G. H., and Goldstein, M. S.: Medical group practice in the United States, Public Health Service Publication No. 17, Washington, D. C., 1951, U. S. Government Printing Office.

titioner, and many are quite competent, do not be shy to assess his qualifications and currency of information. You would do no less in selecting a mechanic for your car.

GROUP HEALTH CARE

Large numbers of salaried people benefit from comprehensive prepaid group practice by virtue of their employment, residence, university setting, or other circumstance. The striking feature of this subsystem is the full smorgasbord of medical resources in combination with an economic arrangement, which makes continual access to these services possible.

In this pattern of medical care the responsibility in preventing and taking care of illness at an early stage is in large measure shifted from the patient to the doctor. Since a fixed annual premium is paid regardless of the individual's rate of illness, the physician has a built-in incentive toward prevention. Liaison among the doctors in the group is fortified by a relationship with patients that is independent of economic considerations. Medical care is potentially continuous rather than episodic, comprehensive rather than segmental.

There are more than 200 comprehensive prepaid group health care plans in the United States. The best known are the Kaiser-Permanente Health Plan and the Health Insurance Plan of Greater New York. The following data on the Kaiser Plan indicates the nature and extent of these group plans.

The Kaiser-Permanente Health Plan is a complex of six major corporate entities and four large medical groups serving 1,507,000 persons (in 1967) in California, Oregon, and Hawaii. It has attracted nationwide attention because it combines the principles of group medical practice and direct service prepayment with the insurance principles of group enrollment. A comprehensive array of necessary medical care services is offered through a single plan.

The Kaiser Plan's first two decades of operation (1945-1965) have seen a transition and a clarification in the purposes for which the plan exists. Initially the Kaiser Plan was distinctly an instrument of the Kaiser Industries; that is, it served as a tool through which the Kaiser Industries could influence their costs of production and gain a degree of competitive advantage, as well as bring about a useful adjunct in employee and community relations. As the plan grew, however, the health objective of employees became more important than its industrial applications to Kaiser Industries. In the past decade the Kaiser Foundation Health Plan has been less oriented to the needs of the parent corporation and more responsive to the membership from which it derives its financial support. As a consequence of this transition to the point where the employee is now the major beneficiary, the Kaiser Plan serves as a model to other less well-established plans in the country.

Table 10-2 summarizes the extent of enrollment by the Kaiser Foundation Health Plan in southern California. This plan serves a diverse population of workers and their families. Benefits are nearly all-inclusive: all services of physicians as requested, including operations, anesthesia, consultation with and treatment by specialists; 125 days of prescribed necessary hospital care each year and an additional 240 days at one-half the prevailing charges; all necessary house calls by physicians employed under the Plan; all prescribed x-ray and laboratory tests and services; full obstetric care; and prescribed physical therapy. Many other services are made available to subscribers at minimal charge.

Two issues, quality of care and utilization of services, are often debated when group health care programs are discussed. Critics claim that quality goes down and utilization goes up, whereas proponents argue the opposite. With regard to quality, the Kaiser Plan employs three techniques to maintain high standards: choice of personnel (a never ending nationwide effort to recruit the best), continued education of physicians (free exchange among colleagues is encouraged and peer review is purposely built in), and internal audit on hospital cases

Table 10-2. Kaiser Foundation Health Plan enrollment, southern California region, by benefit code, March 1965

Benefit code	Subscribers	Total members
XZ (Retail Clerks)	19,042	50,898
WW (Culinary Unions)	12,776	31,997
DD (Longshoremen)	4,456	13,504
FF (Federal Emp.)	22,613	69,941
GG (Federal Retirees)	854	2,168
K (Kaiser Steel)	7,600	27,202
KK (Health Plan Emp.)	3,552	9,657
AA (Group Plan)	45,405	139,084
BB (Group Plan)	15,909	44,644
BC & AC (Group Plan)	16,857	42,459
SS (Supplemental Coverage)	782	2,852
HH (Small Group and Misc.)	3,702	7,158
HH (Conversion)	17,535	38,114
LL (Indiv. or Family Direct Enrollment)	13,170	27,202
Totals	184,253	506,880

From Roemer, M. I., DuBois, D. M., and Rich, S. W.: Health insurance plans: studies in organizational diversity, Los Angeles, 1970, School of Public Health, University of California.

(making it difficult for a doctor or a patient to use hospital space for other than significant medical reasons). Utilization seems no greater and probably is less than average, according to a study by Perrott.* He showed that in admissions and in days of hospital confinement, the Kaiser Health Plan has much lower than average utilization. He points out that if Kaiser patients received the level of hospital service ordered by private physicians, the plan in 1966 would have had to build an additional 500 hospital beds at an average expense of $28,000 per bed, requiring a capital investment of $14,000,000. The operation of those beds would have cost an additional $12,000,000 per year, requiring at least a 20% increase in membership dues.

Prepaid group health care is an important subsystem that seems destined to become more significant in the immediate years ahead. In summary, prepaid group health care (1) makes health professionals assume the risk and expense of illness; thus it may tend to promote individualized preventive medicine; and (2) it is not available to non-

*Perrott, G. S.: Utilization of hospital services, J. Public Health **56:** 57-64, January 1966.

salaried, self-employed, or unemployed persons.

HOSPITALS

The record of hospital development in the early days of our country is sketchy. Apparently, first efforts for the care of the sick were incidental to shelter for the poor and unfortunate through almshouses. The first of these was founded in Philadelphia by William Penn in 1713. The famous Charity Hospital in New Orleans, established in 1737, was originally both a hospital and an asylum for the indigent. The first known hospital in the United States, built solely for the physically and mentally ill, without regard to economic status, race, or creed, was the Pennsylvania Hospital established in 1751. Other early hospitals grew out of a need to provide a place for clinical practice for medical schools in Massachusetts, Connecticut, and New York. These early hospitals were of voluntary sponsorship: public and church-affiliated hospitals developed much later.

Table 10-3 summarizes the growth in both hospitals and number of beds available during the twentieth century. The number of hospitals increased significantly up to

Table 10-3. Number of hospitals and beds, 1873-1967

Year	Hospitals	Beds
1873	178*	unknown
1909	4,359	421,000
1914	5,047	532,400
1928	6,852	893,000
1938	6,166	1,161,380
1963	8,000 (approx.)	1,500,000 (approx.)
1967	8,147	1,631,101
1969	7,845	1,565,908

Data from Health resources statistics, Washington, D. C., 1970, National Center for Health Statistics.
*A crude and inaccurate estimate based on U. S. Bureau of Education data.

1967; but there was an even sharper increase in the number of beds up to 1967 because of the enlargement and upgrading of existing facilities taking place in the previous 20 years under the stimulus of the Hill-Burton Hospital and Medical Facilities Program. Since 1967 a number of hospitals have closed, and the number of total beds has decreased.

For classification purposes hospitals are described as short-term (average patient stay less than 30 days) and long-term (average stay more than 30 days). The 7,845 hospitals in 1969 included 6,715 short-term and 1,130 long-term hospitals. Nearly all short-term hospitals are general hospitals; that is, they provide diagnostic and treatment services for patients who have a variety of medical conditions, both surgical and nonsurgical. About 5% of short-term hospitals offer specialty services only: pediatric hospitals, maternity hospitals, and hospitals specializing in eye, nose, and throat disorders. In long-term hospitals, psychiatric patients occupy 83% of the 576,175 beds; another 7% are occupied by geriatric patients and patients with chronic diseases; and the remaining 10% are devoted to patients with tuberculosis and other patients requiring hospital services.

The number of personnel involved in hospital settings is large. In 1969 approximately 2,800,000 persons were employed in hospitals; nearly 80% of these were full-

time employees. In the same year nearly 32.1 million patients were admitted to hospitals, and the average daily bed occupancy rate was approximately 1,270,000. In addition, many thousands of doctors, volunteers, visitors, and other categories of persons regularly participate in the ongoing activities of hospitals.

Outpatient care

The emerging philosophy of comprehensive care, the real change in morbidity statistics, the concerted efforts to reduce inpatient hospital utilization, and the extension of health insurance (Chapter 11) to cover medical costs outside the hospital have allowed many hospitals to expand the scope of existing outpatient departments. As these services have expanded to include a wide range of diagnostic and therapeutic services to ambulatory patients, outpatient clinics, however sponsored and wherever located, have become established in the network of relationships with other hospitals and community agencies.

Today they serve well over 100 million persons a year. With inpatient costs steadily climbing, there is no doubt that outpatient clinic utilization will continue to increase in the immediate years ahead.

Emergency care

Where would you turn if you suddenly became ill or were injured in a strange city? Would you go to the emergency unit of the local hospital? Perhaps, but could you be assured of the care you felt your due? Would you pay the bill for services received?

The emergency unit of any hospital is a crucial part of the total hospital's operation. Although we seldom consider its qualities, when we do require emergency care we want it to be available and good. Usually the service in an emergency unit is immediate and skillful; sometimes it is not. You can help to improve the quality of emergency hospital care through the following:

1. Use emergency hospital facilities only for emergency reasons. One survey

showed that only 50% of the patients entering the emergency room were classified as emergency or urgent, that 31% were nonurgent, 15% were scheduled visits, and 4% were unclassified.

2. Be sure that your emergency care bills are paid promptly.

3. Voice your praise and constructive criticism of the emergency units in your community to the respective hospital boards, the medical and nursing professions, and the news media.

Nursing homes

Nursing homes are a recent development on the health scene. Prior to 1930 the elderly sick either stayed in long-term wings of local or state hospitals or were placed in public almshouses. Passage of the Social Security Act in 1935, however, made Federal funds available to the needy aged, and the number of proprietary boarding and nursing homes for elderly persons began to flourish. In recent years the growing number of elderly persons, changes in the pattern of illness resulting from advances in medicine, and changes in family living arrangements have resulted in a growing demand for the provision of limited medical and nursing care outside of hospitals. In 1967 there were 584,052 nursing home patients. In 1969 there were 894,490 patients, which reflects the rapid increase in this type of facility. The total number of beds in nursing homes must increase in the immediate years to meet the developing demand.

The Medicare and Medicaid parts (Public Law 89-97, Titles XVIII and XIX, respectively) of the Social Security Amendments of 1965 supplied the much needed financial support to encourage expansion of nursing home facilities. Both Medicare and Medicaid are discussed in Chapter 11.

Related inpatient facilities

Mention must be made of those facilities that accommodate persons not necessarily ill or aged but are classified as "other inpatient health facilities" by the Master Facility Census. Included in this classification are the following:

1. Homes for the blind and deaf
2. Homes for unwed mothers
3. Orphanages
4. Homes for dependent children
5. Homes or schools for the physically handicapped
6. Facilities for the mentally retarded
7. Homes for the emotionally disturbed

Approximately 366,384 individuals reside in 3,817 of these facilities.

PUBLIC HEALTH

Both the purpose and limitations of our present discussion do not permit even a cursory discussion of historic events and persons that influenced the development of public health in America. As with other aspects of life, much of what we did in public health as far back as 200 years ago was influenced by our European heritage. The inhumane and unhealthy conditions of that earlier time caused many responsible people to champion for better things. An excellent review of this period has been written by Hanlon, and more detailed information has been provided by Rosen, Winslow, Richardson, Holmes, and Shattuck.* We also call to your attention the health activities carried on at the international and Federal levels that have an influence on our current health status. The World Health Organization and the many agencies that conduct health programs both

---

*Hanlon, J. J.: Principles of public health administration, ed. 5, St. Louis, 1969, The C. V. Mosby Co.; Rosen, G.: A history of public health, New York, 1958, M. D. Publications, Inc.; Winslow, C. E. A.: The evolution and significance of the modern public health campaign, New Haven, 1923, Yale University Press; Richardson, B. W.: The health of nations: a review of the works of Edwin Chadwick, vol. II, London, 1887, Longmans, Green, and Co.; Holmes, O. W.: Writings IX, medical essays, Boston, 1891, Houghton Mifflin Co.; Shattuck, L., and others: Report of the sanitary commission of Massachusetts: 1850, Cambridge, 1948, Harvard University Press.

nationally and regionally are indispensable.* You may wish to locate the three references cited for further information. Since health activities at these levels are not of a direct personal nature, however, we will not discuss them in detail here.

Public health is preventive medicine, which is primarily carried on in a face-to-face relationship. When anyone has reason to seek a public health service, he will seldom travel to Washington, D. C., or even to the state health department usually located in the state capital, but will turn to his local health department. Depending on its location, this may be a neighborhood public health clinic (now found in most densely populated urban areas), the city health department (as for example the Portland, Oregon, City Health Department), or a joint city-county public health facility (as found in the Weld County Health Department, which serves that county and its largest city, Greeley, Colorado).

Most counties and large cities in the United States today are serviced by a local health department. In sparsely populated areas a single health department office may serve two or more counties covering a large geographic area but relatively few people, such as the health department office in Clinton, Tennessee, which serves approximately 125,000 people in Anderson, Morgan, and Roane counties. In densely populated areas a single health department may require subunits and even sub-subunits in order to reach the total population. An example here is our largest, the New York City Health Department with 5 boroughs, 22 district health centers, and several neighborhood health clinics within each of these

districts to accomplish the necessary face-to-face delivery of service. The local telephone book is a good place to start (usually listed as Health Department under your city or county government offices) when seeking information or assistance on a health matter.

Responsibilities and functions of local health departments

In 1963 the American Public Health Association (A.P.H.A.) issued a policy statement indicating that the fundamental responsibilities of a local health department are: (1) to determine the health status and health needs of the people within its jurisdiction, (2) to determine the extent to which these needs are being met by effective measures currently available, and (3) to take steps to see that the unmet needs are satisfied.* This statement also places emphasis on social planning, particularly in the areas of medical care, regional planning of health resources, effective use of natural resources, and efficient delivery of traditional services. The emphasis on planning seen in the position taken by the A.P.H.A. in 1963 served as a stimulus to subsequent health planning programs of the late 1960's and now in the 1970's.

The functions of a local health department described by the A.P.H.A. in 1950 continue to be valid today, with the caution that health department personnel remain alert to new program thrusts. The following, therefore, are the traditional functions of a local health department.

I. Recording and analysis of health data
   A. Recording and analysis of reports of births, deaths, marriages, divorces, and notifiable diseases
   B. Maintenance of registers of individuals known to have certain specific long-term diseases and impairments
   C. Conduct of special surveys to determine the prevalence and resultant disability from various diseases

---

*The World Health Organization, Geneva, 1967, Division of Information, World Health Organization; American Association for World Health: American review of world health **14**(3), New York, 1966, The Association; Mountin, J. W., and Flook, E.: Guide to health organization in the United States, Washington, D. C., 1953, Public Health Service Publication No. 196 (with updating in Hanlon, J. J. [see previous Hanlon reference], pp. 226-231).

---

*The local health department—services and responsibilities, an official statement of the American Public Health Association, adopted November 10, 1963.

D. Collection and interpretation of morbidity data from such sources as clinics, hospitals, organized nursing services, prepayment plans, industry, and workmen's compensation and disability insurance programs

E. Maintenance of continuing records on the number and qualifications of all types of health personnel, the quantitative and qualitative resources of available facilities, and the types and extent of health services provided through various voluntary and public programs

F. Periodic evaluation of community health needs and services

II. Health education and information

A. Stimulation of the public to recognize health problems that exist, to study the resources available for meeting the problems, and to develop and put into action programs designed to solve them

B. Cooperation with and assistance of official and voluntary organizations such as departments of education and civic, youth, and other community groups in the development of their health programs.

C. Provision of individual instruction by public health nurses and other personnel, as in the case of families in which communicable disease has occurred, of mothers attending well-baby conferences, or of diabetic and other patients who are taught to follow the regimen prescribed by the family physician.

D. Organization of lectures, classes, and courses, such as mothers' and fathers' classes, courses for food handlers, classes for diabetics, and lectures to community groups

E. Use of mass educational and informational media such as newspapers, magazines, pamphlets, movies, radio, and television

F. Development of a well-rounded program of professional education, designed to assist the local health professions to maintain and improve the quality of service

III. Supervision and regulation

A. Protection of food and water and milk supplies

B. Control of nuisances, sanitary disposal of wastes, and control of water and air pollution

C. Prevention of occupational diseases and accidents

D. Control of human and animal sources of infection

E. Regulation of housing

F. Inspection of hospitals, nursing homes, and other health facilities by means of

1. Public education and individual instruction
2. Issuance of regulations
3. Laboratory control
4. Inspection and licensure
5. Revocation of permits and, as a last resort, court action

IV. Provision of environmental health services (as necessary)

A. Construction of pit privies

B. Drainage, and larvicidal treatment of mosquito-breeding areas, residual spraying of homes for insect control

C. Rat proofing of buildings, and other insect and rodent control measures

V. Administration of personal health services

A. Immunization against infectious diseases and other preventive measures such as the application of fluoride to children's teeth

B. Advisory health maintenance service, as in child health conferences, prenatal clinics, parents' classes, and public health nursing visits

C. Case-finding surveys of the general population, such as chest x-ray surveys, serological tests for syphilis, cancer detection programs, and school health examination. Adult health inventories and "multiphasic" surveys for the detection of various groups of diseases may also be included

D. Provision of diagnostic aids to the physicians, such as laboratory services and crippled children's, cancer, cardiac, and other diagnostic and consultation clinics

E. Provision of diagnostic and treatment services for specific diseases such as syphilis, tuberculosis, dental defects in children and expectant mothers, and orthopedic, cardiac, and other crippling impairments in children

VI. Operation of health facilities

A. Operation of health centers and clinics

B. Operation of general or special hospitals (as necessary)

VII. Coordination of activities and resources

A. Provision of effective leadership in meeting community health needs

B. Encouragement of coordination of various official and voluntary agencies to avoid duplication and overlapping and to assure efficient and economical administration

C. Participation on interdepartmental or regional boards dealing with public water supplies, sewage, and refuse disposal, control of atmospheric pollution, housing, city planning, hospital planning, zoning regulation, development of recreational areas and other public programs which

Table 10-4. Percent of total man-hours divided by a typical department to various health programs

	Percent		Percent
Home nursing service	3.24	Mental health*	6.23
Homemaker-home health aide	.79	Occupational health	.41
Cancer control*	1.10	Narcotic addiction control*	.21
Heart disease control*	.89	Air pollution control*	1.48
Diabetes control*	1.11	Eating and drinking inspections	9.76
Other adult health services*	2.52	Milk control, all phases	4.04
Crippled children	2.89	All other food safety	2.40
Child health	13.81	Housing hygiene	.89
School-age child health	9.24	Radiation control*	.30
Maternal health	8.26	Refuse and solid waste	1.58
Family planning*	2.29	School and public building inspection	1.09
Tuberculosis	5.33	Sewage	1.60
Venereal disease	6.16	Swimming places	.21
Accident control*	.59	Vector control	3.21
Alcoholism control*	.38	Water systems	.83
Dental health*	6.24	Barber and beauty shop inspections	.36
Enteric disease control	.37		
		Total	100%

From Palumbo, D. J., and others: A systems analysis of local public health departments, Amer. J. Public Health **59**:678, April 1969.
*These are innovative programs as defined by the researchers.

have significant implications for community health.*

Analysis of current programs at the local level

We expect that you are interested in more than official policy, however. What are local health departments doing today? What are their programs, and how much emphasis do they give to each?

A pilot study of a national sample of 14 local public health departments (drawn from a list of the 114 largest in the country) has been made to determine the proportion of men, money, and materials spent on each program.† Key personnel in each of the 14 departments were interviewed and a profile of 33 different ongoing programs was developed. Not all 14 departments were conducting all 33 programs, but

*The local health department—services and responsibilities, an official statement of the American Public Health Association, adopted November 1, 1950.

†Palumbo, D. J., and others: A systems analysis of local public health departments, Amer. J. Public Health **59**:673-679, April 1969.

the composite reflected, in the authors' minds, how the typical local health department in the United States today allocates its resources. Table 10-4 shows the distribution of man-hours among these 33 programs in the typical department.

An interesting dimension of this study is an analysis of what the researchers describe as innovative programs. These are shown in Table 10-4. Innovation is defined as more than doing what is considered to be new programs; it also means doing old things in new ways. For example, an innovation might be characterized by the time a department spends trying to organize community resources, especially through getting people in the community involved in health programs. The twelve starred programs in Table 10-4 total 23.34% of the total man-hours of effort by the typical department.

Family planning clinics. A striking example of a rapidly expanding innovative program is that of family planning. One local health department (not included in the study cited) has described the extent and purpose of its Family Planning Clinic as follows:

Our clinic currently serves more than 1300 women five days a week from 8:00 A.M. until 4:00 P.M. Our consulting doctors are available Tuesdays and Thursdays.

Any patient is accepted on a referral basis from her private physician (non-private mothers delivering locally receive information about the clinic and are eligible to attend).

Each woman is counseled individually concerning birth control methods and provided the necessary contraceptives. Should she miss a clinic appointment a public health nurse contacts the woman to determine any problem which might make it difficult for her to attend, such as lack of transportation. The continued interest of the district public health nurse in addition to that of the clinic personnel greatly strengthens the program.*

Automated multiphasic health testing. A further example of innovation that moves beyond even those cited by Palumbo and his associates (Table 10-4) is that of automated multiphasic health testing. Multiphasic screening is an extension of the mass screening technique and was first proposed around 1947. It is a means of administering more than one test to a large number of persons and reporting the results back efficiently and accurately. Although many experts have endorsed multiphasic screening during the past two decades, it has not spread as expected. However, new expectations are currently being raised with the prospect of automating the data. Automation, it is argued, will relieve many physicians of routine examination procedures, provide more examination in less time for less money than previously possible, and reduce the cost of a complete health and medical examination.

We argue the case for a periodic medical examination (Chapter 11), yet as medicine is now organized we hope that everyone never suddenly decides to be examined at the same time. If they did, every practicing physician in the country would have to perform 3 examinations a day, 5 days a week, year-round to cover the population. When would they have time for the many other aspects of medicine? Obviously, something has to give, and it is argued that we should sacrifice the benefits of preventive medicine to meet the more pressing problems of acute health needs. Automated multiphasic health testing might permit us to have the best of both preventive and curative medicine, but an important point must be kept in mind if and when it becomes more prevalent than it is today. Both the periodic health examination as performed by special medical groups and the periodic automated multiphasic health testing procedures conducted outside the personal physician's office are screening examinations. Diagnosis, interpretation, and follow-up still remain the responsibility of the personal physician.

What tests are included in multiphasic screening? Over forty programs were reviewed, and the following elements were included in one or more of these programs.

General questionnaire for family history and past medical history
Chest x-ray and pulmonary function tests
Anthropometric measurements
Hearing test
Hematologic test
Cardiovascular examination
Visual acuity and tonometry test
Cancer detection (including Papanicolaou smear, breast examination, and thermography)
Oral and dental examination
Serologic test
Blood chemistry (approximately 30 different blood chemical analyses can now be performed by an AutoAnalyzer)
Stool examination for occult blood
Urinalysis
Other examinations (x-ray of abdomen, Achilles heel reflex test, pain response, proctosigmoidoscopy, gastrointestinal x-ray series, gallbladder x-ray, rectal examination, and pelvic examination)*

No one program includes all of these, and it is not necessary that any should. Multiphasic screening tends to be age specific; certain tests are indicated for one age group or persons in a particular geographic loca-

*A report to the people, Knoxville, Tenn., 1970, Knox County Health Department.

*Gelman, A. C.: Automated multiphasic health testing, Public Health Rep. **85:**361-373, April 1970.

tion, and other tests are indicated in differing situations.

On the question of cost, the Kaiser-Permanente Health Plan, discussed earlier, provides us with some insight.* A study of multiphasic screening under that plan showed a per unit cost, including data processing, to be $21.32 per patient with a work load of 2,000 patients per month. For 1,000 patients the estimated cost is $40 to $50 per examination. If the load were raised to 3,000, the estimated cost could be reduced to $15 to $17 per patient. These figures, even the larger ones, are far less than what a private physician would have to charge for a similar workup. Automated multiphasic health testing will become widespread in the future. Perhaps many local health departments will soon implement a few components and then add to these as they are able.

We said earlier that public health is preventive medicine. Family planning and automated multiphasic health testing provide us with only two examples of innovative programs being conducted by local public health departments today that are designed to preserve and enhance health. There are many others.

State health departments

For the purpose of showing relationships, brief mention should be made of state-level health department activities. Although all 50 states have state health departments, the primary purpose of these is to stimulate and assist local health departments to perform their tasks well. Five common units of state health departments encompass most of their activities: administration, preventive medicine, environmental health, local health services, and laboratories.

An official statement by the American Public Health Association lists the following general functions of a state health department.

1. To represent the public health interests and goals of the state to the elected governing body of the state
2. To promulgate and enforce public health rules and regulations applicable throughout the state
3. To determine state public health policy and to provide a state-wide coordinated public health program with clear objectives for the guidance of local health departments
4. To promote the establishment of full-time local health units
5. To develop an appropriate plan for the coordination of local health services with related hospital and medical programs which may be developed on a regional basis
6. To provide financial assistance to supplement the resources of local health departments
7. To make consultation and other special services available
8. To assist localities to set up demonstrations on a temporary basis
9. To establish minimum and stipulate optimum standards of performance
10. To develop a recruitment and training program for local health department personnel
11. To delegate certain legal responsibilities of the state health agency, insofar as feasible and practical, to well-organized and adequately staffed local health departments
12. To carry on all relationships with local citizens and groups through the medium of or in cooperation with the local health department
13. To carry on a state-wide program of health education
14. To evaluate continually or periodically existing state and local programs*

The service function of the state health department to local health departments is clear. Other obvious categories of program activity are statewide planning, state and Federal relations, interstate agency relations, and certain statewide regulatory functions.

Although one agency in each state is charged with primary responsibility for the public health program in that state, one study made by the Public Health Service in 1950 showed that more than 60 different

*Collen, J. F., and others: Cost analysis of a multiphasic screening program, New Eng. J. Med. **280**:1043-1045, May 8, 1969.

*The state public health agency, an official statement of the American Public Health Association, Amer. J. Public Health **55**:2011, December 1965.

types of state agencies contributed in some way to state health programs.* Fig. 10-3 is a diagram of a very few of these; it also indicates the cooperative influence of other state-level organizations—the medical, dental, and nursing societies; voluntary organizations; state universities; licensing boards; and so on.

VOLUNTARY HEALTH ORGANIZATIONS

Voluntary health organizations are supported by private funds and are directed by persons employed by each autonomous board. They have flourished because of their appeal to altruism.

Voluntary health organizations originated with the Anti-Tuberculosis Society of Philadelphia, established in 1892. In the decade that followed, more than 20 other local tuberculosis groups were formed, and in 1904, 23 of these bodies joined to form the National Association for the Study and Prevention of Tuberculosis. From this meager beginning the National Tuberculosis Association, or N.T.A. (now officially the National Tuberculosis and Respiratory Diseases Association), grew rapidly.

At the dawn of the twentieth century in this country, social unrest was widespread. The labor movement under the leadership of Samuel Gompers was gaining strength in the face of the advancing industrial revolution. The medical profession, as seen earlier in this chapter, was finally beginning to rise above the hocus pocus and patent medicine era of the nineteenth century. Tuberculosis caused one in every ten deaths, and many concerned people saw no organized effort to combat it unless they joined together in a voluntary effort. To eliminate tuberculosis substantially was viewed as a government responsibility, but the need to alert the public and educate it as to the extent of the problem was seen as a voluntary responsibility. Continuing with this interpretation,

the national association grew to include 50 separate state associations and approximately 3,000 local affiliates. Gompers was one of the original six lay members of the National Tuberculosis Association's board.

Since support for voluntary health organizations is derived from donations, a fund-raising campaign is necessary. Again the N.T.A. pioneered in this. Tuberculosis Christmas Seals were first used in Denmark and proved effective because they gave all people an opportunity to contribute to the cause. By 1914 most of N.T.A.'s funds were obtained from the single mailing at Christmas time. Today its continuing appeal is reflected in the 35 to 40 million dollars raised this way across the country each year.

As the N.T.A. demonstrated success other groups were quick to follow. Today we are inundated with over 100,000 organizations at national, state, and local levels that include health in their appeal for funds. The American Association of Fund-Raising Counsel estimated that in 1964-65 voluntary fund raising for health exceeded 1.4 billion dollars. More than 500,000 persons contribute time and money to serve on the boards of these organizations, and more than 2 million others assist in the fund-rising activities. The number who give money in response to the many appeals is, of course, in the millions.

The need for standardization was soon apparent. In 1918 the National Information Bureau developed the following guidelines for organizations desiring approval by that agency. These continue to serve effectively today:

1. Board—an active and responsible governing body (must maintain direction of the agency), serving without compensation, holding regular meetings, and with effective administrative control.
2. Purpose—a legitimate purpose with no avoidable duplication of the work of other sound organizations.
3. Program—reasonable efficiency in program management, and reasonable adequacy of resources, both material and personnel.
4. Cooperation—evidence of consultation and cooperation with established agencies in the same or related fields.

---

*Distribution of health services in the structure of state government, 1950, Washington, D. C., 1952, Public Health Service Publication, No. 184, Part 1.

5. Ethical promotion—ethical methods of publicity, promotion, and solicitation of funds.
6. Fund-raising practice—in fund raising:
   a. No payment of commissions for fund-raising
   b. No mailing of unordered tickets or merchandise with a request for money in return
   c. No general telephone solicitation of the public
7. Audit—annual audit, prepared by an independent certified public accountant or trust company, showing all income and disbursements in reasonable detail. New organizations should provide a certified public accountant's statement that a proper financial system has been installed.
8. Budget—detailed annual budget, translating program plans into financial terms.*

As the number of voluntary health agencies has proliferated, they have divided into several discretely different groups. The first and largest includes those organizations supported directly by citizen contributions and donations. These may be further categorized by type as follows:

1. Agencies concerned with specific diseases, such as the American Cancer Society, the National Foundation (formerly for Infantile Paralysis), the American Social Hygiene Association, and the American Diabetic Association
2. Agencies concerned with certain organs or structures of the body, such as The National Society for the Prevention of Blindness, the American Society for the Hard of Hearing, the National Society for Crippled Children, and the American Heart Association
3. Agencies concerned with the health and welfare of special groups, such as the American Association for Maternal and Infant Health
4. Agencies concerned with specific aspects of health and welfare, such as the National Safety Council and the

*Lear, J.: The business of giving, Saturday Review, December 2, 1961. Copyright 1961 Saturday Review, Inc.

Planned Parenthood Federation of America

A second group of voluntary health agencies consists of private foundations, such as the Rockefeller Foundation, the W. K. Kellogg Foundation, the Commonwealth Fund, the Milbank Memorial Fund, the Rosenwald Fund, and the Markle Foundation. From 1920 to 1950 these groups supported many new local health departments and a wide variety of child health study projects. More recently they have been active in their support of national study projects, such as the W. K. Kellogg support of the National Commission on Community Health Services, Inc., from 1962 to 1966.

A third group of voluntary health agencies is comprised of professional organizations, such as the American Public Health Association, the American College Health Association, the American Medical Association, and the National League for Nursing. These organizations have been especially influential in raising the standards of professional health workers and in providing a forum, through publications and meetings, for the exchange of ideas.

Health councils and community chests comprise a fourth group of health agencies. The primary example at the national level is the National Health Council. Formed in 1921, the National Health Council today consists of more than 50 national voluntary health organizations and is influential as a coordinating body. It has played a key role in the development of a uniform budgeting process to which most responsible health agencies now adhere.

The fifth group, although not strictly voluntary in the sense previously used, nonetheless deserves mention. An increasing number of commercial organizations, usually with promotional and public relation interests as their incentive, have developed health programs that are significant. Insurance companies provide the best example. A number of these currently engage in health and safety projects that are extremely valuable at the local level. Several industries manufacturing products such as soap, milk, meat, and orange juice have demonstrated an interest in health that occasionally goes beyond the immediate sale of their products. Nonetheless, the profit motive influences in large part what these industries do in the interest of health, and their materials and programs must be examined closely in this light.

Functions

One study lists eight functions of voluntary health organizations:

1. Pioneer—uncovering new ways to meet existing health needs
2. Demonstrate—developing experimental programs to improve existing health practices
3. Educate—carrying the health message to all people by all means and mediums available
4. Augment official activities—directing or assisting in a program until public funds are available to take it over completely
5. Protect public interest—complimenting and criticizing public health programs and personnel when appropriate and necessary
6. Promote health legislation—organizing citizen support for crucial and timely health legislation
7. Plan and coordinate—bringing many health organizations, voluntary and official, together in the best public interest
8. Develop comprehensive health programs—combining all functions into a total community effort to enhance and upgrade health*

In whose interest?

There is considerable feeling among health professionals that the voluntary health organization has outlived its usefulness and that with society's greater complexity today new mechanisms are needed to meet the multitude of health needs. It is obvious that seldom does a volunteer group solve its original stated objective and then quietly close its doors. Instead, the chain of events described by Hochbaum usually takes place.

In a young organization, almost all its activities are geared to deal with the very objectives

and purposes for which it was created—nothing matters as much as its self-avowed mission. Later, however, increasingly strong concerns develop to maintain and strengthen the organization for its own sake, to expand its activities, to stake out a scope of goals and activities, and to protect this domain against intrusion by other agencies.*

A prime example of the shift described by Hochbaum is found in the National Foundation, Inc. This organization began in 1932 with President Roosevelt's Birthday Balls and was incorporated, with Basil O'Connor, Roosevelt's law partner, as its president, in 1938. Its express purpose was to conquer poliomyelitis, but its greatest appeal came in the direct patient service it rendered to all polio victims. In its peak fund-raising year, 1954, it collected more than 65 million dollars, and most Americans gave something—time, money, or both—to the annual March of Dimes campaign.

The Salk vaccine, field tested in 1954, subsequently approved, and distributed widely during the 1955-60 period virtually eliminated polio. Although at its peak, the disease caused over 50,000 deaths and more than 200,000 cases per year, today the disease is seldom seen. Such dramatic results from the vaccine might have prompted the National Foundation for Infantile Paralysis to close its doors after it had turned the care of its long-term patients over to local rehabilitation units. Instead, in 1958 the organization shortened its name to National Foundation and expanded its objectives to become "an organized force for medical research, patient care, and professional education, flexible enough to meet new health problems as they arise." Its emphasis today is on arthritis, birth defects, virus diseases, and disorders of the central nervous system, still including incidentally, poliomyelitis. An organization once created to overcome a highly specific health problem, and undoubtedly quite successful be-

---

*Gunn, S. M., and Platt, P. S.: Voluntary health agencies: an interpretive study, New York, 1945, The Ronald Press Co. Copyright 1945 The Ronald Press Co.

---

*Hochbaum, G. M.: Health agencies and the Tower of Babel, Public Health Rep. **80:**331, April 1965.

cause of that, thus became an organization of more general nature, and remained in business. Was this new program emphasis really in the best interest of the general public?

Voluntary health organizations are more flexible than their official counterparts. The story of the National Foundation is a case in point. Also, they are more free to experiment, and they serve to supplement and stimulate the activities of tax-supported agencies. On the other hand, they are less able than official agencies to undertake longer range and more broadly based direct service programs. Also, each agency is financially responsible only to its own board of directors; this fact has resulted in mismanagement of funds on occasion and quite often in a less than accurate reporting of administrative and fund-raising costs. It is this last concern that raises the question of cost-benefit, to which all organizations should be held accountable, but which the voluntary health agencies, by their very nature, may dodge.

For better or worse, however, voluntary health agencies will remain with us. They are and will continue to be an important part of the complex health system, but their multitude and diversity often causes unknowing persons to ignore them all. Yet responsible, effective voluntary health agencies have a place; you should give your time and money only to these and shun the others out of existence. We hope you will be discriminatingly generous.

THE PHARMACIST AND OTHERS

The fifth subsystem that in various ways affects your health status is that represented by the pharmacist and others of a direct service-dispensing nature. We include in this subsystem clinical laboratory services, dietetic and nutritional services, orthotic and prosthetic technology, pharmacies, physical therapy, specialized rehabilitation services, and vocational rehabilitation counseling. Some you will use on a regular, direct basis, others less regularly, and still others only indirectly. Nonetheless, this subsystem is important and is one in which you may spend considerable money.

SUMMARY OF HEALTH SYSTEM FUNCTIONS

From what we have said, certain obvious and other not so obvious functions of our health system deserve summary.

First, the system exists to cure the sick. Unfortunately, as a species we tend to be crisis oriented in most things we do, including our health care. The health system is primarily organized to accommodate this characteristic.

Second, the system exists to keep people well. Many believe that this aspect of our health system should and could be the most vital. To anticipate a health problem and take steps to reduce its effects or maybe to prevent it from ever occurring certainly makes sense. Education, of course, is the most basic tool here.

Third, the system exists as a sounding board for people to talk intimately with professional health personnel about matters that trouble them. Psychiatrists come to mind immediately, but all health professionals will serve on occasion as confidants for people in need. Talk is a safety valve that appears to be more important as society becomes more complex.

Fourth, the system exists to provide rationality where otherwise folk medicine, hearsay, and superstition would prevail. It provides people with scientific evidence so that they are able to make sensible decisions in health matters. Although we often do not succeed to the degree we would wish—witness the fluoridation battles—this function still exists, albeit less obviously.

Fifth, the system exists to preserve an efficient and effective labor force. America would be at a serious disadvantage, as would any other nation, among the nations of the world if her population were more sick than well. Documentation of this function is found in the recent campaigns to improve physical fitness, the wide attention given to our "deplorable" selective service health statistics, and perhaps most significant, the national health legislation that promises soon to cover every possible health problem from conception to the grave.

PLANNING—PANACEA OR DELUSION?

The problems of personal health can no longer be considered in isolation, if they ever could. Health problems are but part of the larger scene that includes problems related to transportation, agriculture, education, use of leisure time, housing, and many other dimensions. In short, we need to consider all components that are part of life as we know it if we are serious about improving the quality of life.

The greatest category of growth in recent years has been in our cities, and it is here where our most serious problems lie. Urbanization has become a pyramid of paradoxes: magnificent parks and polluted rivers, open spaces and high-rise ghettos, medical miracles and high infant mortality, ignorance and world-famous universities, economic power and psychologic incompetence. Owen's fable tells the story well.

There once was a nation of 200 million people that was the most powerful country in all the world. At the national level the inhabitants were very rich; but at the local level they often turned out to be quite poor. And as luck would have it, they all lived at the local level. Seventy percent of the people were crowded into one percent of the land, which they called cities. One-fifth of the city people were the victims of poverty. Many of them lived in slums where the housing was unfit for living, the schools unfit for learning, and the air unfit for breathing . . . But the cities continued to grow uglier and the frustrations greater . . . And there were riots in the streets . . . "If our Country is so rich, why are the cities so poor?" And to this day, no one has been able to answer that question.*

Only recently have we realized that we are in this mess because we have planned poorly or not at all in the past. We have gerrymandered our political units and tried to fit all aspects of life to these hodgepodge boundaries. For example, we have let time-

---

*Owen, W.: A fable, Washington, D. C., 1967, Urban America, Inc.

worn county lines, incorporation regulations, and the town meeting practices of yesterday, all of which once were meaningful, remain to plague us in a time when they no longer meet a need. We have recognized our developing problems and have turned to planning as the panacea that will solve all of them. But whether this panacea becomes a delusion depends on who the planners are, how they make the plans, and most important, on turning ideas into actions. These are discussed in more detail in the following sections.

From 1940 to 1960 more than 2,000 communities in the United States conducted self-studies to assess their health needs. Many of the recommendations made in these reports were implemented; but the large majority were ignored, and only a few communities met all the health needs they had identified. The dilemma of study without action caused many concerned health officials to ask why. What conditions prevail that prompt many communities to embark on self-study, to identify problems, to set priorities, and then to do nothing about them? Does our bureaucratic structure at local, state, and federal levels accommodate study but resist change? Is the American way of self-study, self-decision, and self-action no longer viable within the complex fabric of American life and democratic process? Can we plan effectively, that is, get results as a consequence of our effort? And perhaps most important, what is planning and who are the planners?

Seeking a solution

In 1962 the National Commission on Community Health Services, Inc. was established as a nonprofit, independently operated organization to collect and study facts about community health services, needs, and problems, and to promote the translation of resulting knowledge into effective community health services. It was cosponsored by the American Public Health Association and the National Health Council and was financed by the Kellogg Foundation, the U. S. Public Health Service, and the McGregor

Fund. It was organized in response to the demand of health leaders throughout the country who felt that something should be done to correct the growing disorganized state of community health services. The problems were crystallized in two general categories:

1. Inadequacies in meeting the community needs for a safe and sanitary environment as well as for meeting the the comprehensive personal health needs of the people living in those communities
2. Inadequacies in the ways and means by which communities attempted to organize and administer the services needed through the many government agencies and institutions

The leaders who recognized the seriousness of the problems concluded that the approach by the Commission could provide the nation with insight as to the principles, standards, and criteria that would enable communities to meet their health service needs for several decades to come.

The Commission approached its work through the organization and implementation of three major projects: (1) the National Task Forces Project, (2) the Community Action Studies Project, and (3) the Communications Project. The first project focused attention at the national level; the second focused attention at the community level; and the third project was concerned with promoting the translation of the resulting knowledge into effective community health services.

The philosophy underlying the Commission's efforts was stated in its terminal publication.

The nature of today's society and the complexities of health and other community services require a broad approach to planning and action which can be fitted to each particular community situation, yet is in harmony with broader trends and is capable of further development and change. The Commission believes that planning is an action process and is basic to development and maintenance of quality community health services. Action planning for health should be community wide in area, continuous in nature, com-

prehensive in scope, all-inclusive in design, coordinative in function, and adequately staffed.

The responsible participation and involvement of all sectors of the community, coordination of efforts, and development of cooperative working arrangements are fundamental to effective action planning. Health service objectives can be met through processes which provide opportunity for citizens to work together to understand, identify, and resolve problems, to set intermediate and long-range goals, and to act to achieve the goals.

The readiness and ability of communities to respond to health needs and problems are dependent, in large part, on the presence of effective mechanisms for planning.*

The Commission completed its task in late 1966 and, as such organizations rarely do, went out of business. Before doing so, however, it stated 14 positions and 98 recommendations that ushered in the new era of health planning. In summary, the Commission felt that every state should have a health policy and planning commission that is responsible to the governor and should maintain representatives of government, private, and voluntary groups. Regions based on what it called the "community of solution" idea should be the base of local administration, with both the providers and the consumers of health care participating in the development of the regional programs. It recommended that every community should have its health planning council and professional leadership, financed from a variety of sources, responsible for health services and facilities planning within the context of the region's total spectrum of health services, and coordinated with the planning of other community, regional, and state planning agencies.

Objectives of health planning

An official statement describing the objectives of careful health planning has been developed by the Program Area Committee on Medical Care Administration and Public Health Administration of the American Public Health Association. According

---

*National Commission on Community Health Services: Health is a community affair, Cambridge, 1966, Harvard University Press.

to this statement, health planning seeks to:

1. Improve organizational patterns for health services
2. Speed development of needed new health services, strengthen existing services, and improve utilizations
3. Discourage programs not needed in the community
4. Improve the quality of health care through better coordination
5. Eliminate duplication of health services among official and voluntary agencies at all levels
6. Reduce fragmentation of health services at the state and community levels
7. Help to achieve better geographical distribution of health services, with optimum utilization
8. Establish priorities among new health programs and services, develop better balance among health programs, and provide services more responsive to the special health needs of the area
9. Foster better use of scarce health manpower and more effective development of training resources
10. Identify health needs and problems and help to set realistic goals, keeping expected changes in the area's characteristics in mind
11. Spur faster application of new health knowledge
12. Encourage closer relationships among health services, research, and training
13. Help to integrate health needs into physical, economic, and other areas of planning for community development*

We ask you to make special note of the last of these objectives, which we shall return to shortly.

Legislative adjuncts

The effort of the National Commission on Community Health Services was extremely successful. It made many recommendations for action that endorsed and emphasized the continued, vital need for community-based study and decision making. Planning, however, takes time, the efforts of skilled people (now called planners), and money. Money appeared to be the primary ingredient needed at state and local levels, and the Eighty-ninth Congress responded with verve. In fact, its response to the Commission's recommendations as well as to many other parallel efforts was so overwhelming that it became known as the most health-minded Congress in our history.* Millions of dollars were made available to states to encourage the development of new, badly needed health programs. We are still striving to accomplish the goals described in the laws passed. A partial list indicates the ranging concern of the Eighty-ninth Congress and makes clear why very little health legislation has been passed since.

The Drug Abuse Control Amendments (P.L. 89-74)

The Federal Cigarette Labeling and Advertising Act (P.L. 89-92)

The Mental Retardation Facilities and Community Mental Health Centers Construction Act Amendments (P.L. 89-105)

The Community Health Services Extension Amendments (P.L. 89-109)

The Health Research Facilities Amendments (P.L. 89-115)

The Public Works and Economic Development Act (P.L. 89-136)

The Water Quality Act (P.L. 89-234)

The Heart Disease, Cancer, and Stroke Amendments (Regional Medical Programs) (P.L. 89-239)

The Clean Air Act Amendments and the Solid Waste Disposal Act (P.L. 89-272)

The Health Professions Educational Assistance Amendments (P.L. 89-290)

The Medical Library Assistance Act (P.L. 89-291)

The Appalachian Regional Development Act (P.L. 89-4)

The Older Americans Act (P.L. 89-73)

The Social Security Amendments (Medicare, Medicaid, Comprehensive Child Health Care) (P.L. 89-97)

---

*Guidelines for organizing state and area-wide community health planning, Amer. J. Public Health **56:**2139, December 1966.

*Rusk, H.: Congress and medicine, The New York Times, November 20, 1965.

The Vocational Rehabilitation Amendments (P.L. 89-333)

The Housing and Urban Development Act (P.L. 89-117)

The Extended Comprehensive Health Planning and Public Health Services Amendments (P.L. 89-749)

The Allied Health Professions Personnel Training Act (P.L. 89-751)

The Demonstration Cities and Metropolitan Development Act (P.L. 89-754)

The Highway Safety Act (P.L. 89-564)

Who are the planners?

So fast did what we call health planning come on the scene that there were few people qualified to be called planners. In order to attract the available money, universities scrambled to define curriculums that would graduate health planners. Simultaneously, many communities moved too rapidly on the planning escalator, employing nearly anyone who called himself a planner, thus creating even greater problems from which they are still trying to extricate themselves.

Planning, of course, is not unique to health. The Joint Urban Affairs Institute sponsored by Harvard and M.I.T. has been underway for more than a decade. Schools of architecture and urban planning are growing rapidly or are being created. Political scientists have joined the foray, as have sociologists, social workers, engineers, and many other groups. Unfortunately, not so long ago many individuals represented themselves as planners, when in fact they were not prepared for the mountain of problems they faced. Who are the planners is a question that we are only beginning to answer.

Integrating the effort

We return now to the last of the objectives of health planning cited earlier: to help integrate health needs with physical, economic, and other areas of planning for community development. No group with a major interest, whether it be health, education, or housing can plan in isolation, although some groups have—resulting in the failure of those many community health studies cited earlier. Success, however, will only come when all the needs of a community or region are considered together and a master plan is developed to meet those needs. This necessitates the integration of planning and planners representing all facets of personal and community life *and* the involvement of the key leaders in the community in the decision-making process. Planners seldom are community leaders with the authority to put their ideas into action, but they depend on such leaders to accomplish the desired goals. The leaders must be involved if planning is to be successful. Without question, the decade of the 1970's will witness a clearer definition of planning by all the groups who bear a responsibility for any portion of it in the complex of the community.

ON BALANCING YOUR BUDGET

Have you been aware that we've been talking about you in this discussion of planning? We have. You can demonstrate your influence by exercising it in your community in many meaningful ways. One effective way to do this is to spend your health care dollar wisely. This is progressively more difficult as health costs rise and the competition for your economic resources increases. We hope Chapter 11 will prove helpful to you in this regard.

Health and your budget

The noticeable improvement in the health status of Americans, evaluated in terms of lower morbidity, greater longevity, and higher effectiveness of health care, largely mirrors the affluent standard of living that has typified the United States during this century. Good housing, adequate diets, sufficient jobs, economic deflation, clean air, pure water, noise abatement, spacious recreational opportunities, and a host of other factors will likely contribute more to the health of the nation than better health care, which too often is more corrective than preventive. More and cheaper health care is not the single, simple panacea to our health care problems. Good health care is multifaceted. The purely medical becomes intertwined with the economic and the social, as in the need of the chronically ill for homes, the poor for jobs, the mentally ill for a supportive environment, and the handicapped for tolerance and opportunity.

Health care is expensive and will remain expensive through the 1970's. The expense will be borne by individuals, cities, counties, states, and the Federal government. Although the major attention of this book is devoted to personal health, it should be remembered that funds spent for pollution control, rat control, medical research, food stamps, rent supplements, and other related problems contribute either directly or indirectly to personal health care.

Americans spent about $38 billion in private expenditures for health care in 1968. This figure represented 7% of the public's expenditures on all personal needs and a 14% increase since 1967. Americans also paid a total of nearly $13 billion for hospital care in 1968. They paid $10 billion for physicians' services and $7 billion for medicines and appliances. The average expense to treat a patient in a community hospital was $62.57 per day in 1968.

In the 12 months between July 1, 1968 to June 30, 1969, the Federal government spent about $10 billion for Medicaid and Medicare for about 19 million people. Its total expenditures for medicine and health care was about $60 billion.

Although school health education and public health education are recognized fields of health, there still exists a great gap between what people need to know and what they actually know of health care and its cost. This chapter explores, in a limited manner, several of the facets of health and your budget. Again, keep in mind that adequate or inadequate income does not, in the final analysis, determine the quality of health care you receive. The biggest challenge is to acquire useful information and subsequently to put that information to work.

COLLEGE HEALTH SERVICES

The responsibility of colleges and universities to provide health services for students has been recognized for many years. No matter what emphases are placed on various phases of college and university health programs, the health service remains one of the strongest phases of the overall program.

The present concept of the job of college health service may be defined in terms of the goals of an ideal program. The following goals are proposed by the American College Health Association.

1. To find ways to assure individuals in the college community a quality of medical care which is personal, humane, and comprehensive despite institutionalization, mechanization, and communication problems.
2. To enhance the desirable methods of delivering personal medical care to the college community, and to change the undesirable aspects.
3. To assure that the provision of personal health for members of the college community is effectively coordinated, utilizing resources both on and off campus. This requires the development and maintenance of communication systems to equip health professionals on campus and off campus with the necessary information to provide quality clinical health care.
4. To bring to the college community health program new developments, new ideas, and improvements in the delivery system for personal medical care to enable the academic community health program to optimally serve the human needs of the community. It should also present to the public examples, models, and recommendations based upon careful planning and evaluations.*

The health services department in your college may or may not be similar to most, for departments and programs vary greatly. Some are huge operations that are similar to major hospitals, and others are very small operations with only a part-time physician and one or two nurses. In terms of organizational structure, some programs are autonomous with a medical or lay director responsible for the overall administration of the program; he in turn is responsible directly to the president or a vice-president of the college. In other colleges the director of the program may be responsible to the director of student affairs or to a manager of auxiliary enterprises. Whatever happens to be the size or organizational structure, the program's primary purpose for existing is not altered.

Since there is so much variance in the types of programs, a few of the ideal standards are presented below.

1. A full-time medical director should be in charge.
2. Male and female physicians should be on the staff.
3. Registered nurses should be on duty at all times.
4. Major specialists should be available to students.
5. A health committee should be functioning.
6. The health service should serve as a resource and educational agency for questions relating to medical matters.
7. Student health insurance plans should be available.
8. Preadmittance and recheck health examinations should be required.
9. Students who would be a health menace to the college community should be refused admittance to college.
10. Adequate facilities, supplies, and equipment should be provided.
11. Campus sanitation should be a cooperative responsibility of the college and other official health agencies.
12. Complete, up-to-date records should be kept of all students.

The preceding items are representative of a much more extensive list of criteria. If your college has an elaborate health facility, you are indeed fortunate. If your college has a small facility on campus, you may still be fortunate if your college has provided for the necessary services to be obtained in the local community.

How many times have you visited your health service? Do you know what services are offered? What procedures would you follow in receiving emergency medical care? How much do you know about your college health service program? The health facilities, personnel, and services are for *your* use.

---

*American College Health Association: Personal health services, Position Paper—Task Force II, presented at the Fifth National Conference on Health in College Communities, Boston, 1970, The Association, p. 5.

COST OF MEDICAL CARE

Medical care costs have jumped tremendously during the past few years. Reasons for the acceleration of costs are many: inflation, supply and demand of and for medical personnel, new drugs, more sophisticated medical equipment, and the cost of hospital services.

In 1969 Americans paid $15 billion for hospital care, 217% more than in 1959.

Table 11-1. Differences in distribution of personal expenditures for medical care, United States, 1960 and 1969 (billions of dollars)

Expense item	1960	1969	Difference
Hospital services	5.1	14.6	+ 9.5
Physicians' services	5.3	11.5	+ 6.2
Medicines and appliances	4.9	7.9	+ 3.5
Dentists' services	2.0	3.9	+ 1.9
Health insurance	0.8	1.7	+ 0.9
All others	1.0	2.1	+ 1.1
Total	18.6	41.6	+23.0

Data from Source book of health insurance data, New York, 1970, Health Insurance Institute.

Table 11-2. Consumer price index, United States

Year	All items*	Food	Apparel	Housing	Transportation	Medical care	Personal care	Reading and recreation	Other goods and services
1960	103.1	101.4	102.2	103.1	103.8	108.1	104.1	104.9	103.8
1961	104.2	102.6	103.0	103.9	105.0	111.3	104.6	107.2	104.6
1962	105.4	103.6	103.6	104.8	107.2	114.2	106.5	109.6	105.3
1963	106.7	105.1	104.8	106.0	107.8	117.0	107.9	111.5	107.1
1964	108.1	106.4	105.7	107.2	109.3	119.4	109.2	114.1	108.8
1965	109.9	108.8	106.8	108.5	111.1	122.3	109.9	115.2	111.4
1966	113.1	114.2	109.6	111.1	112.7	127.7	112.2	117.1	114.9
1967	116.3	115.2	114.0	114.3	115.9	136.7	115.5	120.1	118.2
1968	121.2	119.3	120.1	119.1	119.6	145.0	120.3	125.7	123.6

Data from Source book of insurance data, New York, 1969, Health Insurance Institute.
*1957-1959 = 100.

Table 11-3. Medical care indexes, United States

Year	All medical care items*	Physicians' fees	Dentists' fees	Eye exams and glasses	Hospital room rates	Prescriptions and drugs
1958	100.1	100.0	100.2	100.0	99.9	100.6
1959	104.4	103.4	102.7	101.1	105.5	102.2
1960	108.1	106.0	104.7	103.7	112.7	102.3
1961	111.3	108.7	105.2	107.0	121.3	101.1
1962	114.2	111.9	108.0	108.6	129.8	99.6
1963	117.0	114.4	111.1	109.3	138.0	98.7
1964	119.3	117.3	114.0	110.7	144.9	98.4
1965	122.3	121.5	117.6	113.0	153.3	98.1
1966	127.7	128.5	121.4	116.1	168.0	98.4
1967	136.7	137.6	127.5	121.8	200.1	97.9

Data from Source book of insurance data, New York, 1969, Health Insurance Institute.
*1957-1959 = 100.

Payments for doctors' services reached $12 billion, a rise of 130% since 1959. Expenditures for medicines and appliances amounted to over $8 billion, an 88% increase over the costs 10 years earlier. The amount of money spent by the public for all types of medical care (excluding dental care and net cost of health insurance) increased 133% since 1959. Table 11-1 shows the distribution of medical care dollars spent between 1960 and 1969.

The Consumer Price Index shows that

over the years medical costs have increased faster than any major category of personal expenditure. The base index is 100. Figures shown in Tables 11-2 and 11-3 indicate the changes that have taken place since the 1957-1959 standard of 100. The Consumer Price Index is presented in Table 11-2; the Medical Care Indexes, in Table 11-3.

Hospital services represent the major increase in the proportional share of dollar expenditure for medical care. This increase was over ten times as much as was paid for

Table 11-4. Personal consumption expenditures by type of product, 1967

Type of product	Personal consumption expenditures (billions of dollars)	Percent of total
Food (including alcohol)	$109.4	22.3%
Housing	70.9	14.4
Household operation	69.9	14.2
Transportation	63.5	12.9
Clothing accessories and jewelry	50.7	10.3
Medical care*	33.1	6.7
Recreation	30.6	6.2
Personal business	25.7	5.2
Tobacco	9.2	1.9
Personal care	8.5	1.7
Religious and welfare activities	6.9	1.4
Private education and research	7.9	1.6
Foreign travel and remittances—net	4.0	0.8
Death expenses	1.9	0.4
Total	$492.2	100.0%

Data from Source book of health insurance data, New York, 1970, Health Insurance Institute.
*Includes expenses for health insurance.

Table 11-5. Personal consumption expenditures for health by component, age, and sex, United States, 1968

	Expenditures per person (dollars)					
	All services*	Physicians	Hospitals	Drugs and medicines	Dentists	Other medical
All persons	94	31	22	19	14	8
under 6	48	21	11	14	1	1
6 -17	49	16	7	9	14	3
18-34	98	35	27	13	17	5
35-54	108	35	22	22	19	10
55-64	129	40	29	31	15	14
65 and over	177	55	49	42	10	21
Males	77	24	18	16	12	7
Females	111	38	26	22	16	9

Data from Source book of health insurance data, New York, 1970, Health Insurance Institute.
*Totals do not always equal the sum of components because of rounding.

hospital care in 1948. The Health Insurance Institute states that the factors accounting for the increase are:

1. The general rise in the U. S. economy
2. The improved quality of hospital services
3. The use of new and more expensive drugs
4. The broader scope of newly developed health insurance policies
5. The public's greater utilization of hospital care made possible by today's health insurance programs

Americans as never before are using and abusing hospital services. You no doubt know persons who insist that it is more economical to be admitted to a hospital for a medical examination, since in-hospital costs are covered in part or in whole by insurance, rather than submit to a routine examination in a physician's office. From the standpoint of thoroughness, this may well be more prudent, but at the same time it helps inflate hospital care costs. Supply and demand assists in dictating the overall costs of hospital care. As more people are admitted to the crowded facilities of hospitals, the demands for services of hospital personnel increase. With a strained supply of facilities and personnel, the cost rises for both patients and insurance companies.

Table 11-4 presents an overview of the total expenditures by type of products consumed by the public. Medical care ranks sixth among the fourteen products cited. This rank may be questioned, however, when thought is given to the fact that there are thousands of Americans who need medical care but do not seek it until it is absolutely necessary. Realistically, it may be ranked about number five. Where is it ranked in your personal expenditures?

Table 11-5 shows the health expenditures by category, age, and sex. Note the steady increase in the expenditures for all services. The 35 to 54 age group experienced a decrease in hospital expenditures and a subsequent increase at the age of 55. For the same age group, dental expenditures steadily declined. The decline may be attributed to the loss of all teeth and the fitting of dental plates.

CHOOSING A MEDICAL ADVISOR

Your health must be cared for by well-qualified individuals. Since health is your most precious asset, a great deal of thought and attention has to be given to selection of those who will care for it. If you are healthy, you may feel that any physician will serve your health needs. If this is your point of view, your medical care may be expensive and disappointing.

One of the rewarding aspects of American life is that you have a choice of the physician who is to attend to your health. Unfortunate indeed is the plight of people in many other countries where this is not possible.

Not all physicians are good physicians. Some finished medical school many decades ago and have not had advanced instruction, nor have they kept abreast of the phenomenal advances in their respective fields. Others are interested primarily in the volume of patients and personal finances rather than the health welfare of individual patients. Nevertheless, you should not be overly sensitive about the credentials of the majority of physicians, surgeons, and dentists, for most of them are excellent practitioners. The important factor is that you should appraise objectively and logically the qualifications of the medical, surgical, and dental personnel who are to care for your health.

There are many ways to judge a physician's qualifications. The following are suggested guidelines to assist you in selecting a physician, surgeon, or dentist.

1. Do not procrastinate in making your choice. Far too many people wait until an emergency occurs and visit the first physician who may be available at the moment of need. Under such circumstances the choice may be excessively expensive and treatment haphazardly administered.
2. Determine the kind of services you need. Do you need a specialist or general practitioner? Chances are that

your first consideration would be a family physician and/or dentist if an emergency does not exist.

3. Consult valid references for the qualifications and locations of the advisor needed. Some of the references are:
   a. Telephone directory for location. How far would you have to travel to secure services? How complicated is the traffic problem? How long would it take you to get there?
   b. The local medical and dental societies. What are his or her specific professional qualifications in terms of education, experience, and certification?
   c. The nearest accredited hospital. Is he or she on the staff? In what capacity? How long has she or he been associated with the hospital?
   d. The opinions of friends whose judgment you respect. Does he have a good reputation of outstanding services? What are his personal relations with his patients? Does he keep you waiting for long periods of time when appointments are made?
4. After the preceding references have been investigated and you have formulated a priority list of two or three advisors, make an appointment with the one at the top of your list for a medical consultation concerning the services you need. At this time be very careful in observing your response to the personality of the advisor. Confidence in the health advisor goes a long way in dealing with any subsequent health problems. Notice the professional climate of the office. Is it well organized? What about the personality of his assistants? Finally, decide whether he is the advisor you would like to have. Although it may take more than one visit to do this, a firm decision should be made.
5. If your personal contact with the advisor at the top of the list is unfavorable, carefully decide who you should

see next. You must not become a "patient bum," for your reputation of needlessly running from one physician to another soon gets around. When this occurs, the physician-patient relations are negatively affected.

PHYSICIAN-PATIENT ETHICS AND RELATIONSHIPS

The American Medical Association has established a code of ethics as a standard for physicians to follow. The Association's "Principles of Medical Ethics" are:

Preamble: These principles are intended to aid physicians individually and collectively in maintaining a high level of ethical conduct. They are not laws but standards by which a physician may determine the propriety of his conduct in his relationship with patients, with colleagues, with members of allied professions, and with the public.

Section 1. The principal objective of the medical profession is to render service to humanity with full respect for the dignity of man.

Section 2. Physicians should strive continually to improve medical knowledge and skill, and should make available to their patients and colleagues the benefits of their professional attainments.

Section 3. A physican should practice a method of healing founded on a scientific basis; and he should not voluntarily associate professionally with anyone who violates this principle.

Section 4. The medical profession should safeguard the public and itself against physicians deficient in moral character and professional competence. Physicians should observe all laws, uphold the dignity and honor of the profession, and accept its self-imposed disciplines. They should expose, without hesitation, illegal or unethical conduct of fellow members of the profession.

Section 5. A physician may choose whom he will serve. In an emergency, however, he should render service to the best of his ability. Having undertaken the care of a patient, he may not neglect him; and unless he has been discharged, he may discontinue his services only after giving adequate notice. He should not solicit patients.

Section 6. A physician should not dispose of his services under terms or conditions which tend to interfere with or impair the free and complete exercise of his medical julgment and skill as tend to cause a deterioration of the quality of medical care.

Section 7. In the practice of medicine, a physician should limit the source of his professional income to medical services actually administered by him, or under his supervision, to his patients. His fee should be commensurate with the services rendered and the patient's ability to pay. He should neither pay nor receive a commission for referral of patients. Drugs, remedies or appliances may be dispensed or supplied by the physician provided it is in the best interests of the patient.

Section 8. A physician should seek consultation upon request; in doubtful or difficult cases; or whenever it appears that the quality of medical service may be enhanced thereby.

Section 9. A physician may not reveal the confidences entrusted to him in the course of medical attendance, or the deficiencies he may observe in the character of patients, unless it becomes necessary in order to protect the welfare of the individual or of the community.

Section 10. The honored ideals of the medical profession imply that the responsibilities of the physician extend not only to the individual but also to society, where these responsibilities deserve his interests and participation in activities which have the purpose of improving both the health and well-being of the individual and the community.

These principles are generally administered by a local or state medical society. If, as a patient, you feel that you have been wronged by a physician, you should first attempt to absolve any differences of opinion with that physician. If you do not receive satisfaction, your next recourse would be to make your complaint to the local medical society. Accused physicians may also be heard by the state medical society. If the physician is found guilty of misconduct, he can appeal the local or state decision to the judicial council of the American Medical Association.

The patient also has certain obligations to the physician, for the physician and patient share a relationship that carries obligations for both parties.

Your obligations to the physician

Some of your obligations to the physician are:

1. Refuse to engage in self-diagnosis and self-medication.
2. Have regular checkups in order to assist the physician by providing a frame of reference when something does go wrong.
3. Encourage cooperation among all your physicians. If you are receiving services from two different physicians at the same time, inform each about the other.
4. Answer all medical questions frankly and completely. The slightest abnormality covered up or misrepresented may be the key to successful diagnosis and treatment.
5. Be frank about fees and consultations.
6. Follow the specific instructions of your physician. If you feel that you can't, tell him.
7. When instructed to revisit, do so.
8. Make all appointments as much in advance as possible.
9. The physician's time is valuable. Don't waste it by requesting unnecessary appointments.
10. Be on time for your appointment. If you cannot be on time, cancel the appointment early so that other patients may be scheduled.
11. When your bill arrives, pay it. If there are questions about charges that were not previously discussed, bring them to the immediate attention of the physician.
12. Refrain from negatively criticizing one physician to another. If you are impelled to criticize, do it personally to the physician involved.
13. Report all obvious violations of medical ethics to the appropriate agencies or authorities.
14. If you should lose confidence in a physician, consult another.
15. Your cooperation with the physician helps to develop good physician-patient relations and generally assures good results from the services he provides.

Malpractice and the patient

When you enter into a patient–medical advisor relationship, you generally do so on the basis of trust. It is assumed that the physician, surgeon, or dentist possesses adequate knowledge, skill, and experience in his specialty. But regardless of the care with which you select your health advisors, there is a danger of malpractice. Malpractice consists of an inappropriate diagnosis, treatment, or professional action by a physician, surgeon, dentist, or other health advisor.

When a legal wrong has been committed, the law must protect the damaged patient. However, the patient must recognize that legal wrongs, as far as the law is concerned, are weighed against the overall health and social values of the acts of the medical, surgical, and dental professions. Also, if a physician is excessively affected by the fear of legal wrongs, he readily becomes restrained in his usefulness to his patients.

A physician, surgeon, or dentist is generally not liable for an honest error in judgment, where the appropriate course to be followed is open to reasonable doubt. This principle may be applied to the basketball official who errs in a judgment about possession of the ball on a close play. His error does not necessarily mean that he does not know what he is doing nor that he is negligent in his actions, for he, like the physician, has been certified to practice his profession on the basis of his knowledge, skills, and experiences. The physician is held to the standards of his profession and association unless he claims more ability (such as the specialist) or less (such as the new graduate) than the average practitioner.

Understanding between the patient and the physician could reduce the possibility of malpractice suits and charges. Nonetheless, malpractice litigation continues to increase at a significant rate.

To be sure, most medical specialists are well qualified and rarely susceptible to medical malpractice. If you ever contemplate bringing forth a malpractice charge, you must be absolutely sure of the particulars.

Physicians refusing to make house calls or those who pass up traffic accident victims may do so from fear of being burdened by financial and professional damages. The same is true when a surgeon refuses to perform an operation without the consent of the person to receive the operation, unless it is an emergency condition that means saving the life of the patient.

Many patients, however, do suffer because of their physician's errors. Carter summarizes this side of the malpractice problem as follows:

Rarely mentioned in medical discussions of the malpractice problem is the fact that the volume of malpractice complaints is hardly an indication of the amount of malpractice that actually takes place. Unless a patient is crazy for lawsuits, and some people undoubtedly are, he is not likely to file formal complaint about medical treatment except when he not only has been obviously butchered, but has found out that he need not have been butchered. Most people do not know when they are victims of malpractice, and those who may suspect the physician's performance usually do not know what to do about it . . . The reason that malpractice is hard to prove is made immeasurably harder by what lawyers call the medical profession's "conspiracy of silence." The malpractice plaintiff needs expert testimony to prove his case, but he can seldom find a physician to testify for him.[*]

THE SPECIALTIES

The health care of people has become so sophisticated that it is nearly impossible for one person to excel in a general area of medicine, surgery, or dentistry.

Many years ago the general practitioner was the medical man of note. He was qualified and capable to diagnose and treat patients, deliver babies, perform surgery, make home visits, and a number of other things. He was generally qualified to practice after three or four years of formal medical training, one year of intern work, and, rarely, a year or two of residence in a hospital or clinic.

Today many medical students look forward to preparing for one of the many specialties open to them. The same generally holds true for dental students. Specializing benefits the public as it does the medical person. The specialist has more time to de-

*Carter, Richard: The doctor business, New York, 1958, Doubleday & Co., pp. 234-235. Copyright © 1958 by Richard Carter. Reprinted by permission of Doubleday & Co., Inc.

vote to a specific area, and his concentration results in better service to his patients.

The family physician is usually an internist or a general practitioner. He is the medical advisor for approximately four out of five Americans. Most patients contact medical specialists who are referred by the family physician. Family physicians are cognizant of the limitations of their professional services and rarely hesitate to refer their patients to the proper specialist. A list of some of the dental, medical, and surgical specialties follows.

Dental specialties

Specialty	Area of concentration
Oral pathology	Study of disease of the mouth
Oral surgery	Surgical procedures for correction of injury, disease, or malformation
Orthodontia	Malocclusions
Pediatric dentistry	Children's teeth
Periodontia	Treatment of gums and other tooth-supporting structures
Prosthodontia	Artificial teeth and appliances
Public health dentistry	Education and other means of promoting the public's dental health

Medical specialties

Specialty	Area of concentration
Allergy	Allergic disorders
Anesthesiology	Anesthesia and pain relief
Cardiology	Heart and blood vessel disorders
Dermatology	Diseases of skin
Endocrinology	Diseases of growth and metabolism
Gastroenterology	Diseases of the stomach and intestines
Geriatrics	Disorders of old age
Internal medicine	General diagnosis and treatment
Neurology	Diseases of nervous system
Pediatrics	Care and treatment of children
Pathology	Study of disease processes
Physical medicine	Use of exercise and other forms of physical therapy in treatment of disease or in rehabilitation
Psychiatry	Mental disorders
Public health	Community health

Radiology	Diagnosis and treatment of disorders by x-rays and other radioactive substances
Syphilology	Syphilis

Surgical specialties

Specialty	Area of concentration
Gynecology	Disorders of femal reproductive system
Neurosurgery	Brain and nervous system
Obstetrics	Pregnancy and childbirth
Ophthalmology	Diseases and disorders of the eyes
Orthopedic Surgery	Bones, joints, muscles, and tendons
Otorhinolaryngology	Diseases of ear, nose, and throat
Plastic surgery	Repair and restructuring of defects
Thoracic Surgery	Chest
Urology	Urinary and reproductive system
Vascular surgery	Circulatory disorders

The preceding specialties are only representative of many. All of them require that the individual earn the Doctor of Medicine (or of Dental Surgery) degree before going on to specialize. After earning his degree the medical doctor spends one to two years as an intern. After graduation from medical school or after his internship he must pass the state board examination. Once this is passed, he is licensed to practice medicine in that state. To become certified in one of the many specialties the licensed physician works for two or more years as a resident physician or fellow in an approved hospital for that specialty. At the termination of his residency or fellowship and after a certain amount of practice, he takes a specialty board examination. Upon passing it he becomes a board-certified specialist in that area.

The American boards responsible for accrediting the various specialists are:

American Board of Anesthesiology
American Board of Dermatology
American Board of Internal Medicine
American Board of Neurological Surgery
American Board of Obstetrics and Gynecology
American Board of Ophthalmology
American Board of Orthopaedic Surgery
American Board of Otolaryngology

American Board of Pathology
American Board of Pediatrics
American Board of Physical Medicine and Rehabilitation
American Board of Plastic Surgery
American Board of Preventive Medicine, Inc.
American Board of Proctology
American Board of Psychiatry and Neurology
American Board of Radiology
American Board of Surgery
American Board of Thoracic Surgery
American Board of Urology

In addition, there are subspecialty boards. For example, under the American Board of Internal Medicine are Boards of Allergy, Cardiology, Chest Disease, and Gastroenterology.

Nurses

To meet the ideal ratio of 380 nurses per 100,000 patients, the United States will need 975,000 nurses by 1980. The situation indeed looks hopeless if one stops to consider that the population of the United States is expected to increase by approximately 70 million in 1980. At the present time there are approximately 298 nurses per 100,000 people. This low ratio is a very serious matter, for nurses are the primary assistants to the medical men. They are primarily responsible for executing the orders of the physician, which frees him for other duties. Nurses are trained to perform many duties that cut across many health areas.

Nurses may be generally classified as registered professional nurses or as practical nurses. The difference is determined by the quality and quantity of training. Registered professional nurses are trained to be responsible for planning and executing the nursing care of patients. Their formal instruction consists of two to four years of education, usually in a college associated with a teaching hospital. Upon successful completion of a state-supervised licensing examination, the person becomes a registered nurse, or R.N. Some colleges and universities provide additional academic courses, which qualifies the nurse for one of the academic degrees. She may be employed as a:

1. Hospital staff nurse
2. Office nurse
3. Occupational health nurse
4. Private duty nurse
5. Public health nurse
6. School nurse

Practical nurses generally assist the registered nurse or the physician. They may be responsible for the care of a patient who does not need the immediate supervision of a registered nurse or physician. These persons must successfully complete the curriculum of an approved practical nursing school that provides for clinical experiences and must also pass a state licensing examination. The most general designation for the licensed practical nurse is L.P.N.

Since the need is so great and the supply of adequately qualified nurses so short, other persons are qualified to administer to patients by completing very limited training and becoming nurses' aides or nursing assistants.

Other health care personnel

Space does not provide for a discussion of the many other professional persons involved with your health care. Some of these are laboratory technicians, x-ray technicians, pharmacists, optometrists, dental hygienists, chiropractors, psychologists, chiropodists, osteopaths, and dietitians. Depending on the need for their service, each contributes significantly to the health care of individuals.

HOSPITAL CARE

Much has been written about the plight of hospitals, the scarcity of hospital beds, and the caliber of hospital care. Many of the critics are appalled with the quality of the personnel, facilities, and services. You no doubt have read and will continue to read of the problems. But in spite of what may be said, our hospitals are the bulwarks of successful and essential medical services, especially since these services relate to serious illnesses and disorders of human beings. It is here that the medical team takes over in attempting to diagnose and treat our major health maladies, and it is here that most surgery is performed, that the more complicated laboratory tests are performed, and that most babies are born.

Approximately one out of every seven Americans was hospitalized in 1968. An average of 75,000 persons entered community hospitals each day, for a total of about 28,000,000 admissions over a 12-month period. This was an increase of nearly 289,000 hospital admissions since 1967 and represented a 26% rise since 1968. On an average day in 1968 there were 630,000 patients, or 3.2 persons per 1,000 population, confined to hospitals. The annual admissions were 138 persons per 1,000 population. Projecting these facts into the 1970's, one can conclude that the availability of hospital beds is a critical issue that must be coped with in positive terms.

The problem of solving the availability crisis may not be as crucial as it seems. This is especially true as it relates to the duplication of services, overutilization, and other factors. You could assist in solving the problem by making more intelligent use of hospitals, when possible. Particular attention is directed to overutilization of hospitals for diagnostic checkups. Thousands of beds are filled each day with persons who are simply having medical examinations. This in itself may or may not constitute misuse by the patient; the decision about the necessity of hospitalization lies with the physician or the hospital. Some of the hospitals are strict about needless admissions. When this is the case, patients and physicians may be tempted to fabricate the real reason for admission.

The hospital you will generally choose will be that recommended by your physician or surgeon. If you have chosen your medical advisor well, you need not worry about the wiseness of his preference.

Accreditation

Hospitals generally fall into one of two groups: the accredited and the nonaccredited. Reference is not made here to the specialty hospital nor to the kind of control. The accredited hospital is one that is approved by the Joint Commission on Accreditation, which represents the American Medical Association, the American Hospital Association, the American College of Physicians, the Canadian Medical Association, and the College of Surgeons. The standards of the Commission are extensive, covering everything from the qualification of staff to the sanitation of the kitchen. Unfortunately, only slightly more than one half of the hospitals in the United States are accredited.

Being admitted

Being admitted to a hospital can be very pleasant or absolutely fearful. Your physician generally tries to prepare you through a discussion of the details. He will call the hospital agreed on and arrange a space for you. At this time you must decide on the type of accommodations and the time of arrival. The common types of accommodations are wards, semiprivate rooms, and private rooms. The ward is least expensive and the private room most expensive. Many people have gone excessively into debt, living in a private room when a bed in a ward would have been adequate.

If the situation is not an emergency, you should make all of your financial arrangements before going to the hospital. This is especially helpful if your stay in the hospital is to be lengthy. Ascertain the manner in which you will take care of your bill. Check all health insurance policies closely for benefits related to your admittance diagnosis. Doublecheck with the admittance office about these benefits.

You are not going on a vacation, so you should not load down with a lot of clothes, radios, and books. Take along the things you really need, such as slippers, robe, pajamas, and toilet articles.

Report to the admittance office at the designated time. It is here that you will have to be formally admitted. Once officially admitted, you are taken to your room.

Peace and quiet is a necessary ingredient for recovery; therefore, hospitals must adhere to strict regulations that ensure peace and quiet. The patient who is not seriously ill has an obligation to control noise and activity in his immediate area or room. He should keep his radio or television volume down and discourage the excessive gathering of persons in his area or room. In essence, he acts as he would want other patients to act toward him.

Once a patient is officially admitted, the hospital staff is responsible for his welfare until he is officially dismissed or granted a leave. A leave of absence or dismissal is granted upon the approval of the attending physician and the business office. Because they are held liable for possible negligence, hospitals generally adhere rigidly to the regulations of dismissal. It is important that a patient not be allowed to take leave or dismiss himself as he pleases.

Another consideration is the time that the bill must be paid. The bill may be presented to the patient weekly or when he is officially dismissed.

Visiting the patient

Visiting sick friends in the hospital requires that the visitor adhere to all principles that make the visit pleasant. You should arrive on time in a pleasant and optimistic mood and talk in cheerful tones about something appropriate for the moment. You should not lead into a discussion of the patient's problem; if the patient does, attempt to divert his attention from his problems. Unless there is some special reason, do not stay more than 20 to 25 minutes. Do not bring with you into the hospital, either as patient or visitor, any possibly objectionable or harmful habits such as alcohol, tobacco, or heavy perfume. You should never come to the hospital late at night.

HEALTH COSTS AND PROTECTION PLANS

Earlier in this chapter the breakdown of your health dollar was reviewed. It was concluded that you will spend more in the future than you earn now for medical, surgical, and dental care. Be that as it may, the bills for health services must be paid as any other bills. Naturally you would rather be healthy than ill. You probably do not accept the fact that you may at some time

experience cancer, a cardiovascular disorder, or have to undergo major surgery, so you are probably not too interested in planning for such possibilities. However, these matters must be thought of and dealt with far in advance of the moment of immediate need. The problems of health care and protection plans must be dealt with so that you and your family will not be excessively burdened with insurmountable financial obligations.

Paying for health care

You are spending more money today for health care because of the following reasons:
1. Your standard of living is more complex than in the past.
2. You demand more and better health services.
3. Health specialists are having to spend more time and money for training.
4. The supply of physicians, surgeons, and dentists cannot meet the demand for their services.
5. The quality of health services has improved.
6. The services of more health specialists to treat individual patients have increased.
7. Wages paid to hospital personnel have increased.
8. The cost of hospital beds has increased tremendously.

Health is a very unpredictable state, which, when lost to a great degree, exposes you to the risk of losing money, time, or both. Risks in this instance means the extent of uncertainty about the outcome or the cost. There are several ways of remedying the problem of unpredictable cost.

Prevention of loss. In order to prevent the loss of money and time, you have to remain healthy and not need health care. However, it is almost inevitable that you will need health care that will have to be paid for in money and/or time lost from work. Therefore, other methods to offset the eventuality of a health loss must be practiced.

Assumption of risk. You can admit that the risk of loss is real and attempt to make some provision for meeting the costs of health care. The average college student is generally not fully aware of the magnitude of the risks involved in illness nor of the responsibilities that must be met. The individual in assuming the risk of loss for himself does so strictly on a personal basis. Some persons save for "a rainy day" by establishing personal health care funds. Unfortunately, many people do not have the means to take on such a burden under such a plan.

Transfer of risk. You can shift your health loss risks to another individual or organizations. Public health clinics, which care for the indigent, accept much responsibility for their patients' health care.

Combining independent exposures. Since there are millions of Americans who are exposed to risks of health loss, it is believed that some prediction could be made of the degree of exposure to the risk by combining them. Once this is done something can be said, with a relative degree of certainty, about expected losses. The most common example is health insurance, in which the possible losses of a few people are distributed among many. The great majority of health care costs are covered by voluntary health protection plans. Approximately 80% of the U. S. civilian population was covered by various forms of health insurance in 1968. Others paid their bills through assumption of risk plans or transfer of risk plans.

Voluntary health protection plans

Comprehensive major medical insurance is a plan designed to give protection offered by both a basic and major medical health plan. It generally contains a coinsurance provision and a voluntary deductible amount. The maximum benefits are high.

Dental expense insurance is designed to protect against the costs of dental care and treatment. This type of insurance is still relatively new and is most generally sponsored as a group plan. Good individual, comprehensive policies are difficult to find at a reasonable premium. Most of the plans available on an individual basis provide primarily for traumatic injuries that result from accidents.

Hospital expense insurance provides for

Table 11-6. Percent of persons with hospital expense insurance who also have surgical expense insurance, regular medical expense insurance, and major medical expense insurance, United States*

End of year	Surgical expense	Regular medical expense	Major medical expense
1960	90.2	66.8	21.1
1961	91.5	69.5	25.4
1962	91.2	70.0	27.5
1963	91.3	70.8	29.4
1964	91.3	72.6	31.7
1965	91.7	72.9	33.9
1966	91.6	73.7	35.9
1967:			
Under 65	92.9	75.9	39.4
65 and over	83.3	65.0	18.0
Total	92.4	75.3	38.2
1968:			
Under 65	92.4	76.6	40.8
65 and over	83.4	69.4	17.9
Total	91.9	76.2	39.4

Data from Source book of health insurance data, New York, 1969, Health Insurance Institute.
*The "Surgical expense" and "Regular medical expense" categories represent coverage provided by insurance companies, Blue Cross, Blue Shield and medical society-approved plans, and independent plans. The "Major medical expense" category represents insurance companies only.

protection against the costs of hospital care resulting from the illness or injury of an insured person. The benefits include room and board at a specific rate for a maximum number of days and a set amount for all other nonsurgical services performed by the hospital. This plan commonly includes a physician expense clause providing a specified amount for a maximum number of visits.

Loss-of-income insurance provides benefits to help replace any income stopped by a lengthy illness or accident. The terms of the policy determine the three basic obligations of the company: the waiting period before payments will commence, the amount of the payments, and the number of payments.

Major medical expense insurance or catastrophic medical insurance is a plan designed to offset excessively high costs of health care resulting from prolonged illness or injury. Like the comprehensive medical insurance, it contains a coinsurance clause and often a deductible amount, which influences the amount of the premium paid. The deductible amount may range from $50 to more than $500. The policy holder has to pay a percentage of 20% to 25% or more of the cost above the deductible amount for which he is responsible.

Surgical expense insurance provides benefits to pay the cost of operations. The specific benefits are predetermined in terms of the maximum payment for each operation.

Regular medical expense insurance provides payment of doctor fees for nonsurgical care and treatment. The service may be rendered in the home, office, or in the hospital.

Medicare

Medicare provides health care benefits for persons over 65, increased cash benefits, liberal social security programs of old-age survivors, and disability insurance. The basic plan is financed by social security taxes and covers the costs of hospital and nursing home care and home nursing services. A supplementary plan is financed by monthly premiums of $4 and matching Federal contributions to cover physicians' fees and other specified medical costs.

It does not provide payment for:
1. Cost of private-duty nurses
2. Routine physical checkups and dental care
3. Long stays in nursing homes
4. Custodial care
5. Drugs outside the hospital
6. Routine eye and ear examination
7. Eyeglasses and hearing aids

It does provide payment for:
Regular plan
1. Hospital service for a maximum of 90 days per confinement
2. Maximum of 100 days' care after release from hospital
3. Outpatient diagnostic services at a hospital for a maximum of 100 visits per year

Supplementary plan
1. Ambulance services
2. Doctors' bills for home, office, and hospital visits
3. Home health services, previous hospitalization not required
4. Laboratory and x-ray tests outside a hospital
5. Rental of durable medical equipment
6. Surgical dressings
7. X-ray, radium, and radioactive isotope therapy

Medicare will pay the cost of covered services for up to 90 days of hospital care in a participating hospital during a benefit period. For the first 60 days of care Medicare will pay all but the first $60 of expenses. For the sixty-first through the ninetieth day of care, Medicare will pay all but $15 daily for covered services. There is a lifetime limit of payment for 190 days of care in a mental institution.

Medicare also provides a 60-day lifetime reserve, which can be used after the individual has exhausted his 90 days of hospital care in a benefit period. The lifetime reserve days are not replaced after one uses them. Medicare pays all but $30 a day of one's covered expenses during the reserve days.

Table 11-7. Number of persons using Medicare services, United States

	During 1967	
	Number (000 omitted)	Percent
Total persons enrolled under Part A, Part B, or both	20,460	100.0
Meeting Part A and/or Part B deductible	9,190	44.9
Total persons enrolled under both Part A and Part B	18,890	100.0
Meeting Part A and/or Part B deductible	8,960	47.4
Meeting Part A deductible only	370	2.0
Meeting Part B deductible only	5,040	26.7
Meeting both Part A and Part B deductible	3,550	18.8
Total persons enrolled under Part A only	1,570	100.0
Meeting Part A deductible	230	14.6

From Source book of health insurance data, New York, 1969, Health Insurance Institute.

Up to 100 days of care in a participating extended care facility are covered during each benefit period. Personal insurance will pay for all covered services for the first 20 days of care and all but $7.50 daily for the next 80 days. Extended care facility services are covered only if one has been in the hospital for 3 days or longer and enters the facility within 14 days after he leaves the hospital.

College students obviously are not eligible for the services offered under Medicare. Nonetheless, it is important to remember that there are many people who are eligible but need the assistance of well-informed relatives or friends to assist them in obtaining these health services. You should take time to inform your parents, relatives, or friends when the need dictates. Additional information may be obtained from your local Social Security office.

Table 11-7 summarizes the number of people who used Medicare services in 1967. During the 1970's, the number of persons using Medicare benefits will significantly increase.

Medicaid

Title 19 of the Federal Social Security Act, commonly called "Medicaid," is a program wherein the states may expand, with Federal matching funds, their public assistance programs to persons regardless of age whose income and resources are con-

sidered as insufficient to pay for health care. To be eligible for Federal funds, states were required to establish a Medicaid Program by the end of 1969. The law gives the states broad latitude in defining medical indigency. Thus the number of eligible persons varies from state to state, depending on the income limits fixed by the state.

The Title 19 program became effective January 1, 1966. By the end of 1967, 37 states had placed medical aid programs into effect. Total benefits paid on behalf of indigent persons under the program as of June 30, 1967, was $1.9 billion.

How many are insured?

Table 11-8 summarizes the number of people who held the major types of health care insurance policies between 1960 and 1968. Several of the types of health protection plans discussed above are not included.

REVIEW OF HEALTH CARE STATUS

More information about the types of plans discussed above may be obtained by consulting your family's insurance agent or the materials published by the health insurance companies. Once you have learned about the different plans available, you must decide which kind is best for your needs. The traditional comment of persons being "insurance poor" is often true. Thousands of Americans waste insurance dollars need-

Table 11-8. Number of persons with health insurance protection in the United States, by type of coverage, 1960-1968 (000 omitted)*

			Type of coverage†		
End of year	Hospital expense	Surgical expense	Regular medical expense	Major medical expense	Loss of income
1960	130,007	117,304	86,889	27,448	42,436
1961	134,417	122,951	93,466	34,138	43,055
1962	139,176	126,900	97,404	38,250	44,902
1963	144,575	131,954	102,302	42,441	43,927
1964	148,338	135,433	107,686	47,001	44,751
1965	153,133	140,462	111,696	51,946	46,347
1966	158,022	144,715	116,462	56,742	49,372
1967	162,853	150,396	122,570	62,226	51,230
1968	169,497	155,725	129,105	66,861	54,955

From Source book of health insurance data, New York, 1969, Health Insurance Institute.

*Net total of people protected eliminates duplication among persons protected by more than one kind of insuring organization or more than one insurance company policy providing the same type of coverage.

†Hospital, surgical, and regular medical expense includes coverage provided by insurance companies, Blue Cross, Blue Shield and medical society-approved plans, and independent plans. Major medical expense includes insurance companies only. Loss of income coverage includes insurance companies, formal paid sick-leave plans, and coverage through employee organizations.

lessly simply because they do not take time to determine their needs. Your needs are influenced by many factors: the family income, your savings, the number of persons in your family, the benefits you receive through special sources free of charge, and the special health problems of you and your family.

The following questions should help you in reviewing the health protection policies you have or plan to purchase:

Hospital expense:

How much does the policy pay toward room and board and other related services?

What is the maximum period of payment?

How much does it pay for laboratory tests, medication, x-rays, etc.?

Is the room and board rate sufficient in relation to the rates of your local hospitals?

What are the waiting period stipulations?

Is there a deductible amount? Is it too small or too large?

When does a new benefit period commence following a confinement?

Major medical expense:

What is the maximum benefit period?

What are the conditions of reinstatement?

What is the deductible amount? Is it for each claim or for the calendar year?

What percentage are you expected to pay on a coinsurance basis?

What benefits are given for various kinds of physicians?

Are there certain types of expenses not covered?

Physician expense:

What is the maximum benefit per visit for the physician?

How many visits are allowed per confinement?

Are house calls and office visits covered? How many? How much?

Other provisions that should be checked, since they relate to various policies, are as follows:

Coverage of dependents

Inpatient and Outpatient benefits

Benefits for special nursing care

Specific exclusions

Normal maternity benefits

Clauses related to preexisting conditions

Cancellation and renewal clauses

MANAGING HEALTH CARE COSTS

Throughout this chapter it has been continually emphasized that the costs for health

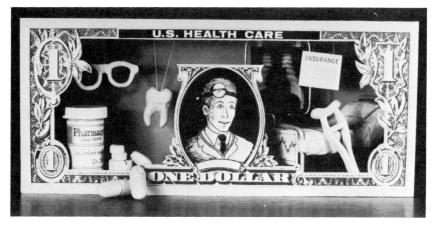

Fig. 11-1. The stress placed on our health care dollar today is severe. In the face of sky-rocketing medical costs, preventive measures regularly taken are far less expensive than curative measures that leave no alternative. (Courtesy Martin Webster.)

care are relatively high for the average person or family. Needs and ability to pay for such services vary a great deal. Most people hold health insurance policies to cover the expenses of a great portion of health care services. Rarely is it true that a person will have insurance to cover all of his medical expenses; therefore, consideration must be given not only to paying health insurance premiums but also to taking care of those expenses not covered by insurance.

Budgeting for health care need not be a haphazard procedure that could lead to possible disastrous financial consequences. You should take time to plan a workable budget that meets your present and projected health care needs. Some of the basic factors that must be considered are:

The cost and coverage of health insurance policies

The size of your family and the age and sex of its members

The cost of medical services in your community, your income, and other expenses

Free public health services available to you

Special health problems in your family

Cost of possible medical services for relatives outside your immediate family

Very often young adults are unexpectedly obligated to defray the expenses of a parent who is incapable of taking care of major expenses for health care. A newly wed couple with family development plans, working on a limited income, may suddenly find that they are morally obligated to take care of a mother or father. Much to their dismay, a financial setback results. Such a problem need not be disastrous if you plan for unexpected costs. How it may be done and whether it is necessary to give this matter serious consideration now must be based upon what you know of your parents. You might begin to solve this problem by asking yourself the following questions:

Is there a family history of poor health?

How old are my parents?

Do I know that they hold good health care policies that are in force?

Do they qualify for free or nominal cost tax-supported health services, such as those under Medicare?

What is their economic security status?

Are my brothers and sisters in a position to assist in paying for unexpected costs?

When the preceding questions have been answered, you must make a decision about your probable personal commitment. If you are to be solely responsible, it is suggested that a comprehensive health insurance plan be obtained for your parents and paid for by you. The cost of the premiums will be high. Before doing so it may be wise, if you have brothers and sisters, to attempt to get them to share in the cost of such coverage.

Paying insurance premiums on time guarantees continuous coverage. Insurance companies usually allow a grace payment period of 31 days after the premium due date. If the payment is received after the grace period, the company is not liable for claims unless otherwise provided for in the terms of the policy. Once the policy is out of force, you stand a chance of either not being qualified for reinstatement or having to adhere to a new waiting period for certain benefits.

THE MEDICAL EXAMINATION

The medical examination is indispensable to good health. Regardless of your physical condition, age, and sex, you should have a medical examination regularly. When you are young, as most of you are, you should have a thorough examination at least once every two years. Ideally, it is better to have one each year. As you grow older, however, you should have them more frequently.

A good time to have your routine medical examination is on or near your birthdate, since you rarely forget this date, and it may also serve to remind you that age is increasing both chronologically *and* physically.

Table 11-9 is a guide recommending the frequency of medical examinations. These recommendations are not absolute. They should, however, serve as a general guide for you, your children, or parents. Obviously, if a noticeable abnormality occurs, you should get a medical checkup even if the previous one was the preceding week.

Table 11-9 shows that the frequency of checkups should be greatest for the very young, least for those 5 to 15 years of age, and increasingly greater for those 35 years of age and older.

The merits of the routine medical examination are significant and well supported. There are a multitude of case histories of the abnormalities uncovered in such an examination. This is especially true in relation to chronic and degenerative diseases. The great majority of the abnormalities detected early are minor and may be treated before they become major.

The extensive examination may include all of the following and more:

Blood pressure	Heart rate
Blood typing and analysis	Hernia
Cancer tests	Medical history
Dental survey	Physical appearance
Electrocardiogram	Posture
Electroencephalogram	Sight and eyes
Gynecologic survey	Sigmoidoscopy
Hearing and ears	Urinalysis

EUTHANASIA

Nor dread nor hope attend
A dying animal.
A man awaits his end,
Dreading and hoping all.

W. B. YEATS

Euthanasia is derived from a Greek term meaning merciful, easy, or happy death. There are several forms of euthanasia; withholding treatment from a patient, ceasing treatments that prolong the patient's life, and administering a potent anesthetic or sedative.

The problem of letting patients die as a merciful release is a relatively new one. It is caused largely by our phenomenal success in medical technology and science. Not too many years ago, when the point of death

Table 11-9. Recommended frequency of health examinations

Age	Frequency
First 6 months	Biweekly
Second 6 months	Monthly
1 to 2 years	Every 3 months
2 to 5 years	Every 6 months
5 to 15 years	Every 2 to 3 years
15 to 35 years	Every 2 years
35 to 60 years	Every year
60 years and older	Every 6 months

Data from American Medical Association: Periodic health examination: a manual for physicians, Chicago, 1947, The Association.

was reached, there was rarely anything that could be done about it. But today medicines and medical and surgical procedures can keep people alive for an extended period of time, whereas in past years these same people would have died much earlier.

For many physicians and patients the question of prolonging life or terminating it is very real. These cases usually involve excessive pain, predicted death, and extremely high medical costs. The patient experiencing a terminal case of cancer may wonder why it is necessary to continue to suffer the traumatic pains or to cause undue financial obligations for the family and friends. Causing one to die, however, is contrary to ethical, moral, and humanitarian principles. Who knows what tomorrow might bring in terms of cure through medical discoveries? As long as there is life, there is always the hope for longer life.

The ethics of physicians have previously been discussed. Physicians are obligated to save the life of a patient and by no means to assist in taking or attempting to take that life.

THE PRICE OF DYING

Death by any cause is a traumatic experience to those close to the one who has died. Whether death was anticipated or not, the survivors are rarely prepared to deal with the related emotional or economic problems. All too often persons who are responsible for burying the dead resort to the "do all I can for the dead" attitude in making funeral arrangements. Case histories reveal that each year many people go into great debt burying their loved ones. This is obviously a personal matter. Nonetheless, it is important to know the particulars relating to the costs of funerals.

Simple funeral services are usually favored, partly because of the belief that money should be saved for the bereaved and partly because of the maintenance of both dignity and religious feeling. A close friend or a relative can often make more objective funeral arrangements than members of the immediate family. But no matter who makes the arrangements, it is prudent to obtain funeral costs in writing, including all auxiliary costs.

The basic price charged by a funeral director generally applies to a casket and minimum funeral costs. For example, in 1970 one undertaker in Louisiana said that he could provide a funeral for $325, but that it would be a very simple one: a pine box with simple covering for display, possibly no embalming, no reposing room accommodations, and direct delivery to a cemetery in the local area.

There is hardly any limit to the extent of funeral expenses. One of the surest ways to ensure that the funeral costs of one for whom you are responsible will be reasonable is to preplan and check excessiveness. In preplanning, it is necessary to give thought to and take steps to ensure economic body disposal.

The body may be disposed of by earth burial, cremation, donating parts of it to patients, or willing it to science. Earth burial, or interment, is the most common means and also the most expensive. Cremation, or incendiary disposal, is less frequently used than earth burial, although in recent years cremations have increased. The major reservation in considering its use is that of certain religious orders. Cremation is less expensive than earth burial, although some crematoriums and funeral directors may insist that a casket be used for the ashes. Some persons may choose to donate parts of their bodies to patients who are in need of transplants. The usual procedure is that the body is willed to a medical school or a specific hospital. Parts of the body may be transplanted or the body may be used as a cadaver in a gross anatomy class of a medical school.

If the body is to be buried, one must consider several factors while deciding on the burial place. Americans are typically people on the move. The native home town is frequently considered the ideal place for burial. Nonetheless, it is important to remember that the costs to get a body to one's home town may be excessive. Consider, for example, the expense of transporting a body from New York to El Paso, Texas.

HEALTH QUACKERY

It is essential to become acquainted with the pseudophysicians of our society who seek to become rich through meaningless verbal exchanges, medications, body-contact experiments, intellectual inquiry, and even extrasensory techniques. These persons are quacks. A quack is one who fraudulently misrepresents his ability and experience in the diagnosis and treatment he offers, or a person who pretends to have medical knowledge and experience when he does not.

Health quackery includes health cults, misleading advertising, and a variety of lures that cause patients or potential patients to waste money and risk their health.

Many centuries ago the demonic theory of disease explained how man became diseased and was cured. This theory asserted that disease was caused by demons, devils, or evil spirits. Any diseased person was thought to be possessed by the demons. Treatment and cure was thought to be effected by driving the demons or evil spirits from the body. The techniques employed were many. The "witch doctors" or the "medicine men" employed rituals, sacrifices of the lives of lower forms of animals, and other techniques to bring about health. The quacks of today do not adhere to the demonic theory. They are pseudoprofessionals who look and talk like the professionals they misrepresent.

In the past, deformed persons, such as hunchbacks, rulers, such as kings and high priests, mystics, and emotionally disturbed persons were believed to possess special powers in healing disease.

At the time of the American Revolution, a quack named Elisha Perkins invented "metallis tractors" to draw disease out of the body. The tractors consisted of two rods of brass and iron about 3 inches long, one of zinc, copper, and gold, the other of iron with some other metals; they cost about a penny to manufacture and sold for $5. James Graham in England set up a temple of healing in which he used the principle of electricity, promising cures and rejuvenation. Just as these two used the discovery of electricity to prey on the emotion and ignorance of people, so have other charlatans used drugs, radium, foods, and general physiology.

People today are conditioned to believe in medical miracles. Some of the modern medical drugs and machines are lifesaving. The quack knows this and takes advantage of public interest. Electricity, radiation, and magnetism are generally mysteries to most of us, and we are to some extent vulnerable to the promotion of worthless gadgets that claim one or more of these properties, especially if they look impressive and professional.

The fraudulent behavior of quacks, though diminished somewhat today, is still supported by far too many Americans. As long as there are customers, there will be quackery vendors. The customers are the ignorant, the nonbeliever, the gullible, and the miracle seeker.

The ignorant victims often accept testimonials or statements as facts without further investigation. To them a doctor is a doctor whether he is an M.D., D.M., or any kind of D. Fortunately, this type of quackery victim is rare.

The nonbeliever has little faith in anything that the majority of people believe. If the majority of the people are for physicians, fluoridation, law and order, ecologic controls, or comprehensive hospital services, he is against them. He is also the type of person who will tell a physician to do something now or he will go somewhere else.

The gullible victim may or may not be ignorant or misinformed: he is compulsive. He cannot seem to resist buying the meaningless nostrums recommended by quacks for various health results. The chances are that his home is well stocked with worthless "health" gadgets and drugs.

The miracle seeker is often an intelligent victim who may or may not have logical reservations about his involvement with a quack. He is primarily characterized by the hope that something good will quickly happen to his poor state of health. He is one who has been told that nothing more of a curative nature can be done for him, such as someone with terminal cancer. In final desperation he seeks someone who will tell him that it is not so—and he usually finds a quack. His philosophy is simply that if all is in vain, why not try the person who promises good results.

Among the quacks' victims are the old and young, the rich and poor, and the ignorant and well informed. Most of the victims are miracle seekers, among whom are included physicians, teachers, business executives, and religious leaders.

MEDICINES AND APPLIANCES

Americans spent about $7.5 billion for medicines and medical appliances in 1968. This cost of medical care is exceeded only by the costs for hospital and physicians' services. It is encouraging, however, to know that the consumer price index for medicines and medical appliances was 98.1 in 1968 as compared with 98.9 in 1956. All other medical care items showed significant increases in consumer prices indices. The greatest medical price index increase was in hospital room rates: from 200.1 in 1967 to 226.6 in 1968. The outlook during the 1970's for the purchase of prescriptions, drugs, and medical appliances is good, especially if the health-educated citizen uses good judgment in health-consuming practices.

Many dollars may be saved by understanding the basic economics of prescriptions and drugs. The Kefauver-Harris Drug Amendments of 1962 stated that your physician can prescribe, and you can use, drugs purchased under their generic names at lower prices than those purchased under brand names. The same law also gave the Food and Drug Administration more power to control the manufacture of drugs to assure their safety, purity, and identity. The savings are great if your physician prescribes a common drug. For example, a certain drug, often prescribed for patients with high blood pressure, sells at a retail price of $6.50 to $7 per 100 under its brand name. But equivalent drugs under their common, or generic, names occasionally sell at a retail price of $1 to $2 less.

In most cases your pharmacist can dispense only what your physician prescribes, even when he stocks a less costly variety of the same drug. But before castigating your physician, it is important to note that:

1. Your particular prescribed drug may be available only under the brand name of the company that compounded it.
2. Generic drugs may not be as cheap as you think. When they are ordered, the druggist may add a markup fee to help cover his overhead.
3. Many brand-name drugs are manufactured to a high standard of quality, whereas generic drugs may not be. Physicians invariably have much more confidence in known brands.

If your physican will not prescribe generic drugs, you should shop around for savings at a large chain store. In the final analysis, it may be best to seek out a physician more concerned about your health and your budget. In any event, you should speak up and let your intentions be known.

There are authoritative volumes that provide up-to-date drug standards. The most commonly used are the *United States Pharmacopeia* and the *National Formulary*. The former, usually designated as the U. S. P., is published at 5-year intervals by the private, nonprofit, United States Pharmacopoeial Convention, Inc. The U. S. P. lists only those drugs that reflect the best practice and teaching of medicine, with the decisions based on creditable and firmly supported scientific fact. The best thing that can happen to a manufacturer's drug is its approval by the U. S. P. or the N. F. When shopping the shelves of the drugstore, the health consumer does well to look for the initials U. S. P. and N. F.

THE CONTEMPORARY HEALTH CARE ENVIRONMENT

Health care and your budget have become important problems of your time. Our country today is experiencing accelerated changes in traditional methods of organizing, administering, delivering, and financing health services. The problems of meeting the health care needs of everyone are often overwhelming.

During the 1970's great shortages may continue in personnel, nursing homes, various essential drugs, hospital beds, and other health products, services, and facilities. Your expenditures for health care will continue to mount.

Among medical economists there is ever growing recognition that the social and economic problems of health care are critical and must be solved on a comprehensive, national scale. Hence, there will continue to be an increased emphasis in health planning that will involve all segments of the community—private and voluntary as well as public and governmental—to determine how to provide good health care as effectively, efficiently, and economically as possible.

PART V

Not man apart

. . . the greatest beauty is organic wholeness,
the wholeness of life and things,
the divine beauty of the universe.
Love that, not man apart from that . . .

ROBINSON JEFFERS

I think health is as much a
right as the right to schooling
or decent housing or food, and
the people have begun to perceive
it as a right.

JOHN H. KNOWLES

This home of ours we call Earth is beautiful—but it may not be for long, and in many places it no longer is. A healthy human being is also beautiful and capable of great accomplishment; but many are unhealthy because of inevitable misfortune, unwise personal habits, or someone else's negligence.

We have talked of ecologic perspective. A proper understanding of this concept must go beyond the notion that ecology is a synonym for conservation or a euphemism for antipollution. Jeffers tells us clearly that we must move from our past and present attitudes of "man and nature," that is, man as separate from nature, to an emerging attitude of "man in and of nature," man as an integral part of the world, as custodian of the Earth, not subduer.

The physical circumstances of our world today demand that we act responsibly, not negligently. Similarly, the delicate homeostatic balance under which we each maintain our personal health also demands that we act responsibly, not negligently. We are in and of our environment; it is impossible to abuse one thing without doing damage to another ("Love that, not man apart from that").

Health is a right—but is is also a responsibility we have to ourselves and to others. Only when we grasp this fact in ecologic perspective will we truly understand it, and only then will we be able to act appropriately. Chapter 12 speaks of right, responsibility, and perspective.

Health: personal right and Everyman's responsibility

Consider Everyman: an average person in search of health. His personal right, health is also his responsibility: to himself, to a family, a community, a nation, a world; for none of these owes Everyman a living. Everyman has got to cope! If he does not, his own failings will echo into the larger social orders. A chain, even an ecologic chain, is only as strong as its weakest link.

Everyman has come a great distance, supported by several thousand years of learned human behavior, passed down through unnumbered generations of forbearers. There was a time when hunting and scavenging were vocations for his ancestors, themselves not far removed from killer apes. Later, farming and tending herds were added, and lately industrialization with urban living have tested Everyman's adaptability (Part I, Introduction). New ideas and devices now press upon him before he has mastered their understanding. If ever there were a time for deliberate and thorough education and training, calculated to promote self-confidence and wisdom, this is it for Everyman.

Partial health is not Everyman's goal. He wants and needs total health: physical, emotional, social, economic, and political. Now more than ever before in history is this so, because in the 1970's Everyman shares his world with 3½ billion souls—a far cry from the few million roaming the earth in 6,000 B.C. Perhaps in the "good old days" he could just move on when threatened by neighbors who carried disease or had de-

signs upon him, but not any more. Space may have been a necessity for the D. Boone family. Today such wide open spaces are wasteful luxury. Or are they? Might wide horizons still be essential to Everyman's total health? Can we so quickly divorce ourselves from the notion of "elbow room"? If we do, can we expect to maintain a satisfactory level of health? Or does Everyman still carry more than 6,000 years of genetic information favoring scavenging, hunting, herding, and farming? All these activities take much space and time, and both are being bartered away today by Everyman!

PAUSE FOR STATION IDENTIFICATION

In this chapter we shall speak of space and time, and the quality of both, as critical determinants of personality. At each juncture, and perhaps between the lines, we shall emphasize quality over quantity in regard to health. We do reserve the right to be wrong, to change our mind later. None of us has the complete picture of Everyman's predicament.

You may or may not agree with psychologists who tell us that sublimation (Chapter 2) is the only solid ego defense mechanism by which anxiety may be truly relieved. Perhaps you will not agree that mental-emotional illness and psychosomatic disease, family breakups and breakdowns, alcoholism, drugs, wars, crime, and waste reflect anxiety throughout Everyman's society; you may feel that these symptoms do not account for a majority of time lost from work and money spent toward recovery of health. Who knows? Possibly anxiety makes us even more efficient. Without trying to be oversimple, however, we suggest that energy expended in an unsettled society is apt to find diminishing returns.

Most of you will reach mature adulthood shortly. Some will be parents, some teachers and leaders. Having come this far, it is unlikely that any of you will be loafers or deadbeats. As you evaluate this final chapter, consider what education should be available to Everyman in your community to equip him so that, pursuing his own instincts, he may still find new adventures, new worlds to explore, new mastery of skill and talent. Remember that if, after graduation, he runs down like a spring-wound clock, he cannot claim to have nailed down any useful education. The educated are those who are self-motivated and keep right on learning. Literacy, open-minded doubt, and honest perseverance strike us as the measures of real education. Is this what you want for yourself and for Everyman? How will your community proceed toward the goal?

THE MYTH

In *Animal Farm* George Orwell brings out the truth observed by Jesus Christ: the poor are always with us. Orwell further points out that men are not created equal at all; even at birth, as we have seen in previous chapters, they are unequal. By the time a starvation diet has taken its toll of brain cells in the human fetus,* Everyman's most human part—his brain function—will have been permanently impaired. This is not to relegate such a personality to subhuman status; on the contrary, we know personally of a case in which not only malnutrition but also viral encephalitis wrought fearsome brain damage in infancy and childhood (as proved by a postmortem examination years later); yet the person himself

found gait and speech impairment no deterrent to the breeding and breaking of work mules for his community. Nevertheless, in general, childhood infections, emotional deprivation, educational inadequacies, and social pressures can cast Everyman ill-equipped into the world of adult responsibility.

Subsistence diet and housing may make it possible for Everyman, as an adult, to live out an average life span for his area. Such measurement in quantity makes nothing seem amiss. However, in the United States in the early 1970's we have many adult males unemployed, representing low-income, large family groups without visible means of support for several weeks out of each year. In addition, a spiralling inflation (robbing Everyman of his buying power), coupled with irrationally apportioned income taxes (exemptions not keyed to cost of living or long-term national needs), easy credit, and widespread, socially encouraged overextension of personal debt, send more and more families into breakup and penury yearly. The search for food used to separate family members many years ago; now it is the search for jobs, not just any job, but high-paying jobs that will keep Everyman's head above water in these hard times. Today's migrant laborer resembles yesterday's slave in that each has been victimized through no fault of his own; each is a low man on his social totem pole.

COUNT THE COST

We have calculated that in the early 1970's and assuming no further inflation a family of four with a six-room house and a single car will have to earn at least $9,000 yearly to avoid undereducation, disease, and excessive debt.

Annual cost to own and operate one car	$1,000.00
Annual cost to feed four people	$2,000.00
Annual home furnishings cost: hard and soft goods (purchase, cleaning, maintenance)	$1,000.00
Annual clothing purchase costs for four	$ 500.00

---

*Winick, M.: Fetal malnutrition and growth processes, Hospital Practice **5:**38, May 1970.

Annual cost to rent or own, including
utilities, exterior maintenance, and
lawn care if any $1,500.00
Annual insurance, education, retirement, and local taxes costs $1,000.00
Federal taxes on $9,000.00 $2,000.00
         Total $9,000.00

Accepting this as a subsistence standard, so as not to burden any other segment of society by failing to handle his own expenses, Everyman may well feel pinched. Should illness, ambition for further education, or excessive taste for either luxury or altruism prevail, Everyman and his family may lose ground, sinking rapidly into the ranks of the poor.

To earn more than is spent is to be rich in 1970, 1980, or anytime; what is true at the individual level is true for the nation. Needless to say, most of the world's people would feel wealthy if each individual received an annual income of $9,000, but we are speaking of the United States.

Nations throughout the world, whose populations were static in the ecologic context existing prior to World War II, have suffered very real problems in the wake of well-meaning but short-sighted American gestures of assistance. Foreign aid problems, with infusions of life-prolonging food and medical care, brought about by virtue of Western technology, have indeed reduced death rates and lengthened life spans. Without a corresponding drop in birth rates, and without increased sustained autonomous agricultural productivity, countries such as Ceylon are in real trouble. It is as if the missionary fervor of church and state, when added to the entrenched habits and ethnic values in favor of as many babies as possible, might be "the invention of the devil."

We must recognize that not only more, but poorer poor, shall be with us according to present trends in the early 1970's. "The bigger the better," you say? "Always room for one more"? Of course you don't say this; nor do we. Do you believe that those countries with fewest poor might entice Everyman to consider emigration, as in the past? Alaska, perhaps? Emigration is not so easy in today's world; for example, Alaska

has asked that all immigrants backtrack (referring to unskilled labor), according to newspaper reports of June 1970.

IRRESPONSIBILITY INDICES

One can find several parameters of substandard living if one looks: the age of an exterior paint job in a city's public housing development, the incidence of rodent and roach allergy in inhabitants of a slum, the many incidences and prevalence of misdemeanors and crimes, infrequency of garbage and trash collection, visibility of solid waste along highways and streets, the prevalence of noisy vehicle engines and smoky exhausts, divergence between assessment laws and actual practices in regard to private property, low school attendance and graduation rates, divorce rates, and suicide rates. But there are other indices one might use: a community's per capita alcohol or tobacco consumption, use of sedatives and tranquilizers and analgesics and narcotics, or its bankruptcy rate.

We recall further how small a proportion of adults in some states has even a high school diploma. This means there are few families able to keep accurate financial records, understand political issues, read "the fine print" in contracts and guarantees, or follow modern health practices. The result is frustration, misunderstanding, emotional breakdown.

We have lost count of those human problems that we have seen in our practice of medicine and in our teaching careers. Human circumstances change; the problems remain much the same. We ask ourselves: is a trailer park really better than a tenement highrise? Is it fair to babies to bring them into a stuffy nursery while mama works in the mill and daddy looks for seasonal construction work? Is it any wonder that mental and physical disease is rampant in this vast population? We see such diseases of neglect as early loss of teeth, athlete's foot, gastritis, malnutrition ("I just never ate any breakfast at home, and now I'm too tired to get up and fix it for the kids"), battered children, and alcoholism. Neglected throats still bring rheumatic fever; neglected precautions still bring household and automobile accidents. Suicide, schizophrenia, and divorce are serious health problems. Present-day legal and medical management of these ailments makes as much sense as a Band-aid for lung abscess. Is it good for Everyman to stand by and deny responsibility for his sick neighbor? How many cripples will we be subsidizing in a total world population of 7 billion?

THE MAJOR EMERGING PROBLEMS

"The major emerging problems of the present generation are not related to health statistics in the more traditional sense, but to national and international crises that will arise out of rapid population growth."* "To a starving man, four slices of bread mean more than the four freedoms." Who said that? Does it matter whether Adlai Stevenson or Mao Tse Tung? Either way, it has an ominous ring. Today's hungry children may be tomorrow's patrons of totalitarianism, no matter whether they enter by the rear door or the front.

Not only population pressures may wither the leaves of Everyman's tree of life, but: "the roots, they may die: they'll all be forsaken, and never know why," as the story goes, in the ballad "On Top of Old Smoky." Perhaps saddest of all our human plights in the United States today is our loss of that resource considered most valuable in many mature societies: our elderly. Charles Stevenson wrote in the June 1970 *Reader's Digest* that at Hastings College of the Law, "you have to be retired to be hired," and that competition for admission is keen. Here, older citizens continue productive, as teachers, as they should be. But too often have we wasted the ripe fruits of life's tree. Our elders—the best sources of continuity, stability, wisdom, experience—have been relegated to early retirement and obscurity, whether in lonesome distant colonies, separate apartments, nursing homes, or worse.

A factor in the waste of this resource has been our population mobility. Grandchildren may be hundreds of miles away from the best housekeepers, nursemaids, tutors, story-tellers, and advisers, when these are needed. Who can deny that, regardless of cause, it is wasteful to operate two separate households, each handicapped without the other? The loss is mostly to children and grandchildren: to miss the family history, and its sense of belonging; to miss useful advice born of hard, long experience, gained by one's own family; to miss the good feeling of knowing one is needed, even as a child, in helping Grandma or Grandpa day after day to do the things ancient eyes, ears, or joints will not permit; in short, to miss the chance of learning and earning genuine love and respect.

We know that it is not so simple. The elderly may not be willing to take a back seat when they have to; their children may not know how to make them comfortable in it. But careful efforts to work out these problems at the personal and family level would pay large dividends in terms of lasting health and happiness, for Everyman.

Plan ahead

Since many of our failings result from premature leaps, we think Everyman would be well-advised to begin early in planning ahead. If it is possible for him, by virtue of innate capability or by education and training, he ought to pursue further training in a trade, craft, or profession. The larger society owes itself the responsibility of making it not only possible but pleasant for a youthful Everyman to grow educationally. In return, the recipient might be required (by prearrangement, as in a few states already) to practice his skills for a few years where the state feels they are most needed, perhaps in rural areas, perhaps in the ghetto.

No man can perfectly serve two masters simultaneously. Educational pursuits are not often honored when Everyman is at the

---

*Linder, F. E.: The health of the American people, Scientific American **214:**21, June 1966.

same time trying to raise a family and support a wife, but it can be done with planning. Without planning, a healthy, happy family is an impossibility. With some planning, not only can grant money be found, or part-time jobs, or loans, but fatherhood can be delayed until Everyman is better prepared to devote himself to his wife and children.

It is advisable that couples planning marriage first be assured of a combined income of $9,000 in the early 1970's. It surely makes no sense for the customs of society to push Everyman into a premature marriage predicament and thus subsidize the seeds of its own discomfort and disease.

Family planning ought to take into consideration the numbers of babies and children eligible for adoption. It can be advantageous to everyone to remove a child from public wardship. Much expense and discomfort for the larger social order could be spared if this policy were consistently encouraged; unfortunately, it is not given sufficient premium in our society. A reasonable way to limit family size while providing for homeless children might be to deny income tax exemption after a second birth per family but give extra annual tax exemption for any adopted children.

"Love suffers long, and is kind," we are told. Genuine respect and affection between two spouses can mean a good deal more than money in the bank and will not falter when the latter is inadequate—at least, not right away. We do know of examples in which a wife has been put through school by a husband, with the wife, upon graduating, reciprocating for her husband until he was through his first phase, then he again paying for her education, each helping the other until both had completed their desired level of formal training. But unless one parent can be home with the children at all times, this schedule is not the best one by which to try to raise them.

Everyman must choose to plan or not to plan. Look within for your own decision. What is best for a laborer will obviously not satisfy the needs of a skilled professional person. The one will have begun to master tools of his trade by age 18 or 20; the other will need 10 to 12 more years. Society needs both, of course, and they need each other.

Mistakes will be made: impetuous actions may cause hardship; but if dealt with honestly and with love, they are rarely fatal. In education, one can always look ahead, having missed the fast express, and catch the slow train of correspondence or evening classes, available in most cities. Fortunately, state colleges and universities have long provided for the needs of adults in search of further education.

THE POLLUTION PROBLEM

Indirectly and directly, the oceans make up a prime determinant of our ecologic balance. They influence our rainfall, climate, and our food chain. Thor Heyerdahl tells us he has witnessed oil pollution the breadth of the Atlantic between Africa and tropical America, as he crossed by papyrus raft in 1970. In recent years, few Florida beaches have been free of oily debris. It is easy to see the oil, easy to guess whence it came, but more difficult to know the extent of damage to ocean life—so critical within a few meters of the surface—by this and other debris or invisible pollutants. Nor is it easy in a democracy to come to grips with the problem. Oil and industrial interests have been parlayed all the way to our country's highest office and its cabinet posts in recent years. It will take strength to answer the challenge of cleanups and prevention of soilage in today's Petroleum Age; the task is likely to be too much for one in the oil industry itself. Our democracy—our bureaucracy—will confront the test as it deals with this already far-advanced situation. Are we ourselves ready for the test? Is Everyman? Have we the courage to support a definitive solution?

Land, too, has been critical in our ecology, and critically abused, and with it, air and inland watersheds (Chapter 6). In some areas dangerous pollutants have already brought sickness and death in epi-

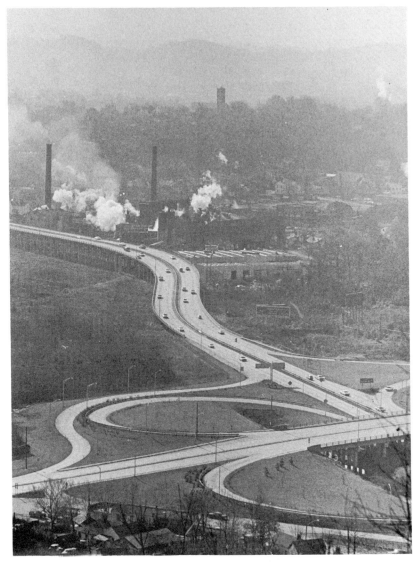

Fig. 12-1. Our cities may soon be concrete tombs unless we are able to control the atmosphere pollution from automobiles and industry.

demic proportion to fish, wildlife, plants, and people. One of our states announced in 1970 that not a single stream within its domain ran pollution-free enough to provide safe water for swimming. Continued pollution means certain illness; we must admit there is no space available for practices that breed wastes not further processed for reclamation. We must speed the day, individually and collectively, when no person or agency will be permitted to exceed his or its own capacity for self-support. Retrieval of waste and recycling waste production into the ecologic chain without polluting air, land, or water must be clearly legislated and enforced.

AVOIDING ECOLOGIC HOLOCAUST

Passing the buck has become routine; too many of us frankly don't want to get involved. Too busy with other pursuits, we "let George do it." Can Everyman afford

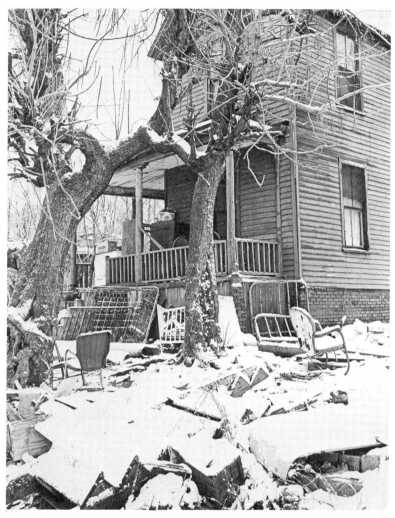

Fig. 12-2. Even the beauty of newly fallen snow is unable to hide the ugliness of neglected refuse.

such mottos? One doesn't need to be a Jeremiah to see famine and disease on the horizon for all of us if Everyman drags his feet in the business of environmental clean-up. After all, by natural unplanned evolution it takes 50 years to introduce a new idea and another 50 to see the results, which spring from the idea itself, become general.* That will bring us to 2070 A.D. and some 25 billion human beings on our plant earth.†

*Gibons, J. D.: From Knoxville News-Sentinel and personal reports of talk given June 12, 1970, Optimist Club, Knoxville, Tennessee.
†Chapin, R. M. Jr.: Fighting to save the earth from man, Time, February 2, 1970.

Without broad and rapid implementation of definitive plans, tomorrow will find us a dead culture, like bacteria planted too thickly on yesterday's growth media in the laboratory incubator. None shall overcome.

Listen to the university coed overheard in a car waiting for the light to change: ". . . so at the dorm they kept asking me and asking me where I was going; and I told them, 'I don't care where I'm going!' " Does she speak for Everyman? We trust the young woman wasn't serious. But one such thought can wreak havoc. We hope the coed suffered little pain in the experience apt to follow, but experience can be a hard teacher. She may not have got off too easily, particularly if her remark reflects habits already firm. It is easy for a young person to reverse course and drop harmful habits, just as it is easy to plunge into self-destructive habits. Changing course is harder for larger social orders.

We shall not all have a chance to live in contrasting societies before chosing our own paths in life. So we have designed some examples—call them fables—for illustration. One society, the young one, changes rapidly and meets trouble just as rapidly; the other, older society has been a good deal slower to work with new ideas and practices until they prove themselves useful. Consider as you read on: in which society will the offspring have ample elbow room, opportunity, and self-respect? In which would Everyman attain a satisfactory level of health?

First fable

There was once a great stadium, carpeted with porous earth and grass, upon which occurred at regular intervals events of the greatest social importance. It was neither old nor new. Festivals, ceremonies, sports events, and even an occasional minor prophet made use of its facilities. The rains came, were absorbed by sod, and made the earth healthy. Cool, green grass continually respired, absorbed heat, cushioned falls, absorbed carbon dioxide and other wastes, resisted invasion by fungi and other organisms, produced oxygen, and lent certain known and varied risks to activities there, all of which enhanced the enjoyment of all within the stadium.

There came a day when the stadium's arena was transformed into something much different. A brand new turf replaced the old one. Results were prompt and marked: a greener green and no mowing required at all. Pride of ownership was rampant all about the stadium; people came from far and near to be among the first to see, feel, taste, smell, and hear the difference. The rains came again, and the arena was flooded. Tons of water unable to soak into sod or to evaporate did not immediately disappear. Sunshine after the rains raised, by several degrees, the temperature at ground level; the new turf grew much hotter than the old grassy sod, and more humid; molds flourished upon the plastic blades of green until the green grew gray and black. Other molds grew apace between blisters that covered those punished soles that trod the turf on Saturdays. Some thoughtful people began to fear that a mistake had been made; they were hushed by the drummers dispatched by vested interests from within and without the campus. Score: prophets, zero; profiteers, 100.

Again prevailed a hasty remedy: it was decided to let the stadium be among the first to gain an air-conditioned, plastic bubble dome by which, of course, the turf would be protected against both rain damage and overheating. But it happened that on the very day when all the seats were filled, a severe electrical windstrom appeared (unrecognized and unpredicted by the official weather bureau at the airport).

With electrical power failure the bubble dome contained and concentrated the smoke from thousands of cigarettes; photochemical smog was formed, which poisoned respiratory mucous membranes; tornado winds smashed the plastic bubble, sending splinter fragments into human flesh as missiles. Souvenirs of the mishap were long treasured by the town's surgeons; the medical men worked around the clock against chemical bronchitis and eye damage, and the pharmacists doubled the price on cortisone. Lawsuits were rapidly translated into losses for the stadium ownership far exceeding the gate receipts. No one lived happily ever after. The stadium was condemned and left as a landmark.

Second fable

A couple of newlyweds, honeymooning in Europe by courtesy of the United States Army, decided to play the game as they found it. Strategic washing once daily and hot tub bath once weekly (using water heated the night before, when power rates were lower) became habit after a short period of adjustment of notions. Heat was used sparingly and not at all at night. Extra clothing and bedcovers proved more practical than it had seemed back home in America. Not even the newborn baby grew ill in such Spartan surroundings. The couple were very much in love with each other and with the country visited; thus it was no hardship for them to adapt to a new situation. Daily shopping for fresh produce eliminated much need for canned foods, whose containers would only have been burdensome. Reusable string bags served for shopping, and never broke or tore. Daily shopping permitted use of a tiny refrigerator and rapid rotation of its content; there was no spoilage nor waste space. After being read, the newspaper served as tinder for the apartment stove (coke-fueled and clean). Toilet and bath facilities were shared with other tenants for, with proper scheduling, it was possible to get along well with much less than they thought possible. Kitchen facilities were also shared with another family, and small periods of deliberate overlapping use served for regular socializing over tea or coffee. Language class evolved spontaneously, if not perfectly. Tea leaves, coffeegrounds, hulls, peelings, and egg shells became garden compost. Bacon drippings unused otherwise served to fuel patio lanterns. Table crumbs fed birds on the balcony.

There was no need for owned automobiles; buses and taxis were available for those rare occasions when legs and bicycles could not serve conveniently. Trains were dependable, comfortable, and inexpensive. For the very wealthy, superhighways served superbly and carried intercity commerce as well; standardized careful construction left nothing to chance; interchanges were perfectly cloverleafed, and emergency telephones regularly spaced on both sides of the road. Signs were liberal, legible, and attractive. Outings on bicycles revealed many secrets: how European women keep trim and sleek of limb, how motor traffic may be kept out of congested areas, how a

country may preserve its beauty and space (no dumping, no littering, frequent cleanup enforced at homeowner level, and enforced pride in upkeep of few possessions). With so much material to do without, the Army earnings of our young husband sufficed for his venture into professional life upon return to the United States, and all did live happily ever after.

Who goofed?

Can it be that we have spent our time studying the wrong things? Has it profited us to try to find absolute lessons in history and social studies? Recalling Chapter 7, one is reminded that no cure is possible when causes are unknown. The social scientist, who must satisfy himself with description only, is in much the same position as a traditional pathologist who looks at diseased tissues. What first began the disease process is often obscure or missing altogether. Unable to design controlled studies, the sociologist is therefore limited in accounting for each human variable and is unable to observe humankind through a succession of generations. It might be better to ask experimental psychologists to use their rodent colonies to provide basic answers for us and to check these against the impressions of our own "senior citizens."

THE MEDIA, OR THE MIND POLLUTED

It may be that we have allowed too much falsehood (the Japanese call it "fancy talk") to condition our thinking and goal setting. What do you think of bacon ads for a product that "won't burn," of roof treatment "guaranteed not to leak for the lifetime of the house," and many more claims by an equal number of product pushers? What happens to the person who in good faith purchases the products and finds his false hopes dashed to pieces upon unrecognized facts? Have we encouraged mental health and economic stability by this sort of approach? Madison Avenue techniques now extend to government programs of health insurance, not to mention policies offered by other underwriters on every imaginable aspect of human risk. We wonder whether such a policy may be terribly wasteful of the quality of human living in the long run.

What of the myriad little half-truths in our culture, such as the "milk is good for you" philosophy? We know of more lives damaged by adherence to this slogan than lives enriched. Consider the ills of milk-fed tots, anemic from this iron-poor food; of those with lactase insufficiency, unable to use milk for anything but a laxative; of those with brain damage because of leucine intolerance and low blood sugar from a diet of milk; of those allergic to casein and lactalbumen; of those with milk as the cause of their ulcerative colitis.

There is also a hedonistic decoy technique "pleasure above all else": the tobacco industry is fond of it. What honest person could think that it is not damaging to use tobacco? Bring into contact with human mucosa the raw or partially combusted leafy debris from a tobacco farm, with all its earthy admixtures, such as the spores of gram-positive bacilli (that bacterial genus giving us food poisoning, tetanus, gas gangrene, botulism, and hypersensitivity lung disease). What happens? Every physician learns to recognize "smoker's nose," "smoker's throat," precancerous leukoplakia, chronic bronchitis, emphysema, and lung fibrosis. These diseases are rules, not exceptions, in chronic users of tobacco. It is the cigarette that smokes; man is just the sucker. But "there's a sucker born every minute," as well they know in the tobacco industry.

There is another maxim: "you can't cheat an honest man." Would we really have so much waste and ill health if we had not, by our very permissiveness and attention loving, encouraged the attentions of the advertisers? Would we have so much waste waiting for recycling and disposal if we had not permitted ourselves to be pushed, pulled, persuaded, and panicked into purchases and habits we could have done without? Does "planned obsoles-

cence" (prototype: combustible cigarette) give you more, or less value received for hard-earned dollars? His neighbors probably will not worry about either his mind or his bank account if Everyman happens not to smoke, drink lavishly, buy new outfits and a new car every year; but his friendly Pontiac dealer and some other product pushers may manage to convince him that the neighbors have their doubts.

BUREAUCRACY'S SAGGING SOFT UNDERBELLY

The next misdirection concerns organization. Efficiency is lost when more people are added, after some point of diminishing returns. In a rigid, military unit the point comes later than for a less-defined and overlapping bureau; but sooner or later operations bog down under weight of numbers. Gideon took pains to avoid this event at the Battle of Midian,* releasing the thousands who never really understood what they were supposed to do. In many of our public and private agencies it often takes nearly all of the money poured in just to sustain the superstructure; actual delivery of services is reduced commensurate with the organization's internal communications problems. As a result, a given agency almost never solves its original mission, and the continuing presence of the problem, instead of provoking just wrath of taxpayers and abolishment of the agency, is inappropriately regarded as "evidence" that the agency should continue to be funded.

Providers of services are also consumers, of course (Federal definitions to the contrary notwithstanding). It also seems unfair that poorer, less educated people never qualify for lasting positions within the agencies (since the job specifies literacy).

Then there is the second problem having to do with a services strategy. Out of the most self-less beginnings, vested interests of the most troubling kind seem to evolve. The purveyors of services acquire an interest in the maintenance of demand—even the expansion of demand—for

---

*Judges: 7.

their particular product as much as does any commercial interest, and this typically is exacerbated by the conviction of the service class that it is uniquely absolved from anything so sordid as self-interest. I wish this weren't so, but I fear it is.*

It should be apparent that any good operation must have responsibility at each level vested in a single individual, with strict lines of communication, no overlapping authority, and strict standards of performance. When we see in our society a host of professional and amateur social servants promoting a patchwork of exercises in planning, advertising, employing (with Federal funds—our tax moneys) and competing with all other agencies duly established earlier at state and national levels, we are not much encouraged. The older agencies at least have some sort of internal communications scheme and some external liaison going for them. It seems useless to muddy the waters with more agencies. We can see an even more useless solution ahead, however, as frustrated groups "throw the baby out with the bath water" and revolt. That is anarchy; it is a very real danger.

POSSIBLE SOLUTIONS

Give the mission; insist on performance; fire any deadwood on hand; reward efficiency and initiative; use what we have on hand already. "Make it do, with spit, glue, and bamboo." "The difficult we accomplish immediately; the impossible takes a little longer." These are probably corny mottos, but they helped us win a couple of wars. Should we give up what already works pretty well? Of course, these things are not so simple as they sound; no war was ever won within a 40-hour week.

That everyone has the right to live is agreed; the right to loaf is another matter altogether. But let's not punish the wrong guy. Deserted or widowed wives and orphaned children need help, not blame or

---

*Moynihan, D. P.: One step we must take, Saturday Review, May 23, 1970, p. 21.

advice. Ghettos in Appalachia and in metropolises need more than just "operation bootstrap," though this spirit is essential. What about widespread individual commitment to back up words with actions undiluted by the superstructure of middlemen? There are not enough wealthy benefactors to go around; the job will fall on our great middle class, too. What about a negative income tax? What about tax exemption for those families who play host to the needy neighbor while her urban ghetto is undergoing renewal? Is anyone for that kind of "slum clearance"? We understand your lack of enthusiasm, for this is not a definitive approach, only a stopgap.

We submit that we do care where we're going; that we need an exercise in success and self-confidence for the larger social orders; that now is not too late to dig in and make a good start, but tomorrow may be otherwise; that direct, definitive action is cheapest in the long run; that for Everyman, example is better than precept.

NOISE IN THE SYSTEM

If dedications were in order for chapter sections, this one would acknowledge Dr. Eugene Stead, the great teacher of physicians. Stead has ever been deaf to all trivia that detract from the pursuit of excellence. To those who do not know Dr. Stead, it may suffice to explain that if deluged with sewage, he would not turn his brain toward ways of making it edible or speeding its removal; he would, if it were the best alternative, locate the tap and turn it off. We commend to our readers this direct approach. Consider the following distractions that have plagued Everyman.

Newsworthiness

Placing premium on the new, the untried, the different, is now a habit throughout our society. We are bored with the same old things; we take on sophisticated unconcern toward any subject, object, or person with which we have superficial familiarity. We disregard, if not actually slander, the exceptional person who troubles to scratch beneath surface appearances. On the other hand, we prick up our ears at even the least substantial rumor, least promising trend, impractical gimmick, or seasonal sensation.

We behave similarly toward news reports, smothering them in ads, then watching them unravel, bit by bit, on the radio, on television, and in the newspaper. For items of genuine importance we find no prime time nor prominent space. There is too much to sell. At the end of each report, we still are cheated: a lick and a promise, rarely more. It is as if news media and its bosses were afraid to face day-to-day reality close to home, to stay with problems until clarified, to present the usual, or to recognize the norm.

It is hard to say whether any one group is to blame for the above situation. Which would you say: the providers or consumers? Caterers and patrons are in the same boat; indeed, they are one and the same person. Still, the piper plays as he is paid, and so do the media. We feel that as long as consumer goods constitute the major index of our gross national product, we shall continue to suffer a reasonable chance of incomplete story telling by news media (as influenced in turn by their patrons, the advertisers). We would be far healthier if quality education were the major index of national worth and were so recognized and rewarded by the media.

Household opiates

It is the nature of opiates to dull useful senses while consuming time and energy and heightening useless sensations. Note how television, at the heart of the home entertainment center, has usurped the place of the devotional corner, the unabridged dictionary on its pedestal, and the music stand. So captivating is it that television is more habit forming than was any of the other diversions. Its intrinsic multimedia approach (sound and sight) make it a Pied Piper and Pandora box all in one. Such a medium might better be reserved for the aged or ill who require passive entertainment and have better sense than to try to ape the actions depicted there.

Recalling Chapter 2, one can easily postulate other mass opiates. An unhealthy personality tends to embrace any of several unhealthy ego defense mechanisms. Thus, a projector-rationalizer may join the Black Panthers or the Ku Klux Klan. Militant cultism gets him either way. Another sample: when one identifies with the "beautiful people" pictured in ads for tobacco or alcohol, while denying the risks of using these products, one may join the vast average segment so highly prized by demographers; but denial and identification are still unrealistic solutions. What does it take to change Everyman from the patently ridiculous into the sublime? Would it help if his family recognized and rewarded his better nature and more useful habits? Might the news media help here? No doubt public reward means more to many than family gratitude. It is a shame that we cannot all peek into the future, seeing our own "mug shots" year after year as caught in the act of devotion to habits we employ, although it is pretty hard to embarrass some of us. Wise physicians often tell us what will happen, but scant heed is paid.

SOLUTIONS?

Education, if it brings a spirit of lasting inquiry and healthy doubt, is a safeguard against falling prey to such opiates. Education is primarily in the hands of individual teachers; to us, this makes teaching our society's highest calling. But education is not apt to occur if teacher and students outwardly distract each other, or if there is too much "noise in the system." Overstated or neglected appearances may spoil the message, and its reception as well.

Education aims for behavior change. When a sane mind performs self-evaluation and sees illogical habits, anxiety will result until bad habits are replaced with good ones. Education, then, repays temporary distress with ultimate ease and greater competence.

Rough, but still jewels

At home, at work, and at play we have idols: they are our thoughts, words, and actions. "Twinkle, twinkle, little star; what you say is what you are," said a child we know, as reported by her second grade teacher.

Thoughts take time; actions require more time. Thoughts come first, since actions depend on them; but without actions, thoughts are worthless. Consider the words of Paul Ehrlich, the great scientist: "Waste not a single hour, for life is too short to accomplish the things demanded of us by humanity." That sentiment came from a healthy, self-respecting, disciplined man. With planning and care Everyman can attain to a like status. Ehrlich may have passed up most of what an average person would call opportunities; no doubt he was marching to the beat of another drummer than that audible to patrons of whatever consumer products his age provided. He possibly owned no real estate; he may not have hunted, fished, or golfed. He may have missed some meals and shaves for the sake of an experiment. It doesn't matter; he made no fetish of appearance.

Many gifted persons have had handicaps. Beethoven was deaf; Stephen Foster a pauper and eventually an alcoholic. Yet their acomplishments, achieved in spite of the burden of such social and physical handicaps, were great. You can think of others: Woody Guthrie, for instance.

Little idols

Vehicles vie with wars nowadays in dealing death to Everyman. Still we worship them. Outwardly full of violence, inwardly serving sexual fact and fancy to many (automobiles now come equipped with hot pink upholstery, stereo music, soft lights, reclining seats). Our cars will kill many, many more of us before we wise up. Even for Americans with an average income the family car is a huge overstatement of design; its accessories seem to encourage even nuttier "nuts behind the wheel," year by year. In Germany our American cars are derisively labelled "Strassenkreutzer" (literally, "oceanliners of the streets"). Con-

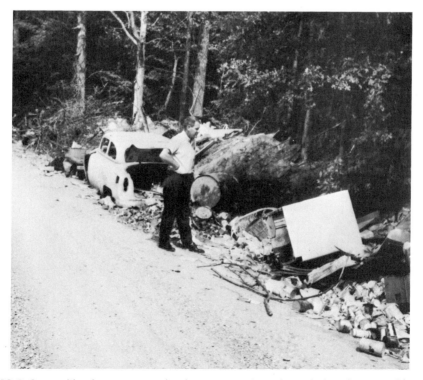

Fig. 12-3. Scenes like this across our landscape remind us of our disdain for natural beauty. We will not be a healthy culture until, through education, we learn to appreciate and respect the world in which we are but short-term guests.

sumption, we remember, was once the name of a disease; now it pertains to rate of dollars or gallons of fuel expended in operation of one of these mobile, nondisposable hulks whose obsolescence is foreordained. Consumption remains a disease: to consume without recovery of wastes is to be consumed by them, if one is not first struck dead on the highways.

It is disease to throw into mass production a moving source of pollution and physical trauma. Our housing patterns may be as sick as our transportation. Certainly the two are interrelated. It is just as sick a practice to permit human single-story construction to sprawl over the landscape, mile after endless mile, so that mind and eye are cluttered by the evidence of social cancer and transportation becomes impossible except by private vehicle. It is disease to pattern ourselves after neighbors who own several internal combustion engines, operating many of them simultaneously: cars, boats, motorbikes, lawn mowers, and tractors. It is disease to put all the blame upon the manufacturer, whose products still must be purchased and operated by some responsible person.

How short-sighted to abandon the railroads, with their grand potential, existing tracks, and right-of-way, for the alternatives to rail transit. Never will there be a real solution when moving sources of pollution are involved; but a stationary source, such as an atomic power plant in place of an electric railroad engine, can be effectively safeguarded, inspected, constrained, and shut down; responsibilities can be fixed and defined. By contrast, the mobile internal combustion engine, from power saw to jet plane, is about to bring us to the end of our collective wits, as well as to the end of physical health for Everyman.

Name your poison

One of our cherished fallacies is that every homeowner or renter must also be a homesteader: so much acreage, with so much "land improvement." What Everyman is after, of course, is elbow room. But instead of sparing the countryside for hunting, camping, fishing, and hiking, he carves it up into small individual pieces of the pie. Instead of preserving the ecology of estuaries and tidal basins, so vital to the seafood chain, he dredges and fills, canalizes and drains. Instead of preserving inland watersheds, he scalps the earth with mines and subdivisions, to the immediate detriment of natural beauty, and soon to the detriment of his own person.

Actually, most of us spend all sleeping and the majority of waking hours within four walls. It should not matter whether our living units are stacked up, down, or sideways, from the practical standpoint. When apartment high-rise design includes thick walls and fast elevators, one can easily enjoy the best of two worlds: preserving weekend and vacation-week outdoor space and beauty—even large parks within easy walking distance of home and office—while enjoying the economy of a compact municipality. Utilities, fire and police services, schools and shops, and factories and businesses can all live close together in harmony, as we can witness from experience in other societies. The cliff dwellers of old were on to a good thing in their living quarters: erect, safe from tornadoes, on barren ground, with all the horizon unspoiled. Need new housing? Tear down the crumbling one and build a higher hogan. Need a car? Who needs even a horse, since all needed recreational and retail facilities are within walking distance?

But consider the present situation. With acreage (even one-half acre) to tend, multiplied by hundreds of similar neighbors, comes loss of water table, as trees are cut, stream banks cleared, and acceleration comes in surface runoff and evaporation. Less ground water means more expensive water supplies, from municipality down to lawn sprinkler. Did you ever notice how the tap flow slows to a trickle when all good citizens are washing dishes and taking baths? Consider how much water it takes to shower, to flush, and to run a dishwasher.

In the evening the paterfamilias is apt

to be found riding herd on his domain: cowboy hat, chewing a blade of grass, holding a hose or riding a baby tractor as the sun sinks in the west. This is great relaxation—if he has the time to spare—but expensive for Everyman. Every week the baby tractor chews up one of the neighbors in our community: how about yours? Was it any worse to get pawed or stepped on by a horse?

Gardens, moreover—and garden clubs, God love them—are enjoyed by all of us. They comfort the soul. Where else can we watch our labors bear fruit so quickly? How better can we lose frustrations than by breaking clods of ground? But even gardening can get out of hand pretty quickly. Aching backs, asthma from the organic dusts stirred up and inhaled, blisters, and insecticide poisoning are all preventable with planning, but all predictable without planning. Hopefully our private wars on weeds and insects will be safe and relaxing pursuits, or at least serve to keep us out of greater mischief.

With lawn and gardens next door to other lawns and gardens, it is natural for neighborly competition to emerge, for both quantity and quality. There are other hazards: roaming dogs do not understand property lines; human feuds may be a consequence. Seasonal invasion by elm beetles, box elder beetles, and a host of other arthropods may arouse the ready ire of a fastidious neighbor. Gossip follows: "Why doesn't that lazy Mr. Jones spray his trees?" is heard at the next meeting of the garden club. The next thing we know, not one, but several neighbors are out for blood. No doubt there are those who object to cottonwood fuzz, to pine pollen, and to dandelions. You know the reaction; we generally respond in kind, but go one better if possible: "What about the shabby television aerial of yours sticking up like a sore thumb?" "Why don't you cover up the noise from your heat pump so I can get some sleep in my hammock?" These are all valid objections; we merely want to emphasize how nice life can be when neighbors can get lost in a planned wilderness or retreat behind thick apartment walls.

So it goes: a natural hunter versus his suburban neighbor, the natural farmer. Never have the twain existed peaceably together. Mature societies have legislated the dog and cat into houses and kennels. Mature societies have set aside community garden space within reach of the bicycle. Mature societies have spelled out carefully the areas of interneighborhood responsibility. Even in the suburb Everyman finds that free enterprise carries the seeds of revolution. The inhibited, average fellow would pull up stakes and move, or remain and go gradually crazy, before revolting against the system or searching for the heart of the problem.

LARGER COWS AND MORE SACRED

In the South, as in other areas of the United States, we adore colonial appearances: columns, verandahs, plantation-size space, bucolic grace. For a long time, we have permitted ourselves these luxuries. But times are changing rapidly, and with less acreage per capita we indulge ourselves in other ways. For example, in the upper middle income brackets it is not unusual to find 300 light bulbs per house, 6 to 10 switches per room, and 3 to 6 electrical appliances running on a 220 volt circuit. The family will probably have a lake or mountain cabin, or farm, or both; time will be distributed among them, but not equally; upkeep will sag here and there. A few head of cattle or horses remain to keep us in touch with the grassroots of our culture. Perhaps this is good; perhaps the hazards outweigh the benefits, for Everyman's community.

Interestingly, our conveniences of modern living are inconvenient. Good appliance service is nonexistent. If advertisers and salesmen were legally liable for the malfunction of products sold, there would be a great cry and much disturbance on Madison Avenue; but with settling of the dust there, we would predict a much more liveable world.

KEEPING UP WITH JONES

Added to the forces of inner greed nibbling at our budgets is the force of outward fashion. When shapes change every year, from clothing to cars, the manufacturer is free from responsibility for craftsmanship and product warranty; his item doesn't need to be very good, since it will be sold, swapped, or discarded before long. Basically, this may be what has happened to Everyman's buying power: he has been buying bubbles. We submit that national pressure against inferior quality and changing fashion would make a good deal more sense than price and wage controls. In the final analysis, though, we cannot escape some blame ourselves; we have been less than eternally vigilant to prevent these things. As Pogo says, "We have met the enemy, and they is us."

THE SPORTING LIFE: GAMES THAT PLAY PEOPLE

Participator sports, if left to participators and kept away from spectator influence, would probably be unreproachable. Athletics is a most important feature of Everyman's personal development program. Organized sports, such as the Little League, intercollegiate sports programs, and the AAU, offer regular exercise with motivation, teamwork, fellowship, competition under rules of fair play, recognizable and attainable goals, gratification through perennial improvement, well-being, and recognition. None of these values is peculiar to organized sports, but the chances are that Everyman and his children will find it more convenient to rely on organized sports for meeting many needs of a growing personality.

But disadvantages do exist in organized athletics, and at times they outweigh the advantages. To acquire and maintain a good golf game may take $500 annually, exclusive of club membership. (And if the latter leads to wasted time at the bar or waiting for a tee, then a golf game is scant recompense for the harm done.) Also, few of us can afford 4 hours and 9 holes, three times weekly, to keep up a high degree of skill at the golf game. Hopefully, most of us have better things to do.

Other sports can be named: tennis, handball, swimming, and many team sports; in short, any participator sport in which injury to an opponent is not the object. Participation is the other sine qua non for a useful sport. Spectators—if the sport is subject to their influence—are often best understood in terms of mob psychology. Just as Roman citizens grew more and more bloodthirsty as stadium spectators, so also with soccer and football fans, and now, even with basketball fans. Unsportsmanlike conduct is not only condoned on many college and university campuses today, it is even made "strategy" by opposing coaches. If fans have been chiefly responsible for this trend (as we think they have been), then there may be a lesson for us in many nonathletic human experiences. The consumer, granted his request, may end up with an inferior product; in the long run, everyone suffers. A lot has to do with the quality of each consumer—with Everyman—and not so much as one might think, with the provider—again, Everyman.

In the formative years of personality, it sometimes can be deadly to turn to Little League activities. Recently, an entire newspaper page was devoted to candid photographs of miserable, broken, defeated little contestants. These children, and others we could name, had been pushed past the breaking point by overly ambitious parents and coaches. The adults involved were perhaps a bit immature in their own personalities, giving in to denial, rationalization, and identification. We agree that pursuit of excellence, for many youngsters, is best learned on the sports field; we applaud the self-sacrificing adults who invest time and love into these youth activities; but for Everyman's sake, we should not forget that athletics is only a game. It is far better in sports to have travelled pleasantly than to have arrived, at least in the learning years. Who has ever learned his lesson well in an atmosphere of fright, disgust, or anger? It seems far better for the community to recruit only mature, understanding fathers and older boys, and to ensure that everyone plays often, no matter what the skill level.

We can scarcely justify team sports for youngsters if they destroy self-confidence. One must remember that athletic ability is ultimately a product with slim market in the adult world; but courage and confidence are for all time. It might be better for most communities to invest leadership talents and time in Scouts, the 4-H Club, YMCA, Campfire Girls, Future Farmers, Future Homemakers organizations, and school and instrumental music for the youth of the area, if it seems that more harm than good is coming from the more highly prized sports organizations.

TIME FOR REFLECTION

We have not intended the intrusion of either optimism or pessimism. We are not clairvoyant; we have tried not to color our opinions. It remains important for Everyman to try to see where he has been, where he is, and where he is going, if he would ever reach a worthy goal: be it merely survival, or survival with health.

A COMPLEAT CITIZEN

Like parents, educators have the mission of training each new generation in the best attributes of the past while pointing them toward promising future avenues. Learning to live is a bit like learning to play chess. Chess teaches us to make haste slowly, to develop every member of the team individually, to plan well ahead, and to consider every alternative. The rules of chess we can learn; the skilled game we get only through practice and through correction of past mistakes.

We have tried to indicate that many changes on a broad social scale call for time, and that time is running out fast for nations caught up in burdensome, deep-rooted habits. We have stated that it is probably wasteful to try to single out scapegoats other than Everyman for blame, or agencies other than Everyman for correction. We feel it is nonsense to expect government, organized medicine, science, technology, religion, or jurisprudence to bail Everyman out of his predicament. However, it seems reasonable to do all possible to encourage in ourselves, our children, and any pupils we might have, a sense of personal responsibility and self-respect, and

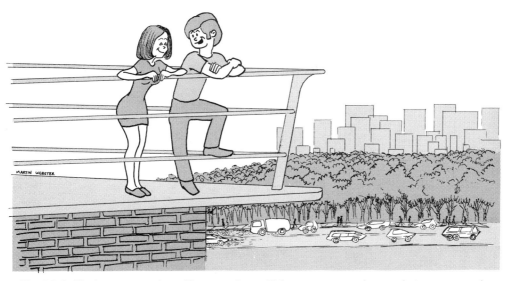

Fig. 12-4. "Let's try not to be self-centered—we'll have to get used to our being concerned about Everyman and not just ourselves." (Courtesy Martin Webster.)

to share with them a continued effort toward self-improvement.

UTOPIAS

We offer these assumptions for your inspection: that it is the individual's responsibility to survive, that he is his own logical and best provider and consumer. At each successively higher level, it is the responsibility of larger social orders to set lateral limits between subordinate units; reward and punish; coordinate and bridge; delegate duty commensurate with ability; and to set the example by following rules more stringent, with fewer privileges than those granted lower social orders, so as not to grow at the expense of the supporting strata. Everyman has functions expected of him at three levels: within himself and with others at his own level, as well as upward and downward to the next level of social order. Those with honest love and energy will move most easily among neighbors, of course. Everyman's health will eventually suffer if negligence is permitted at any of the social levels. Ill health is clearly evident in the United States in the early 1970's.

Second only to parenthood and teaching, politics is among the highest of social callings. It calls also to the inept, to imposters, to egomaniacs, and to exhibitionists (as what profession does not). It is symptomatic of disease in our national society that a recent poll revealed the following to be parameters of a "successful" (that is, surviving) politician in the 1970's:

1. Rapid response to every social pressure
2. "Invisibility," that is, never showing himself in action or revealing his real thoughts
3. Photogenicity on television

May Everyman be preserved from such political successes as these; but in the early 1970's, politics does not look very healthy.

CRYING HAVOC

Bad as they may be, it is not prototype politicians, nor foreign conspiracies that will bury us; it is the growing pile of dis-posable, nonreturnable tools and packaging. We may, of course, need burying soon, considering the growing morbidity and mortality from private and public pollutants, such as petroleum, tobacco, alcohol, television, and others, used and abused so generally and for so long. Life spans in some families are not getting longer; they are decreasing.

THE END IN SIGHT: GOOD HEALTH FOR ALL

We have tried to be realistic. If our society is imperfect, it is because we—individual members—are imperfect. None of us can change the world, true. Many try; they invariably damage the world, and themselves with it. But every one of us can, if we wish, change ourselves. In the final analysis, behavior patterns in human beings are in the hands of each person individually: change is truly a privilege and a duty reserved to the individual.

None of us is completely wrong. Even bad situations have a good aspect, which can be seized upon and enlarged. An open mind permits us to recognize mistakes, brand them as such, and avoid repeated error in the future.

Healthy persons—with healthy personalities—will not give up and feel the need to yield up their personal responsibility for self-determination to some outer population trend of the moment. No matter what demographers preach, we who strive for health can and ought to chart our individual courses. An honest, normal human being has no use for those who would glorify a population trend based on statistical averages. An emotionally healthy adult or teenager knows that his personal worth cannot be downgraded except by the self, and is not troubled by outside pressures to conform.

But from within, to thoughtful human beings, comes the ancient urge to enjoy being ourselves, and especially to know the happiness that comes when we better ourselves: when we push our individual norms onward and upward, always trying to learn what is our full potential, by putting knowledge into practice.

Ecology teaches us that we need other creatures—not just human friends—for continued health. The other part of the blessing is that other creatures need us. Ennobling? Yes! To know that we have help at hand when we ask is to know just as surely that *our* help can and needs to be offered freely to the other creatures that share our part of this earthly spaceship we call home: to our human neighbors, and to all natural resources, living as well as giving life.

Healthy individuals will not hesitate to build solid interpersonal relationships upon what is the best they can give and the best that they can see in their neighbors. Did the mayor do something reasonable and right for a change? Tell him so, and with the easy smile, which comes from frequent practice, thank him. He'll get the message. He's okay. We may not change the other guy, but we can make it a lot easier for him to make the right change himself. And the great thing is that we are apt to get back from life about what we give. If we are healthy men and women, it will not hurt us to take from our healthy selves, each day, and thereby leave things a little better than we found them.

Index

Ophthalmologist, importance of consulting, 63-64
Opiates; *see* Narcotics
Opium, early use, 131
Optic nerve, 63
Optician, function, 64
Optometrist, function, 63-64
Order, importance of, 20-22
Organ of Corti, 68-69
Organic chemicals, synthetic, as water pollutants, 162
Organizations, inefficiency of, 318-319
Orgasm in sleep, 220
Others, guides for understanding, 50-51
Otitis media, 74
Outpatient care related to hospitals, 270
Ova, 207
Ovaries, 207
Overweight, 94-96
Oxygen-demanding wastes as water pollutants, 162

P

Paint, abuse of, information summary, 135
Paranoia, 45-46
  resulting from lysergic acid diethylamide, 140
Parasitic disease, rank as health problem, 7
Paregoric, 133
  information summary, 134
Parent-child conflicts in family disintegration, 259
Parenthood, 246-252
Pathogenesis, 167
Pathogenic organisms in disease, 169-170
Patient, malpractice and, 291-292
Patient-physician ethics and relationships, 290-292
Pellagra, varied complaints in, 187
Pelvis, female, longitudinal section, 206
Penis, 210
Pentobarbital, 135
People, improving relations with, 49
Periodontal disease, 60-62
Personal health, 29-202; *see also* Health, personal
Personal health services, direct, 265-268
Personality, healthy, 31-53
  basic characteristics, 33-34
  guidelines for maintaining or regaining, 48-51
  survival of, 52-53
Personality clashes in family disintegration, 258
Pesticides, 156-158
  biologic magnification of, 156-157
  and ecologic balance, 157
  harmful effects on humans, 157-158
  human deaths caused by, 157
Petting, 220-221
Peyote, 138
Phagocytes in control of disease, 170
Pharmacist, 280
Pharmacogenetics, 189
Phenobarbital, 135
Phenothiazine, 136
Phenylalanine, 85
Phenylketonuria, genetic basis, 244-245
Phobias, 44
Phosphorus, 86
Photochemical smog, 159
Physical differences between sexes, 205-210

Physical examination, premarital
  female, 233, 236-237
  male, 237
Physical fitness
  definition, 99-100
  importance of, 100-101
  rating of sports for, 106
Physical self, understanding of, as element of health, 18-19
Physician(s)
  number and type, 266
  obligations to, 291
  prestige of, upswing in, 266
  quality of health care, 267-268
  specialty fragmentation of, 266-267
Physician-patient ethics and relationships, 290-292
Physician visits in evaluation of health status, 15
Physiologic effects
  of alcohol, 144
  of caffeine, 155
  of theobromine, 155
  of theophylline, 155
Physiologic needs, relation to emotional health, 35-36
Pill, contraceptive, 224-225
Pimples, 57
Pinna, 68
Pinning, 216
Pinkeye, 67
Pituitary gland, 198
Placenta, 247
Placidyl; *see* Ethchlorvynol
Plant nutrients as water pollutants, 162
Plantlike organisms in production of disease, 168
Plaques, 60, 61
Platt, J. R., on crisis of transformation, 23-26
Pneumonia, rank as cause of death, 6
Poisoning
  accidental, 155-156
    emergency treatment, 155-156
  food, 174, 180-181
Poliomyelitis, 180
Pollution
  air, 158-162
    effects of, 160-162
    sources, 159-160
    types, 160
  mind, media and, 317-318
  water, 162-163
    sources, 162-163
Pollution problem, 313-314
Polyneuropathy, alcoholic, 150
Polysaccharides, 81
Posture
  and appearance, 75-77
  deviations in, 76
  good, maintaining, 76-77
  improvement of, exercises for, 79
  mechanics of, 75-76
Potassium, 86
PPBS of personal health, 261-306
Predestination, belief in, and accidents, 114
Pregnancy, 252-255
  complications of, rank as health problem, 7
  development of embryo during, 246-250
Prejudice
  definition, 40